Disclaimer:

This book is not intended as a substitute for medical advice. You should consult a physician in all matters relating to your health for symptoms requiring a diagnosis or medical attention.

This book provides historical information on the subjects discussed. Annotated updates are also included. It is not meant to diagnose or treat a medical condition or provide medical advice in any way. If you are in a life-threatening medical situation, seek medical assistance immediately. Apitherapy and the use of bee-related products for medical treatment are not FDA-approved. Do not feed honey to babies one year or younger.

The publisher and author are not responsible for specific health or allergy needs that may require medical supervision. The publisher and author are not liable for negative consequences or damages to anyone following the information in this book.

"Bee Venom Therapy" is in the public domain. All annotated additions are copyright © 2024 by Giles Gem Publishing, LLC, under number TXu 2-438-854, and may not be reproduced in any form without written permission from the publisher or author, except as permitted by U.S. copyright law.

Annotations by Mindy Giles. Digitized by Giles Gem Publishing, LLC.
The book cover was designed by Rabia Riaz.
Cover illustrations by Anders at SereneDoveDesigns.
First Printing, 2024

ISBN 9798322224679 (Paperback)
ISBN 9798322223825 (Hardcover)

CONTENTS

ANNOTATED NOTES TO THE READER

NOTES TO THE READER

This publication is an annotated copy of the rare 1935 first edition of "Bee Venom Therapy." This literary work is reproduced to ensure future generations continued access to this treasure trove of medicinal and historical information.

Likely due to his beekeeping experiences in his youth, Dr. Beck was intuitively drawn to the magic of bees and their medicinal powers. He was born in Budapest, Hungary. He was multilingual, which made the international medical literature much more accessible to him. Much of the research and medical literature of the era originated in the European countries. Dr. Beck kept a library of books on bees and beekeeping from all over the world. His ability to assimilate medical information in foreign languages further provided him insight into the prospective benefits of bee venom. These works are referenced extensively in his "Bee Venom Therapy" book.

Dr. Beck took great care in compiling evidence of bee venom's efficacy. The "Bee Venom Therapy" book prudently documents many of his patients' improvements seen through the years from Bee Venom Therapy by both Dr. Beck and his kindred international colleagues.

Dr. Beck was a trailblazer and prognostic in understanding how much the world would need bee venom in future generations. In the later years of his life, he worked hard to record and preserve his work for posterity.

An example of how this literature is implicit a century later is in Dr. Beck's chronicles of the root cause of arthritis, which he sought to treat. He elaborates on the cause of arthritis as insufficient circulation.

"I am firmly convinced that the main producing cause of these ailments (arthritis and rheumatism) is merely a local relative state of suboxidation, produced mainly by impaired circulation. A pathological suppression of a normal flow of blood and lymph will produce an inadequate oxygen supply, be it an idiopathic condition or the result or complication of other unfavorable endogenous or exogenous influences. Insufficient circulation and the consequent relative anoxemia are a great handicap, destructive to all living tissues."

"….. suspended circulation means the destruction of tissues mainly due to a lack of oxygen; they simply "suffocate….

i

ANNOTATED NOTES TO THE READER

Now what are the effects and consequences of defective circulation and insufficient oxidation which, at the same time, are the indirect causes of arthritis and rheumatism?

They are:
a- Disturbed local metabolism; and
b- Bacterial growth.

- Dr. Beck, Bee Venom Therapy

The information presented by Dr. Beck related to circulation and carbon dioxide (CO_2) (See Chapter IX, subsection Producing Cause) is profound, considering the publication of his work dates back to 1935. Currently, many forward-thinking medical professionals are recognizing the vital role of carbon dioxide in the whole body system and, specifically, developing an understanding of the effects of carbon dioxide and its relative relationship with oxygen. To be more precise, how oxygen uptake in the tissues is influenced by carbon dioxide versus oxygen and the relative pressure of the vessels. Much of the information in "Bee Venom Therapy" can be evaluated for current ubiquitous conditions plaguing modern society.

Unfortunately, Dr. Beck did not have a myriad of protégés studying with him to continue his legacy. A team of like-minded doctors learning the practice could have changed medicine as we currently know it. Dr. Beck expressed frustration after mentoring other doctors in his practice to later found out they had discontinued the administration of bee venom because of the patient's reaction. It is currently well understood that bee venom can cause a Jarisch-Herxheimer reaction (Herx), a clear sign of bacterial die-off. The Herx reaction was not understood at the time as a positive outcome. Dr. Beck observed initial reactions, which were signs of it working in the body, followed by significant improvements in patient conditions. However, persuading the medical community to appreciate the Herx reaction was challenging. [1]

When Dr. Beck died in 1942, bee venom treatment and research became virtually nonexistent. After World War II, the medical industry focused on high-tech options, and natural remedies were abandoned—that is, until recently.

This book is more relevant to the chronic conditions plaguing populations worldwide now than in 1935.[2,3] Dr. Beck's work must be reassessed in light of the current ubiquitous chronic health conditions and declining life spans.

Many years were lost in appreciating the potential benefits of bee venom and developing clinical applications. It is an exciting time to witness the resurgence of Bee Venom Therapy. The favorable facts that bee venom is anti-inflammatory, anti-oxidant, anti-bacterial, anti-fungicidal, neuroprotective, cancer-protective, liver-protective, etc., are currently available in the scientific literature. Due to its potential to improve a myriad of ailments, research is underway by the pharmacological industry to develop effective means of delivering bee venom without the use of live bees.[4] Dr. Beck pioneered Bee Venom Therapy for arthritis, but evidence is emerging showing potential therapies for many chronic ailments.

Dr. Beck's book is a bit dissonant because language presentation has changed over the last 90 years (e.g. "Let us ascertain now the correctness and accuracy of these statements….. and many words look as if they are misspelled). Regardless, this book is worth reading for those of you who wonder, "Is it safe, and could it help me?" I encourage you to take a deep dive. The evidence from yesteryear, paired with contemporary evidence, is very compelling. Take yourself back in time and appreciate all that Dr. Beck imparted with his "Bee Venom Therapy."

Bee Venom Components

Bee venom has been used in alternative medicine practices for thousands of years. It contains various compounds, including those shown in Table 1. Varying mechanisms of action contribute to the anti-oxidant, anti-bacterial, anti-fungicidal, anti-biofilm, anti-tumor, and liver-protective properties. Bee venom and its components are effective in treating many ailments. The active ingredients likely have synergies that we have yet to understand. Table 1 provides the primary components of bee venom. [4,9,37,45]

Sub Compounds in Bee Venom and Biological Effect	
Melittin	Melittin consists of 26 amino acids and comprises about 50% of the venom's dry weight. It has antiviral, antibacterial, and anticancer effects but is primarily responsible for the pain associated with bee stings. It is a peptide with biological activity. Melittin prevents blood from clotting and provides a bulwark against radiation. It produces anti-nociceptive, anti-inflammatory, and anti-arthritic effects once administrated to the acupoint of the patient. [5]

Sub Compounds in Bee Venom and Biological Effect	
Apamin	A polypeptide that is able to cross the blood-brain barrier, and therefore, they affect the functioning of the central nervous system. They are anti-inflammatory and pain relieving properties [5,37]
Adolapin	Also a poly peptide with properties similar to Apamin. It is an anti-inflammatory, anti-rheumatic, and analgesic.
Phospholipase A2 (PLA2)	It is an enzyme that causes inflammation and cell damage, however, conflicting research suggest it is anti-inflammatory with immune-protective effects. It plays an important role in prostaglandin and leukotriene biosynthesis, as well as catalyzing other biological reactions. The most allergenic and, therefore, the most harmful component of bee venom. New experimental data have demonstrated protective immune responses of bvPLA2 against a broad range of diseases, such as asthma, Alzheimer's disease, and Parkinson's disease. [5,6,7,49]
Hyaluronidase	It is an enzyme that allows venom to enter tissues and causes blood vessels to widen and tissues to become more permeable, increasing blood flow.
Acid phosphatase	Allergen.
Mast cell degranulating peptide	A powerful anti-inflammatory agent. A peptide that degranulates mast cells by releasing biogenic amines.
Protease inhibitor	It has anti-inflammatory and hemorrhagic properties and inhibits the action of various proteases, including trypsin, chymotrypsin, plasmin, and thrombin.
Histamine	It dilates blood vessels and increases capillary permeability. It is an allergen. [8]
Dopamine, noradrenaline	Neurotransmitters that affect the behavior and physiology of the senses.
Alarm pheromone	It puts the colony on high alert.

HEALTH CONDITIONS IMPROVED WITH BEE VENOM

Dr. Beck's work is an admirable testament to the efficacy of treating arthritis and rheumatism with bee venom. Yet, it does not address other conditions currently thought to respond to bee venom positively. The conditions benefiting from bee venom are supported by 21st-century references from published scientific and medical journals, bee venom treatment provider websites, etc. Collectively, seeing the positive impacts of bee venom and the potential it provides to those suffering is awe-inspiring. While the evidence is very favorable for those conditions noted, more research is needed to understand the impact of bee venom. [9,10]

Lyme Disease

Recent attention has been given within the self-help community to Bee Venom Therapy for the treatment of Lyme Disease. When Dr. Beck was alive, Lyme Disease was not known. It was first discovered in 1975, long after Dr. Beck's death in 1942. [11]

Lyme disease is caused by Borrelia Burgdorferi bacteria and possibly several different strains and species coinfections. Once established in the body, it is not generally circulated in the blood. It has chameleon properties and resides in tissues where it causes inflammation. It is difficult to eradicate due to the unique attributes of the bacteria. Upon entry into the body, it is coated in saliva, which hides it from the immune system, so antibody assault may not initially occur. The corkscrew shape helps it penetrate the tissues. Once it inhabits the body, it alters itself from a corkscrew to a round body (cyst), changing its proteins to remain in disguise from the immune system. The body attempts to attack the foreign resident bacteria but isn't successful in killing the infection. As the bacteria proliferate, they can establish residency in the brain, heart, cartilage, etc., and conceal in biofilms. Lyme patient symptoms are variable and dependent on bacteria location, strain, and other contributing vectors the tick introduced. The general quality of the immune system also impacts patient symptoms. [12,13,14,15]

Bee venom has several synergetic means to combat the bacteria. Bee venom penetrates the bacterial outer three layers and destroys it. Additionally, it acts as an enzyme to dissolve the biofilms where the bacteria hide. When biofilms dissolve, the concealed bacteria are exposed to the destructive properties of the bee venom. Finally, bee venom has a paralysis action. Paralysis prevents it from sending off persister cells that would reproduce and subsequently proliferate, effectively halting reproduction. [16,17]

It is well established that chronic Lyme Disease has a relationship to and may be a precursor to ALS, Parkinson's, and Alzheimer's. Just imagine, for a moment, the potential of a mainstream treatment to cure Lyme Disease with respect to these secondary diagnoses. What an opportunity missed by not continuing the bee venom research after Dr. Beck's death.
[18,19,20,21,22,23,24,25,26]

Note from the Contributor: I am an advocate of bee venom for the treatment of chronic Lyme Disease. I was motivated to republish the works of "Bee Venom Therapy" due to my unexpected and profound healing experience with Bee Venom Therapy for Lyme Disease. I want to ensure the healing powers of bee venom are well known and are carried forth into the world. I am forever grateful to the pioneers and advocates of Bee Venom Therapy for helping me find my way to health.

Cancer

Bee venom has been found to have potent anti-cancer properties. Melittin, a primary component in bee venom, is effective at disrupting cancer cell growth. It engages additional cancer-fighting pathways and causes apoptosis (cancer cell death).

While the evidence is very favorable, more research is needed to understand whether bee venom is best suited as a preventive or curative treatment for cancer patients. [9,19,27,28,29,30,31,32,33,34,35,36,37]

Heart Disease

Various in vitro and in vivo studies suggest that bee products may be effective in preventing and treating cardiovascular diseases. Bee venom can attenuate cardiac dysfunction in diabetic hyperlipidemic rats in a dose-dependent manner. Apamin (a component of bee venom) has demonstrated potential benefits in anti-atherosclerosis and anti-heart failure. Additionally, it improves other cardiovascular precursor conditions, such as metabolic disorders. [9,38,39,40]

Diabetes

Bee venom has antidiabetic properties. It has potent hypoglycemic, hypolipidemic, anti-inflammatory, and antioxidant effects and is helpful in combatting metabolic issues (e.g., Type 2 Diabetes). In his book, "Honey and Health, Dr. Beck includes a subchapter titled Honey and Diabetes to elaborate on the fundamental chemical and physiological contrast that exists between ordinary sugar and honey. He comments, "Honey does not ferment in the stomach because, being an inverted sugar, it is easily absorbed, and there is no danger of bacterial invasion." Evidence suggests it reduces blood glucose levels, enhances insulin secretion, and improves lipid profile. It increases antioxidant capacity, and the pancreas exhibits improved β-cell secretion in rats treated with bee venom. [9,40,41,42]

COVID

Bee venom has shown potent antiviral, anti-inflammatory, and immunomodulatory effects, which suggests that treatment could be a promising complementary therapy to prevent SARS-CoV-2 or other similar viral assaults. In Hubei Province in China, the local beekeeper association investigated 5,115 beekeepers (including 723 in Wuhan) from February 23 to March 8, 2020. This was the period when COVID-19 originated in the Hubei Province of China. The results showed that none of the sample population had COVID-related symptoms. Comparatively, at that time, the general population COVID mortality rate in the Hubei Providence was approximately 4%. [9,43,44,45,46,47]

Parkinson's Disease

Bee venom has promise as a treatment for Parkinson's disease. Parkinson's Disease is a neurodegenerative disease involving neurotransmitter abnormalities. A primary component in bee venom (PLA2) has shown neuroprotective effects and could postpone the progression of degenerative diseases. The effects mainly included enhancing motor performance or alleviating memory impairments, inhibiting oxidative stress, decreasing neuroinflammation, and protecting neurons. [19,20,48,49,50,51,52]

· Alzheimer's

Bee venom is promising as an Alzheimer's treatment. Several of its active components are anti-inflammatory, which can be used to prevent and treat nervous system disease. Alzheimer's is also a neurodegenerative disease, and the benefits of bee venom are similar to those described for Parkinson's Disease. [9,19,23,53,54]

Arthritis

Dr. Beck documented extensive evidence of the efficacy of bee venom for arthritis. Recent 21st-century medical literature further substantiates Dr. Becks' findings. Recent scientific literature shows therapeutic effectiveness in treating inflammatory arthritis and musculoskeletal diseases. Treatment decreased arthritis index in RA rats. The primary components, MEL, and apamin, have anti-inflammatory, antioxidative, and other beneficial effects on arthritis. [2,9,33,55,56]

Skin Conditions

Bee venom restored wounded tissue antioxidant enzymes GSH Px, mitochondrial SOD and CAT activities, and the chemokines CCL2, CCL3, and CXCL2 levels, and then rescued wound macrophages from apoptosis induced by mitochondrial membrane potential. The above results provided a new example of bee venom treatment to stimulate angiogenesis and improve the wound healing process of diabetes. [9,19,56]

Multiple Sclerosis

Both clinical trials and lab testing confirmed that bee venom is an excellent form of biotherapy for Multiple Sclerosis. Bee venom either fights off inflammation and destruction of connective tissues (as in the case of rheumatism and arthritis), or returns activity and mobility by supporting the natural body defense (as in the case of multiple sclerosis and lupus). Apamin and bvPLA2, primary components in bee venom, contributed to the control of Multiple Sclerosis. [9,56,57]

ROMAN NUMERAL CONVERSION

Roman numbers were commonly used throughout the book, particularly in Chapter X, Apitherapy, and Chapter XI, Treatments with Injectable Bee Venom, where dosage is provided. This conversion chart assists in converting to modern units.

Value	Roman Numeral	Calculation	Value	Roman Numeral	Calculation
0	NA		11	XI	10+1
1	I	1	12	XII	10+1+1
2	II	1+1	13	XIII	10+1+1+1
3	III	1+1+1	14	XIV	10-1+5
4	IV	5-1	15	XV	10+5
5	V	5	16	XVI	10+5+1
6	VI	5+1	17	XVII	10+5+1+1
7	VII	5+1+1	18	XVIII	10+5+1+1+1
8	VIII	5+1+1+1	19	XIX	10-1+10
9	IX	10-1	20	XX	10+10
10	X	10	Etc.		

BEE VENOM THERAPY

Bee Venom, Its Nature, and Its Effect on Arthritic
and Rheumatoid Conditions

BY

BODOG F. BECK, M.D.

*There proceedeth from their bellies a liquor wherein
is a medicine for men.*

THE KORAN, xvi, 71.

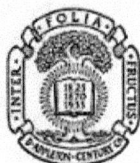

D. APPLETON-CENTURY COMPANY
INCORPORATED
NEW YORK   LONDON

TO THE
PATHFINDERS
OF
BEE VENOM THERAPY
THIS WORK IS RESPECTFULLY INSCRIBED

PREFACE

There is no greater scourge or curse among all human ailments than arthritic, rheumatic, or rheumatic afflictions. The number of sufferers is daily increasing. The extreme agony, excruciating pain, torment and misery which generally accompany these ailments, the hopeless wretchedness of body and mind, the resultant functional incapacities and deformities, are indescribable and appalling. Only the poor pitiful, miserable victims, who are in their pangs, can really comprehend the true meaning of these words. In addition to the physical and mental suffering, the diseases also have great social, economic and industrial importance, since the motive mechanism of the body is disrupted.

In magnis et voluisse sat est.[1] When I try to introduce injectable bee venom to the medical profession as a curative remedy for these conditions, a treatment so far little or almost unknown in the United States but extensively employed in European countries and with great success. I hope this attempt will be received by the medical fraternity, to use another classic expression, *Sina ira et studio*-without anger and partiality.

I fully realize the difficulties of the task. First, there is an unfortunate, regrettable, almost lamentable ambiguity which surrounds the subjects of arthritis and rheumatism; the etiology, pathology, and therapy, even their terminology, are utterly disconcerted and unsettled. It requires a very skilled seamanship to navigate the ship "Therapia" through this rough and turbulent ocean of confusion.

Furthermore, the fact that the remedy and the modernized modification of the venerable, time-honored, ancient, almost prehistoric treatment are practically unheard of in this country adds to the difficulties. Besides, I frankly admit, the remedial agent has all the earmarks of being plebeian, unscientific, and, of course, questionable. I fully anticipate a skeptical and distrustful attitude on the part of the profession-"the acid test of mistrust" -because I confess that my own mind was not any different before I became convinced of the real merit and extraordinary efficacy of this curative substance. But the remedy has already suffered a similar fate, many times, during past centuries.

Quod si deficiant vires audatia certe
Laus erit; in magnis et voluisse sat est.
(Though you should fail, I praise your courage still,
In great attempts enough to show the will.) Propertius, II, 10, 5.

PREFACE

Bee venom is an age-old nostrum in the hands of the laity, but scientifically the substance and its application still remain an almost unexplored field. Possibly, on the surface, the principle has all the semblance of being rather simple, unscientific, almost nonprofessional, but the reader will soon become convinced that he is confronted with one of the most interesting and perplexing medical problems. In fact, I do not know of any other subject in medicine which would involve more branches of the various sciences. It requires a thorough knowledge and wide application of every phase of clinical medicine, organic and inorganic chemistry, biochemistry, physiology, pharmacology and toxicology, pathological anatomy, serology, immunology, anaphylaxy, idiosyncrasy, allergy, in addition to comparative anatomy, morphology, zoölogy, and the history of medicine. The bibliography of the subject, which in itself is extensive, must also be considered.

The subject-matter, I state again, is rather difficult and complex. Systematized sciences, as a rule, are characterized by absolute, settled, authoritative doctrines, but our subject abounds with intricate questions-it is a conglomeration of tangled, vague, almost mystic and occult conjectures, demanding explanation, solution, and orderly settlement. Many confusing riddles have yet to be solved. We know the producing causes, but their consequent phenomena and all other effects often lack apparent support. We have to speculate and interpret them with hypotheses and theories, giving individual views and ideas to elucidate certain obscure actions. The subject is still in an experimental and consequently in a controversial stage.

To invite and secure the coöperation of the medical profession in clearing many enigmatical features was one of the considerations which prompted me to publish the present volume. My primary intention was to give a detailed description of the present definite status of bee-venom therapy, the therapeutic results obtained by innumerable, prominent foreign co-workers, and the complete technic to be employed. Essentially, it is meant to be a condensed textbook of bee venom therapy.

To treat the topic appropriately and make it fully comprehensible, I have had to include several other academic subjects which ostensibly extend beyond the scope of this review. I refer to the chapters: *Animal Venoms, The Chemistry and Production of Bee Venom, The Effects and Treatment of Bee Stings, and, also, to the chapters: Immunity, Anaphylaxy, Idiosyncrasy, and Allergy*. These subjects, however, have such an important and intimate relation to bee venom therapy that I thought it expedient to add them to the material. If occasionally I have been rather didactic, repeating certain, though important facts, I ask consideration for this technicality. Errors are bound to occur, and are almost unavoidable when one adopts a new treatment. To prevent this contingency, I was forced to give more detailed explanations, so as to aid the uninitiated in acquiring the necessary experience, practice and skill.

Concerning the neological and heterogeneous word, *apitherapy*, (do not look for it in the dictionary), which is hybridized from the Latin and Greek language, I would suggest its adoption as it is more euphonic and concise that the correct word *melissotherapy*, and besides the selfsame root has already been employed in several familiar and extensively used words, like apiary, apiarist, apiarian, apiculture, apivorous, apiology, etc.

With all humility and reverence, I dedicate this volume to

Vis Medicatrix Naturae

New York City   B.F.D

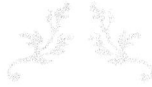

"Il ya donc une action à distance du venin s'exerçant plus particulièrement sur les régions atteintes de rheumatisme. Nous avons entrepris avec scepticisme nos recherches sur l'action antirhumatismale du venin d'abeilles; nous sommes maintenant convaincus des possibilités de succes dans des cas jusqu'alors rebelles aux medications usuelles."

MAURICE PERRIN

Professeur a la Faculté, Nancy, France
(Revue Médicale de l'Est, April 1, 1933)

"There is a remote action of bee venom, most particularly on regions affected by rheumatism. We undertook with great skepticism our researches concerning the antirheumatic effect of bee venom; we are now convinced of the possibilities of success, even in cases which have been so far refractory to the usual medications."

PART I: THEORETICAL CONSIDERATIONS

Chapter I Explanatory Note

Medicus curat, Natura sanat.

An old aphorism in Latin which means that the physician cures
while nature heals.

Since the events and facts of the past were recorded in the oldest
existing annals and chronicles of the world, we find there has been a
universal and generally accepted belief that people suffering from
rheumatoid ailments, when repeatedly stung by bees, have remarkably and
rapidly improved or have been completely cured. This creed has been
conveyed and handed down like an heritage from one generation to another,
from ancestors to descendants, from fathers to sons, by written and unwritten
communication. In addition, there is the well-recognized fact that beekeepers
during their occupation, continuously exposed to bee stings, gradually
become accustomed to their effects and likewise never suffer from
rheumatism, arthritis or gout. If they were afflicted with any of these
ailments prior to their occupation, they are cured without experiencing any
recurrence. There are many reports of similar recoveries from paralytic
conditions and, also, statements that apiarists never suffer from malignant
growths, e.g., cancer. The belief that bee stings promote longevity is very
prevalent.

This age-old tradition is known and accepted in nearly every land.
In Germany (especially Bavaria), France, Italy, Austria, Switzerland,
Czechoslovakia, the Balkan states, in the Caucasus, and even in America,
bee keepers and a considerable part of the rural population firmly believe
that bee stings will cure arthritis, rheumatism, gout and other neuritic
conditions. There are many propagandists of this idea. Lay beekeeper
specialists systematically dispense the treatments, putting on patients daily a
gradually increasing number of bees. In Southern Tyrol, there are several
well-known and extremely popular places to which regular pilgrimages are
made by rheumatics, who travel there from far-away countries, seeking
relief from their painful afflictions. Reports of miraculous cures are
innumerable. Even many members of the medical profession have submitted
themselves to these treatments.

But only a few physicians have undertaken the task of administering
them, exposing their patients and themselves to the stings of live bees. The
procedure was tedious, difficult and burdensome, consuming enormous
amounts of time, requiring skill and courage, as it was not exempt from
personal danger. Only the combination of physician-beekeeper was fit and
competent to accomplish the task. There was another drawback to the

1

proceedings, this time on the part of the patient, namely, the horror of the bees inflicting their painful injuries.

Needless to say, the medical man-even when perfectly qualified to undertake the "job"-hesitated to compete with the laity in this rather undignified occupation, exposing himself to being mocked and ridiculed, not only by members of his own fraternity, but even by the rest of his patients. Undoubtedly, inasmuch as the procedure had all the semblance of quackery, a great amount of broadmindedness and a very firm and liberal spirit were required to confront such an embarrassing and awkward situation, which it inevitably created. No wonder that it has remained almost the exclusive privilege of the lay class.

Meanwhile, in the daily press, in entomologic and bee journals, innumerable scattered articles have appeared about the wonderful and incomprehensible cures of rheumatic and paralytic cases as the direct consequence of bee stings. For centuries it has been a favorite topic of the periodicals.

More than a century ago, in the German *Frauendorfer Blätter*, an article appeared, reporting the occurrence of a peculiar case: a woman with a paralyzed arm was stung by a number of bees and, as a result, recovered the use of her arm. The writer of the article appealed to the medical profession to explain this miracle, suggesting and inviting a thorough investigation.

T. P. Demartis, of Bordeaux, who wrote a series of articles about the use of animal venoms in medicine, published a letter in *L'Abeille Médicale* (July 25, 1859) which he received, in connection with his research work, from a M. De Gasparin, describing his experience. M. De Gasparin was reduced to permanent infirmity by chronic rheumatism and bronchitis. He tried all medicines and various spas without obtaining relief. One day, while walking in the garden, he was stung on his arm. The arm swelled considerably, but his rheumatism disappeared. De Gasparin further stated that with the same method he later cured his chronic bronchitis and, also, a painfully swollen gland. He knew of other rheumatic cases cured on the same principle and, also, two cases of cancer of the face. He complained that, though he mentioned these facts to several of his medical friends, they not only attached no importance to his reports, but absolutely ridiculed the whole idea. He requested Demartis to champion this authentic information and create propaganda for it.

M. Lukomski, Professor of Technology at the Institute of Forestry of St. Petersburg, Russia, published an article in the *Gazette des Hôpitaux* (No. 107, Sept. 1865), reporting cures through bee stings, not only of rheumatic and neuralgic ailments, but of intermittent and remittent fevers and various tumors. He suggested that the medical profession try the method for pest and cholera. Lukomski suggested the technical term "*apisination*" for the procedure.

Several years later, P. Fabre lectured on the subject before the Academy of Medicine in Paris, referring to these publications and also reporting his own experiences. A "poor devil" near Nice, crippled by rheumatism of his legs, exposed them to bee stings and was perfectly cured. Two other inhabitants of the vicinity had similar success.

The *Annal de Société Entomologique* quoted several cases. A veteran, Fernand de Vingeanne, who had acquired a bad rheumatic ailment during the 1870 campaign, was completely cured of it after he had been stung by bees. A retired facteur rural (letter carrier), who for some time had been unable to walk, fully recovered after being stung by about a dozen bees. The *Entomologische Nachrichten* (1878) published similar remarkable cures. A brewer, stung by about half a dozen bees, lost his painful gout, all his symptoms disappearing. A nine-year old, paralyzed child of an inn keeper, in Rettenbach, Oberpfalz, previously unsuccessfully treated for the condition by all possible means, recovered perfectly after having been "exposed" to a number of bee stings.

The *London Medical Record* (XIII, 1885, P. 178) stated: 'El Siglio Medico' relates a singular case from La Paz, Bolivia: A woman suffered so much from rheumatism for six months that she was unable to sleep. Her right arm was absolutely useless, and she could not even dress herself. She heard about cures through bee stings, procured some bees and applied three stings the first day. The result was so surprisingly beneficial that the following night she was able to sleep and her pain soon entirely disappeared." Dr. Packer, of Kansas City, in 1904 reported the case of a man named Gardner, who had been afflicted with articular rheumatism for four years, unable to walk except with the help of crutches. In August, 1903, he was hobbling around the yard when he fell against a bee hive and upset it. The enraged bees pounced upon him and he was nearly stung to death. He became very ill, but after recovering found that his rheumatism had disappeared, suffering no further attacks.

E. W. Ainley-Walker, Lecturer on Pathology at the University College, Oxford, wrote an article in *The British Medical Journal* (Bee Stings and Rheumatism), in which he related his correspondence and gave the answers received to a questionnaire published in several medical and lay papers. He tried to ascertain if there were any truth in the alleged popular belief that bee stings cure rheumatism. The enquiry covered (1) the extent to

3

which this belief was prevalent, (2) the amount and the kind of evidence available in its favor, (3) the amount of evidence which could be obtained to the contrary, and (4) the clinical character of the rheumatics thus stated to be cured.

The questionnaire was inserted in *The Lancet, The British Medical Journal,* and subsequently in *Nature*, a magazine, *The British Bee Journal*, and also widely copied by various newspapers. The doctor engaged in consider able correspondence with persons, both lay and medical, who either reported their own experiences and observations or had sent references and statements of others.

E. T. Burton, of Birmingham, England, wrote as follows:

"Having read Dr. E. W. Ainley-Walker's article in *The British Medical Journal*, I determined on the principle of 'fiat experimentum,' etc., to try on myself the effect of this new inoculation. I was attacked by acute arthritis in my right hip and sciatic neuritis of the same side. Nothing gave me relief. I sent for some bees and when I received the supply put on about eight over the sciatic nerve and the hip joint. Next morning, when I awoke not only was I able to turn about in bed but I could walk across the floor without limping, without pain or without the necessity of holding to the bedpost, as I had done for the last three months. I put on half a dozen more, the same evening six more, and the final instalment two days later. I was then able to run fifty yards without pain. May I add that if I live for three months I shall be sixty-seven, and I have been a rheumatic subject for the last twenty-five years. I intend to continue these applications of bees. There was no other medicine that ever gave me a more 'avaricious' appetite. Of course, there will always be proud skeptics...." Burton later administered bee stings to his own patients and reported many remarkable cures. Surgeon Major-General Johnson, of Virginia, wrote to Dr. Ainley Walker: "The belief is prevalent in the States. I saw treatments applied in the case of Col. W. T., for acute rheumatic fever, with 103° F. temperature, with the result that twenty-four hours later the temperature was normal, joints painless and freely movable. The same patient reported later that he had subsequent attacks which were similarly cured."

Dr. McLay, of Lincolnshire, mentioned in his reply a case of rheumatism of the shoulder, with great stiffness and pain, of two or three months' duration, having been cured by accidental bee stings on the hand.

Dr. Valentine Rees reported that he himself had lumbago for a week, and was absolutely unable to move. A clergyman who had suffered from chronic gout for many years and took up beekeeping for this reason-since having been practically free from pain-applied the bee treatment to the doctor. He immediately recovered.

J. B. M., a layman, wrote to Dr. Ainley-Walker, from Australia, that he had suffered from rheumatism of the shoulder for 25 years. Nothing helped him. At last he decided to try bee stings. He applied the bees every morning to his shoulder and by the end of the week he was free from rheumatism. He remained so for twelve months, when he had another severe attack, which was so intense that he was unable to move. He again applied twelve stings, 48 hours later six more, and the same evening was entirely relieved from pain. After that he was free once more for three years. He had a third attack, which was similarly treated, and since, had had no recurrence. He reported the case of a Mrs. R., whose hands were stiff and gnarled. She could not lift a small plate. Once when she approached a hive, the bees became so angry that they literally covered her hands, stinging them all over. By the end of the week she called on him and said, "Look what the bees have done for me," raising her hands, opening and closing them frequently. Her fingers became almost as lissome as they ever had been. Same correspondent had knowledge of other remarkable cures.

About thirty years ago (May 13, 1905), an article was published in the *Scientific American* which told about the long-standing belief that bee stings cure rheumatism and stated that scientists, on the whole, were skeptical of their value. For many years, little had been heard about the subject. About that time, however, it had been revived-possibly on account of the judicious advertising of beekeepers, as there was a report current that a large chemical firm was buying bee stings, "cornering the supply," and it was expected that 1,000 bees would sell for about $10. According to this periodical, Dr. Benton, Entomologist of the Department of Agriculture, who had been consulted, ridiculed the idea because the supply of bees was so enormous that it was inexhaustible. He admitted that bee stings may be efficacious in some cases, but ineffective in others. Dr. Benton, himself, suffered from chronic rheumatism but, although he was stung thousands of times, the stings did not effect a cure (of course, there is the possibility that his case was not of true rheumatic etiology-Author).

Only a comparatively short time ago (1913), an article appeared in France in *the Journal de la Santé*, relating quite a number of cases cured by bee stings, asking the medical profession kindly to take these facts into consideration and explain them. A farmer, who could hardly move on account of his rheumatism, was stung one day by several bees. He noticed immediate relief and notified his family physician, asking him to continue the "treatment." The physician applied 18 bees weekly. The result was almost miraculous. The same physician had similar success with other cases. For instance, he treated a young girl, suffering from a painful rheumatic condition, and, also, a violinist who for years had been unable to hold the bow in his hand but soon after the treatments was able to resume his profession. Even in chronic cases, this physician found bee stings to be a marvelous remedy. The treatments were started with five or six stings, their number being increased to 24 weekly, according to age and condition. The doctor put the bees on the skin with a forceps and kept them on for about five minutes.

Henry Bouquet, medical correspondent of *Le Temps*, in the January 31, 1924, issue said: "I wrote an article some time ago, about the grave dangers of bee stings and I think it is time now to be fair to the little beasts, to rehabilitate them and speak about the wonderful curative value of their stings. It is rather strange that in spite of all the testimonies in its favor this method is still under consideration by the medical profession." Various other scattered articles were published in the foreign medical press. Marfort of Geneva, E. Monin of Lyon, and Kruger of Nimes reported chronic rheumatism through bee stings. Lamarche, of St. Marcellin, stated that several of his patients assured him they had used this method with great success, while all other remedies failed. Lamarche himself suffered from neuralgia and rheumatism, but after taking up beekeeping, exposing himself to stings, he was cured. He tried the treatment on a woman who suffered from an extremely painful sciatica, spending her nights groaning in She obtained great relief after five stings and was entirely cured in a few more sittings. According to recent reports Dr. Brecher, of Rumania, succeeded in curing forty-two advanced cases of trachoma with bee stings.

The correspondent of the New York Times reported from Kansas City, Mo., in the July 29, 1928, issue, that the oldest resident of Olathe, Kansas, maintained for years that nothing was quite so effective for rheumatism as bee stings, but said of course, the younger generation scoffs at that. He stated that F. B. Haskin, President of the Patrons Bank, who did not class himself a believer of the theory, suffered from rheumatism for six weeks. One day his son called to him that the bees on his farm were swarming. He hobbled out and the medically-inclined bees apparently thought that he had come for treatment, so they stung him on the face, arm and back. Altogether he received five stings. Next day he was entirely relieved from his rheumatism. He said he was not a new man by any means, but certainly a repaired one, and recommended bee stings to anybody who had hardihood, fortitude and... rheumatism. "The little 'buzzers' do the work."

EXPLANATORY NOTE

In the April 28, 1934, issue of the *British Medical Journal* we find the following letter:

Sir, "Can any member of the B.M.A. assist the Devonshire Royal Hospital, Buxton, to obtain standardized bee sting for the treatment of arthritis, fibrositis, and neuritis? From January, 1932, to August, 1933, we have used bee sting at the Devonshire Royal Hospital, made by Wolff, under the name of *apicosan*, and have obtained excellent results; but in August 1933, the Customs notified the hospital that an import licence was required, and the Ministry of Health wrote stating the necessity for a licence. On December 9th, 1933, we wrote a joint letter to the Ministry of Health, stating that we had found *apicosan* of definite value in the treatment of certain rheumatic conditions, and that we wished to continue our investigations. We offered to allow them to investigate our cases. There was no reply to this letter. After waiting three weeks a letter was sent asking for a reply. The Ministry replied to the last letter by asking for particulars of manufacture, and all the available information was forwarded to the Ministry: but we are still not allowed to obtain supplies. It is interesting to note how the Ministry of Health obstructs a genuine attempt at research into the treatment of rheumatism and allied diseases, and prevents the use of *well-recognized remedies* for English hospital patients suffering from the above diseases."

We are, etc.,
(Signed): D. Shipton, M.D.
J. Barnes Burt, M. D.
Buxton, April 16th.   Honorary Physicians

In the May 19, 1934, issue of the same journal Dr. Herbert G. White (Heathfield) writes:

"I was interested to read the letter of Drs. Shipton and Burt in the Journal of April 28th. About twenty years ago an agricultural labourer came to see me who was quite unable to work, being crippled with arthritis and unable to grasp the handles of a wheelbarrow. I recommended him to try bee stings. Accordingly, he went to a bee keeper and received half a dozen bee stings on each hand once a week. In three months' time he was able to return to work completely cured. Surely some of our manufacturing chemists should be able to put up bee venom for treatment of rheumatism;[2] of course it would have to be less painful than the ordinary bee sting. I have frequently

---

[2] Since June, 1934, an injectable bee venom has been manufactured in England (Author).

7

recommended others to try the cure, but have not been able to get them to submit to it."

Recently (1933), during the opening of the last National Honey Show in the Crystal Palace, London, one of the exhibitors, W. A. Whitlam of Thornton Heath, said, "I suffered from rheumatism so acutely that I had to take to bed. I took up bee keeping and like all bee keepers I was stung frequently. The more I was stung the less I was troubled with rheumatism. This year I was stung hundreds of times and my affliction has gone. Sufferers from rheumatism are less subjected to swelling from the stings than normal people and they feel less pain."

The enumeration of all the cases which I have quoted, or the further citing of additional reports appearing in the domestic and foreign press, would have really no scientific significance or value except for the fact that this consistently large number of articles should have been sufficiently important to arouse medical attention.

And still there has been no appreciable response from the medical fraternity. The issue has always received a rather cold reception, mingled with a certain amount of doubt, ridicule, even utter contempt. It was a discovery made and practiced mostly by the laity, and to enter into competition with it, was surely below the dignity and honor of any member of a high and noble profession.

The experiment—if we can call it such-is not by any means a new one. It had already been taken up ages ago, dropped and revived many times. This went on for centuries. Innumerable times, the idea vanished into total obscurity, almost oblivion. It was brought to life for a short while, just to be discarded. It went through these ecliptical stages again and again.

If we give earnest thought and reflect on the repeated dismissal and revival of this traditional practice, we can easily comprehend and explain both occurrences. It was simply set aside on account of the many inconveniences, difficulties, and hardships which anybody was bound to encounter on assuming an obligation for such a venture. It required, also, unusual courage and endurance on the part of the patients to undergo the torture of the exposures. All these circumstances materially contributed to the abandonment of the method. Why it came to life again is also easily explained by the fact that there always has been urgent need for a reliable remedy for such prevalent and obstinate afflictions as arthritis and rheumatism, which cause so much suffering and are so difficult, often impossible, to cure. Both these facts, the discarding of the method on account of the insurmountable difficulties, and its revival, because it accomplished such remarkable results, speak well for its value.

The drawbacks have been manifold. Bees are rather peculiar creatures; difficult for the uninitiated to handle. It requires persistence to try to force them to perform certain methodical tasks and expect their coöperation. They are most furious if you disturb them near the hive and it is prerequisite to use them immediately after their removal, as it is their fury which one must utilize to make the treatments effective. While they are being taken in a container to a bedridden patient, the bees lose their aggressiveness, get sluggish and indolent, and will not sting even if annoyed or irritated. It requires a beekeeper to handle bees. A medical man, if he undertakes to conduct these treatments with live bees, must beforehand acquire enough knowledge to master the situation; otherwise he is likely to get into serious difficulties.

Then there are the seasonal hardships. Their use from early fall to late spring is considered in general so inefficient and unsatisfactory that it is thought hardly worth while to bother with them.

Dr. E. F. Phillips, Professor of Apiculture at Cornell University, Ithaca, thinks otherwise. His opinion is that if one understands how to manage bees and to care for them through the winter it would be quite possible to use live bees throughout the whole year. If they were kept in a house for purposes of easy access, the colony would not last the winter through, but it would be quite possible to replace the colony during the winter even in our climate. In Ithaca, during Farm and Home Week in the coldest part of February a colony was brought in from the apiary for exhibition purposes. No doubt an "unseasonable" application of bees is impracticable, and is more easily said than done.

Of course the possibility that bees may be obtainable during the winter months and their stings utilized for therapeutic purposes, does not literally mean that their venom is efficient. Most authors are of the opinion that the venom is effective only when collected from fresh flowers. In itself the fact that high temperature greatly increases the potency of the venom is an argument against its winter use.

There are also many other obstacles. It is altogether a tedious, tinkering performance and it is no wonder that so many detest and dread the abominable work and invariably wash their hands of it, throwing up the matter in disgust.

Philip Terc, a general practitioner of great repute, in the provincial town of Marburg, Styria, Austria, took up the task most seriously. The reason which influenced him was that he himself suffered from a very obstinate case of rheumatism. One day he was painfully stung by a number of bees, with the result that his ailment was entirely cured. He had heard reports of similar occurrences many times before, but had ridiculed the idea just as much as others still did. His own experience greatly impressed him and changed his mind, as he fully realized that here was a remedy worthy of a thorough trial. But he did not know how to go about it and soon abandoned the idea as thousands of others have done before and after him. The intricacies of the procedure frustrated many attempts.

In 1879, a woman suffering from a severe case of neuralgia in the head and deafness called on him for professional advice. Her ailment had defied all previous treatments in the hands of other physicians, and Terc himself was unable to give her relief, though he used his best efforts and all known remedies. One day the discouraged patient expressed her disappointment and told him that she had depended on his good and great reputation and expected that he would employ some kind of new method to afford her relief. Terc remembered his own experience. Anxious to help the patient in her distressing predicament, he decided to try an application of bees. He called on her daily, putting the bees on her head. The stings had no effect. He applied a total of about 90 stings without either a reaction or improvement. What surprised him most was the fact that the patient suffered no ill effects from the stings. One morning he put 15 more on her neck and shoulders. The patient later sent for him requesting that he call without delay. When Terc arrived at her hotel, he found that her face was terribly swollen and she was unable to open her eyes. The patient was otherwise jubilant, as all her pains, for the first time in a long while, were gone, and she told the doctor that she clearly heard the sound of the church bells. The patient was permanently cured.

This was Terc's first case, but it gave him plenty of material for reflection and great impetus for further experiments. The incident was very instructive but rather puzzling to him. He could not understand why the patient did not react to stings as a normal person would, why the reaction was retarded for such a long time, and when she did respond, why only then the sudden and marked improvement manifested itself. He thought that there must be a peculiar, intimate relationship between bee venom and rheumatic ailments. His later experiences confirmed this supposition-at the time just a guess-that the longer the duration of the illness and the more severe the malady the more stings were required to provoke a reaction. Mild cases reacted to few stings; obstinate and chronic cases demanded hundreds. In other words, rheumatics required more time and a larger number of stings to produce a reaction than a normal person; the reactive symptoms developed less rapidly, were milder, of shorter duration, and disappeared more quickly.

After this initial and surprisingly successful result, Terc decided to continue his experiments. He had no difficulty in securing sufficient material. There were plenty of applicants. He worked continuously for the next ten years to gain experimental and practical knowledge, to familiarize himself thoroughly with the administration of stings, and to study their effects on rheumatics, following up his cases with very careful observations. His difficulties were enormous. He had to devote all his time to only this phase of his practice, in a small provincial town without the comfort of hospital facilities, lacking money to control his cases in a really scientific and systematic manner. Misunderstood and ridiculed by his colleagues, he had a truly unenviable task to carry out the realization of his dreams— namely, to give treatments with what he thought was a powerful, dependable and remarkable remedy. He virtually went through the usual agonies and martyrdom of a pathfinder. On the other hand, the number of his successful cures increased and Terc had the satisfaction of achieving miraculous results in many desperate cases. Terc often expressed the opinion that he was convinced, beyond any doubt, *that almost all true arthritis and rheumatism can be radically and permanently cured with bee stings,* except those cases of many years' standing, where the joints already have been destroyed and ossification has taken place. He thought anyone who would make a statement that bee venom is only a local irritant, like a vesicant, and not a constitutionally powerful and efficient remedy, talked as a blind person spoke of colors.

In 1889, after ten years of uninterrupted and hard labor, Terc decided it was time to arouse the attention of the medical profession and induce them to adopt this indispensable treatment. He succeeded in gaining the interest and confidence of an influential professor of the aristocratic and conservative Imperial University of Vienna and received permission to deliver a lecture on the subject before the ruling medical society. He did so, but the reception was extremely cold. In itself, the fact that a provincial physician, not even a member of the faculty, sine cathedra, should claim the honor and glory of an epochal discovery, a cure of a heretofore refractory disease, arthritis deformans, and with such an "odious nostrum," was received with such scorn, disdain and opposition that the lecture was not even printed, as was customary, in the official organ of the society. Terc said he was glad to run away from Vienna, as he feared that he would be interned in an insane asylum.

EXPLANATORY NOTE

Philipp Terc's experience reminds me of the sad and tragic fate of Ignaz Philipp Semmelweis, which is one of the most pathetic chapters of medical history. It is a rather odd coincidence that the place of the drama was also Vienna and the "hero," his namesake, "Philipp."

In 1847, Semmelweis, at the time in the Obstetrical Department of the University of Vienna, with mortality statistics sometimes as high as 26%, had the courage to announce a new theory; he made a statement concerning puerperal sepsis, namely, that he firmly believed it was not an epidemic disease, as it had been so far considered, but that it was caused by physicians coming from the dissecting room without washing their hands. He gave orders that a bowl of chlorine solution should be placed in every ward and that physicians must wash their hands before attending to a confinement or making a digital examination. This pronunciamento, instead of being hailed as the *birthday of antisepsis*, met with general opposition. Semmelweis was ridiculed and declared a fanatic. Even in 1860, all the obstetrical textbooks stated that it was very "doubtful" whether cadaveric poison was the real cause of "epidemic" puerperal sepsis. The University authorities even refused Semmelweis' request for special linen for his department. He was unwilling to accept the linen which had also been used in the dissecting rooms, and was compelled to buy even bed sheets for his clinic with his own money. How blind opposition can be; he reduced the mortality of his department to almost one-half percent (from 26%) and yet even this achievement could not break the hostility and antagonism.

In 1865, after years of unsuccessful and desperate fighting for this principle, which broke his spirit and deranged his mind, he died, a young man of only 47, in an insane asylum near Vienna. The leading daily of Vienna, the *Neue Freie Presse*, announced his death in several short lines: "Semmelweis had been an able specialist in obstetrics who had certain ideas regarding epidemic puerperal sepsis." A whole generation of physicians was ignorant of a discovery which had such a revolutionary character and magnitude. His enemies and opponents felt so guilty and ashamed that they did everything in their power to silence even the mention of his name. Years after Semmelweis had tried so hopelessly to secure recognition for his theory, Lord Lister advocated surgical antisepsis, and to-day he is considered the father of antiseptic surgery. (In this connection, it is interesting to note that Oliver Wendell Holmes anteceded Semmelweis by several years. On February 13, 1843, he lectured in Boston on the subject of contagiousness of puerperal fever, and made the statement that cadaveric poison, "even" erysipelas, might be conveyed to maternity cases. To avoid puerperal fever, Holmes advocated that physicians should change their clothes and wash their hands with calcium chloride before attending to confinements. He likewise stirred up violent opposition, especially from the Philadelphia obstetricians Hodge and Meigs, and very soon gave up the fight. In 1855, when Holmes heard of Semmelweis' efforts, he repeated his views, referring to the good results Semmelweis had obtained through the application of this "new" method, but opposition remained just as obdurate.)

We frequently observe that pathfinders who make important discoveries not only are not taken seriously by their contemporaries, but also meet expressed antagonism.

That the opposition is not only personal but often objective is best proven by the hostility which a most important drug of our pharmacopoeia, quinine, had to face ere it was accepted. Podolsky, in his interesting book, Medicine Marches On, described the reception given to the cinchona bark when it was introduced into Europe in the 17th Century. The natives of the Peruvian wilds noticed that when certain uprooted trees fell into a pool of water, the water became so bitter that it was unfit to drink. Then some natives who were seized with violent fever and could find no other source to quench their thirst, were forced to drink from these bitter pools, and noticed that their fever disappeared after drinking the magic water, driving out the heat-devil. After a Spanish Jesuit, who had become infected with malaria and had prepared a decoctum from the bark of this tree, fully recovered, the bitter bark was taken to Europe, where it met violent opposition in every country, some fanatics even spreading a rumor that the Jesuits had conceived a scheme to poison the non-Catholic population.

Terc had bad results, too. All the chronic and incurable victims implored his assistance. Many sufferers-impatient in awaiting results-quit their treatments; others were persuaded to do so. Some feared the stings and stopped. A great number, after they were relieved of their pain, gave up the treatments and paved the way for a recurrence. In general, it required a great deal of endurance both on the part of the physician and of the patient to withstand the strain and ordeal of such a fatiguing, wearisome, and painful procedure.

Of course, on account of some unsuccessful cases, Terc was the target for attacks from his colleagues and also from the laity. His good results were silenced by friend and foe. Unfavorable results hurt his reputation more than successful cures helped it. He often intended, in his despair, to give up the struggle, but he had too much confidence in the effectiveness of the treatment. Seeing his once despairing and hopeless patients, whose ailments did not yield to any previous attempts, and were given up by other physicians, looking splendid, happy, and permanently cured, not subjected to recurrences, he felt that it was his duty toward

13

suffering mankind to persevere, and continue the efforts of trying to convey his knowledge and hard-earned experience to his colleagues. He stuck it out, in spite of all difficulties and obstacles, ignoring ridicule which is never a test of truth.

We must really consider Terc as the greatest exponent of bee sting therapy -a real martyr to his faith, principles and profession. The treatments consumed all his energy, will-power, and endurance and for this he was rewarded with constant opposition, contempt, and malice. Terc had to combat distance, time, inconvenience, and ignore even his personal safety. He was stung many times on his hands. Terc found that the bees are more irritable if held between the fingers instead of with forceps, so he utilized this additional improvement in his method of application. He had to carry complicated paraphernalia to his bedridden patients. In the fall, the treatments, by virtue of seasonal exigency, had to be discontinued. This always left many half-cured cases exposed to the exacerbation of the symptoms, and cured cases, to the hazard of a recurrence of the old malady, which was no joy for him, and still less for the patients.

Terc's first important discovery, as I have stated before, was that *arthritic and rheumatic subjects did not react to bee stings* in the same manner as a normal person did. While the average individual will exhibit a fairly violent reaction, a rheumatic seems to possess a decided immunity (pathological immunity). Terc's next observation was that, while he employed enforced and sometimes amazingly drastic measures to provoke a reaction, the delay in the reaction indicated with precise mathematical accuracy the duration and extent of the pathological conditions. Certain groups manifested a similar delay. He considered this circumstance a very important etiologic and also prognostic factor, a true and dependable criterion.

There was another important point on which Terc laid great significance and also considerable diagnostic value; namely, that this *pathological immunity is confined only to true rheumatism and arthritis.* Very often we anticipate treating a supposed rheumatic patient and notice right at the start that not only do we not find an expected state of immunity, but provoke an alarming, violent reaction; in fact, the reaction is more expressed than that of a normal person. Terc called these cases "*pseudorheumatics*" and warned that with very *few exceptions* they would prove to be *tuberculosis, lues, or gonorrhea.* These three pathological states react to bee venom so violently that further treatment is absolutely contra-indicated and must be given up entirely. The diagnostic value and

14

significance of such an incident evident. This may happen when such conditions are not even suspected.

The fact that bee venom provokes, as a rule, a fairly persistent and strong reaction in an average normal individual, but does not produce any reactions in rheumatics and arthritics, is certainly a very interesting and apparently a rather puzzling phenomenon. Undoubtedly, there seems to be an intimate, or rather reciprocal correlation, between rheumatic conditions and bee venom. On the other hand, bee venom produces an unusually violent reaction on luetic, tuberculotic, and gonorrheic subjects.

We know that cutaneous inoculations with tuberculin and gonococcal protein have an important confirmatory diagnostic value. Tubercular or gonorrheic arthritis, tested in this manner, will give a positive reaction in considerable number of cases. It is true that in gonorrheal arthritis a negative reaction does not necessarily exclude gonococcus etiology and that reactions sometimes vary from negative to positive during the interval of a few days, still a persistent negative reaction is usually an argument against gonorrheal arthritis.

If we try to bring into play a process of fair reasoning and deduce the cause of these diametrically opposite manifestations, we have solved a very complex subject which may lead us to the interpretation of many so far unintelligible questions. I will attempt to explain this problem-to the best of my ability-in Chapter VII (Immunity).

I wish to make now a brief comparison between the tedious, inconvenient treatments of the past and the advantages and facilities of the easy, comfort able, and convenient methods at our disposal today.

Terc successfully treated thousands of cases with live bees. His contemporaries used the same method in the administration of the treatments. The patients had to be carried to the hives or the hives to the patients. Accurate dosage was rather difficult. The amount of venom and the bees' aggressiveness vary considerably and the stings are also influenced by many other circumstances. The handicaps and hardships were great, sometimes almost insurmountable. The time consumed by treatments was considerable. The surface of the body which can be utilized for a large number of bee stings is limited. Some space must be left between the stings to make allowance for their spreading tendency. After each treatment, it was necessary to wait sometimes for a week or more until the site of former applications sufficiently healed and could be used again. To provide the bees was often circumstantial and expensive. The treatments could be properly administered only during the summer months, at the utmost during about three months a year. The applications of the stings are rather painful. And then when everything was over, the stings must still be removed.

Today we have injectable bee venom and we can faith fully imitate the sting of the bee. There is no noticeable difference between our injections and natural bee stings except that the injections are almost painless. We can control the correct dosage, the substance is always ready for use, the technic is very easy. There are no seasonal obstacles; we can continue the treatments without interruption at any place and any time. No need today to apply hundreds of stings; all we have to do is to use a higher concentration of the solution. The loss of time, the delay-which means everything in these special types of disease-is nonexistent. The former inconveniences, insuperable difficulties and drawbacks, even the fear of an occasional sting for the operator, are all banished.

There is no reason today why the medical profession should not take this effective remedial agent out of the hands of the laity. We certainly have to admit that there is great need for an efficient remedy to relieve the distress of untold millions of sufferers and incapacitated victims.

Let us hope Terc's wish will be realized. He closed one of his lectures in 1907 with these words: "I trust…. One day…..through a lucky accident… maybe in foreign lands... that the truth of my observations will be recognized and proved... even post meam mortem."

May I conclude these preliminaries with the words of Rudolf Virchow: "We are simply naturalists; as such we demand that every intellectual should contribute to the recognition of natural laws, because only under these laws are satisfactory conditions to be expected. Medicine must go back to Nature and a physician should be the high priest of Nature."

CHAPTER REFERENCES

AINLEY-WALKER, E. W. Bee Stings and Rheumatism, Brit. M. J. Lond., Oct. 1908.

BUCHNER. Repetitorium für Pharmacie, 6, 420, 1857.

BURTON, E. T. Answer to Ainley-Walker, Brit. M. J. Lond., II, 1369, 1908.

DEMARTIS, T. P. Abeille Méd. Par., 30, July 25, 1859.

LUKOMSKI, M. Gaz. d. hôp. Par., 107, Sept. 1864.

EXPLANATORY NOTE

PODOLSKY, E. The Use of Bees in Medicine, N. York M. J., Nov. 1930.

TERC, PH. Über eine merkwürdige Beziehung des Bienenstiches zum
Rheumatismus, Wien. med. Presse, 35, 1888.
Der Bienenstich als Heilmittel gegen den Rheumatismus, Steirischer
Bienenvater, I, 1904.
Das Bienengift in der Heilkunde, Steirischer Bienenvater, V, 1907.
Die Beziehung des Bienenstiches zum Rheumatismus und zur
entstellenden Gelenksgicht, 1910.

TERTSCH, R. Das Bienengift im Dienste der Medizin, 1912.

WALDHEIM, VON, F. S. Ignaz Philipp Semmelweis, Wien & Leipz., 1905.

Chapter II Medical History of the Bee and Its Venom

"The wise man will seek out the wisdom of all the ancients"

A physician, after he discovered in the Library of the College of Physicians of Philadelphia (which he considered, at that time, the center of medical learning in the United States) that Adams' edition of the works of Hippocrates had rested with the leaves uncut for over twenty years, said: "New things are too much in vogue. Beyond question, the medicine of the past is harmfully neglected; few have a desirable taste for its literature and fewer yet a sufficient knowledge." So I do hope the reader will not disapprove if I tender a short historical sketch of the bee and its venom. Bees, bee venom, honey, and wax have been used as remedial agents since remotest antiquity. The practice is as old as Methuselah. Ancient writers, without exception, record the miraculous effects obtained by their application. Hippocrates, Celsus, Galen, Pliny, etc., frequently mention them, referring to their beneficial and extensive use; they were considered popular therapeutic remedies and important healing power was ascribed to them. For example, externally honey with crushed bees was applied for ophthalmia, toothache, sore gums, and carbuncles, and was employed almost exclusively for these maladies. Bees cooked with honey were given for dysentery.

In the writings of archaic cultural states, Babylon, Egypt, Rome, Greece, Persia, and Ethiopia, frequent references were made to the medicinal value of bees and honey. The oldest medical books all praise the bee as a nostrum. Galen used dead bees, crushed them in honey, and said, "If you put them on a bald head, or thin hair, you will see the hair grow." Pliny described at great length the therapeutic value of bees. He burned them, mixed their ashes with oil, and used the substance for almost all kinds of ailments. The diuretic effect of bee-tea is mentioned in every old script of all countries. The directions for preparing it are remarkably similar, just as though all had been copied from one prescription-and in the old ages China, India, Arabia, and Europe were very far apart. The Celtic, Teutonic, and Gallic races, also, used bees as medicine. "Put twelve or fifteen freshly killed bees in water, take one swallow two or three times a day, and it will cure hydrophobia." They dried dead bees, reduced them to a powder, which was used as a principal ingredient of many nostra. The powder, mixed with water and drunk every morning, was an unfailing cleanser of the system. The ashes of burned bees, compounded with honey, was considered an excellent salve for all kinds of diseases of the eye. History mentioned the

18

fact that Charlemagne, the great conqueror (8th Century), was miraculously cured of his obstinate gout by bee stings.

In old accounts of different nations, the use of the bee and honey was described as a traditional home remedy. The "bee cures" advocated were numberless. Freshly killed bees, crushed in honey and rubbed on the gums of infants, were supposed to greatly influence and help the growth of teeth. Internally, they were thought to help digestion. Ashes of burned bees were supposed to grow hair. If you rubbed a crushed bee on a painful tooth, would stop the ache. The sting would cure podagra and rheumatism. In the Slavic countries even today, they cook bees with cereals, like barley and corn, as a diuretic remedy to cure hydrops.

Conradus Gesner, in 1658, published a very interesting book:

The History of Four-footed Beasts, Serpents,
to Which Whereunto is Now Added
The Theater of Insects
or
Lesser Living Creatures
A Most Elaborate Work
by B. T. Muffet.

Muffet described in great detail the use of bees in medicine, "going as far back as the script goes." "Take their bodies as soon as the bees are out of the hive and pound them, drank with some diuretics or wine or milk it will strongly cure dropsy and dissolve stone, gravel, open all passages of urine, cure all stoppages of the bladder, cure griping or wringing of the belly and guts. Bees that die in honey cure impostumes, help the dullness of the sight and hearing, soften hard ulcers of the lip, heal carbuncles and running sores, cure the bloody flux. Honey strained with them helps the curdities of the stomach or specks and red pimples in the face. Dead bees powdered, as Galen already writes in 'Euphorist,' were mixed with honey, and if parts of the head that are bald and thin are anointed, you shall see the hair grow again."

In 1716, Salmon, in the *New London Dispensatory*, told of the beneficial effects of bees on the human system. "The whole Bee in pouder given inwardly provokes Urine, opens all stoppages of Reins, breaks the Stone, they are good against Cancers, Schirrus Tumors, the King's Evil, Dropsie, dimness of Sight, for being taken a good while they waste the Humor and restore Health; so their Ashes, both made into an Oyntment . . . cause Hair to grow speedily in bald places."

MEDICAL HISTORY OF THE BEE AND ITS VENOM

Samuel Dale, in his *Pharmacologia,* 1737, recommended Apis for baldness and as a good diuretic; John Quincy in his *Complete English Dispensatory*, London, 1733; Lewis in his *Materia Medica* in 1768; Motherby in *The Medical Dictionary* in 1776- all described the therapeutic benefits of the bee in a nearly similar vein. In *Die Tiere im deutschen Volksmedicin Alter und Neuer Zeit*, Johannes Jühling, after an extensive search of the oldest German archives, told all about the use of bees in medicine. "In podagra, put the bees on the most painful place; in fluor albus, let yourself be stung by a bee; for loss of hair, kill bees, mix them with honey, and it on the bald spot. If a sterile woman eats bees she will get pregnant. If you have rheumatism, get stung by bees."

In old Germany, we often find references to a medicine made from bees, which had an emmenagogue effect. They called it "Salvemet," and given to women and girls to produce catamenia. It was administered on St. Catherine's day, and it not only promoted the menstrual flow, but had also a beautifying and strengthening effect, for which purpose it was often used. In old Saxony and Bavaria, bee stings were a recognized remedy for podagra. Dried and powdered bees were believed to contain some "highly exalted" volatile oils and salts, which, taken internally, had a diuretic and diaphoretic effect. Mixed with unguents and anointed on the head, it contributed to the growth of hair upon bald places.

At the beginning of the last century Constantin Hering, an outstanding figure in homeopathy and an ardent follower of Hahnemann, in his *American Provings* advocated bees for various ailments. H. Goullon, another homeopathic physician, in 1876 introduced Apis during the World Congress of Homeopathy in Philadelphia. It was the main subject of his address. He said: "It is time to separate the wheat from the chaff, get rid of skeptics and jeerers, and accept this wonderful substance as a useful remedial agent." J. Kafka also gave his experiences with Apis, and, while he didn't consider it a polychrest, he found that it has a strong effect on the skin, mucous surfaces, and glands. He obtained especially good results in erysipelas. Altschul and Hale, others of the school, had great praise for Apis.

In 1858, C. W. Wolf, a prominent homeopathic physician of Berlin, edited his book *Apis Mellifica or The Poison of the Honey* Bee considered as a Therapeutic Agent. The book enumerated in detail the medicinal uses of the bee. In his foreword, he said: "Every physician who has spent many years in the practice of medicine is morally bound to publish his experiences provided he is satisfied that such publication might be useful in the general interest of humanity. In my forty years of experience in the conscientious and philanthropic exercise of my profession, I found that the bee is the best little friend man possesses in the world; it helps to heal all internal and external maladies." He put five live bees in half an ounce of alcohol, shook them three times a day for eight days with about "one hundred vigorous strokes of the arm." This was the "mother tincture." From it he obtained attenuations up to the thirtieth centesimal scale. As a rule, one-third to one-thirtieth potency was sufficient to be effective. He administered the tincture internally, and day after day obtained more satisfactory results. Wolf found Apis the greatest polychrest next to aconite. He considered the introduction of this remedy of brilliant merit and Apis as one of the most deserving apostles of homeopathy.

Most of these homeopathic physicians used Apis internally in the form of tincture and infusum. Their results have been especially satisfactory in the treatment of acute hydrocephalus of children. The more acute and dangerous the condition, the more readily it yielded to the action of Apis. They have never been compelled to resort to any other accessory means. It was likewise found efficacious in ophthalmia, and achieved very rapid cures. Bees have been very extensively employed in all inflammations of the mucous membranes; the tongue, mouth, throat, and larynx; in diseases of the respiratory tract-cough, hoarseness, etc. Apis produced striking results, and the substance has been considered the safest and best remedy in these distressing afflictions. In inflammation of the gastric or intestinal mucous membranes, a specific power was attributed to Apis and it was given extensively for gastritis, nausea, vomiting, distension, dysentery, etc.

Apis was also considered a sovereign remedy by the homeopaths for arthritis, rheumatism, and intermittent fevers. It was supposed to affect every portion of the nervous system, the cerebral, spinal, and ganglionic nerves, by producing a process of "sanguification" on the same principle as fever and ague. No other known remedy in medicine represented such a striking affinity to fever and ague. Wolf asserted that he did not come across a single case of intermittent fever which would not yield satisfactorily to it. He never noticed that relapses ever took place or secondary diseases developed. Wolf considered it more powerful than cinchona. Even cachexia, caused by the long administration of quinine, was cured with Apis. In erysipelas, scarlatina, rubeola, measles, pemphigus, and urticaria, it gave speedy and sure relief.

The remedy was often administered externally. Carbuncles and furuncles were quickly and easily cured by covering them with honey in which bees had been crushed. It promoted suppuration by discharging the decayed cellular tissues, effecting a speedy cure.

Hering warned of the great need for caution in giving the drug during pregnancy, as he did not know a remedy with a stronger abortifacient action than Apis. He gave it to "honest women" who didn't know that they were pregnant, and it was only revealed by a subsequent miscarriage after one or two doses of Apis.

The drug is greatly glorified in the homeopathic pharmacopoeia as endowed with extensive virtues-a deeply and speedily acting drug, affecting the whole muco-membranous tract and nervous system, mainly, as already mentioned, through the important process of "sanguification." Homeopaths depended greatly on it and had unlimited faith in its curative value. F. P. Davis in the *Medical Summary,* 1908, said: "If there is any remedy that will give prompt and expected results, when properly exhibited, it is Apis." The writer considers it rather remarkable, if we assume the venom is the potent component of Apis, that it is used with such success in homeopathy by oral administration when it is a recognized chemical fact that the venom is destroyed by digestive ferments. The ferments destroy the venom and vice versa: they neutralize each other-a certain amount of ferment will destroy a corresponding amount of venom. If we find that Apis, in spite of this fact, still has sufficient effect on the system, the attribute must be due to a surplus in the potency of the venom which is not destroyed by digestive ferments. This ought to be the best proof of its efficiency.

The physicians of the eclectic school, likewise, use bees in the form of tincture, made of two ounces of bees to one pint of alcohol.

We find innumerable mention by some medical men, but more frequently by the laity, of the miraculous effects of bee stings on arthritis and rheumatism. As I have stated previously, there are many places on the Old Continent which have a regular pilgrimage of sufferers, flocking there from faraway countries with the hope of relief from their distress. The treatments are administered by beekeepers, without any medical knowledge, and still many accounts circulate of marvelous results and cures.

Only lately, November 11, 1933, in one of the Duluth, Minnesota, papers an article appeared which stated that August Halgren, 73 years old, who had been badly crippled with rheumatism 17 years ago, started a bee farm at the time because bee stings were supposed to cure rheumatism.

"It worked," he reported. Not only did it work, but it provided Halgren with a prosperous business. He now maintains a farm of 157 bee hives. All comers are supplied with enough bee stings to cure their rheumatic pains. A Duluth grocer, virtually crippled when he first visited

22

Halgren's farm, credits his bees with a complete cure. Halgren charges nothing for the treatments at his "bee clinic." "I was cured by a good will offering and that's the way I will cure you," he tells each patient.

Tickner Edwardes, in his *Bee Master of Warrilow*, vividly described how these treatments were administered. The excerpt is so illustrative that I am loath to omit it:

The long, lithe and sinewy Master of Warrilow, of Sussex, with three score years of sunburn on his keen, gnarled face, and with the sure stride of a mountain goat, describes the physician bee keeper.

It was a strange procession coming up the red-tiled path of the bee garden. The bee-master led the way in his Sunday clothes, followed by a gorgeous footman, powdered and cockaded, who carried an armful of wraps and cushions. Behind him walked two more, supporting between them a kind of carrying-chair, in which sat a florid old gentleman in a Scotch plaid shawl; and behind these again strode a silk-hatted, black-frocked man carefully regulating the progress of the cavalcade. Through the rain of autumn leaves, on the brisk October morning, I could see, afar off, a carriage waiting by the lane-side; a big old-fashioned family vehicle, with cockaded servants, a pair of champing greys, and a glitter of gold and scarlet on the panel, where the sunbeams struck on an elaborate coat-of-arms.

The whole procession made for the extracting-house, and all work stopped at its approach. The great centrifugal machine ceased its humming. The doors of the packing-room were closed, shutting off the din of saw and hammer. Over the stone floor in front of the furnace where a big caldron of metheglin[3] was simmering-a carpet was hastily unrolled, and a comfortable couch brought out and set close to the cheery blaze.

And now the strangest part of the proceedings commenced. The old gentleman was brought in, partially disrobed, and transferred to the couch by the fireside. He seemed in great trepidation about something. He kept his gold eyeglasses turned on the bee-master, watching him with a sort of terrified wonder, as the old bee-man produced a mysterious box, with a lid of perforated zinc, and laid it on the table close by. From my corner the whole scene was strongly reminiscent of the ogre's kitchen in the fairy-tale; and the muffled sounds from the packing-room might have been the voice of

---

[3] Honey wine

the ogre himself, complaining at the lateness of his dinner. Now, at a word from the black-coated man, the bee-master opened his box. A loud angry buzzing uprose, and about a dozen bees escaped into the air, and flew straight for the window-glass. The bee-master followed them, took one carefully by the wings, and brought it over to the old gentleman. His apprehensions visibly redoubled. The doctor seized him in an iron, professional grip.

"Just here, I think. Close under the shoulder-blade. Now, your lordship...." Viciously the infuriated bee struck home. For eight or ten seconds she worked her wicked will on the patient. Then, turning round and round, she at last drew out her sting and darted back to the window.

But the bee-master was ready with another of his living stilettos. Half a dozen times the operation was repeated on various parts of the suffering patient's body. Then the old gentleman-who, by this time, had passed from whimpering through the various stages of growing indignation to sheer undisguised profanity-was restored to his apparel. The procession was reformed, and the bee-master conducted it to the waiting carriage, with the same ceremony as before.

As we stood looking after the retreating vehicle, the old bee-man entered into explanations.

"That," said he, "is Lord H, and he has been a martyr to rheumatism these ten years back. I could have cured him long ago if he had only come to me before, as I have done many a poor soul in these parts; but he, and those like him, are the last to hear of the physician in the hive. He will begin to get better now, as you will see. He is to be brought here every fortnight; but in a month or two he will not need the chair. And before the winter is out he will walk again as well as the best of us."

"Of course," continued the bee-master, "there is nothing new in this treatment of rheumatism by bee-stings. It is literally as old as the hills. Every bee-keeper for the last two thousand years has known of it. But it is as much as a preventive as a cure that the acid in a bee's sting is valuable. The rarest thing in the world is to find a bee-keeper suffering from rheumatism. And if everyone kept bees, and got stung occasionally, the doctors would soon have one ailment the less to trouble about."

One of the greatest exponents of lay apiarian therapeutics was Ernest Lautal of Marseille, France. He was not only an apiarist, but was also considered a philanthropist.

His treatments were not restricted to rheumatism alone, but branched out to various other diseases, several of them considered incurable. He called his procedure "apipuncture." Lautal installed a model apiary in Marseille, with an office, where he treated rheumatism, gout, lupus, eczema, epithelioma and leprosy. He served the destitute gratuitously. Let him tell it in his own words.

"I had no idea that the honey bee would ever prove useful to cure all these ailments because only very few physicians recognized the curative power of bee stings. Many desperate patients, prepared to make an end of their lives, came to me and asked for bees. I gave them all they wanted, often even applying them myself, and they are happy now at being cured.

For many years I suffered myself from an obstinate eczema over the whole body, especially on my hands and forearms. I was under the treatment of many dermatologists but could not obtain any relief. One day while handling bees, I was attacked on my left arm, against my wish, by a great number of bees. The accident caused me quite an anxiety, not only because it caused me great pain, but I was afraid that my exanthema would become worse. To my great astonishment the eczema entirely disappeared from my arm. This incident gave me an idea and I tried the same treatment upon my right arm and exposed it voluntarily to bee stings. The result was, likewise, satisfactory. I continued the experiment and succeeded in curing all my skin trouble. I administered the same treatment also to others with great success.

I then extended the field of my experiments in the treatment of tuberculotic affections of the skin and had unexpected and surprising results. Obstinate and rebellious cases of neuralgia, also, rapidly yielded to apipuncture, and I can see the time when this treatment with bee stings will be an accepted method for rheumatism, eczema, lupus, cancer, leprosy and many other diseases."

Lautal added that he stopped several epileptic convulsions with bee stings. His success as the inaugurator of these treatments aroused so much attention and interest that Dr. Boinet, Professor of the Faculty of Medicine in Marseille and Physician in Chief of the Hospitals, authorized him to install bee hives in the two principal hospitals of Marseille, Hôtel-Dieu and Conception, and entrusted the patients into his hands. The method gradually became more popular and several prominent physicians undertook the treatments, which are described in Chapter XI, under the heading "Dermatoses."

Lautal also suggested bee stings as a control in doubtful cases of death in the absence of a physician. This advice was based on the fact, first, that bees obstinately refuse to sting a corpse, and second, if the stinging act is forcibly induced by strong pressure on the bees' abdomen, it will not elicit any inflammatory reaction as on a living person.

As proof of how unwilling the medical profession was to assume the burden of handling live bees and to have their names associated with the subject, the following incident is a good illustration.

E. W. Ainley-Walker, on June 17, 1907, wrote a letter to editors of *The Lancet*:

TO THE EDITORS:
SIRS:

In the course of an enquiry into the relation which I have been led to suppose may exist between certain manifestations of rheumatism and an abnormal production of formic acid [4]in the tissues, my attention has been called from time to time to a curious belief which appears to be prevalent in various parts of the country. This very interesting piece of folklore is to the effect that frequent exposures to the stings of bees (beekeepers) is both protective and curative for rheumatism. My correspondence leads me to conclude that this belief is widely disseminated and is probably familiar to many of your readers.

---

[4] Bee venom does not contain formic acid.-Author.

May I therefore be allowed the privilege of making the following enquiries (through your correspondence column) of any of your readers who are sufficiently interested in the question to send me such information as has come within their knowledge?

1. Have you met with the belief that bee stings cure or prevent rheumatism?

2. Do you know any case in which a rheumatic subject claims to have benefited in this way as the result of working among bees?

3. Are you acquainted with any reliable evidence which supports or explains the origin of this belief?

4. What were the characters of the rheumatism in question?

I am, Sirs,

Yours faithfully,

(Signed) E. W. AINLEY-WALKER.

You can judge for yourselves the extent of the interest aroused within the medical profession by the fact that hardly more than a dozen replies were received and some of those who answered were too timid even to sign their names, and assumed a sobriquet. One of the answers, which appeared *The Lancet* of June 29, 1907, was as follows:

TO THE EDITORS OF THE *LANCET*:

SIRS:

In answer to the questions of Dr. E. W. Ainley-Walker in your last issue, I can narrate an example of the belief that the stings of bees have a curative effect in rheumatism. Some eight years ago, when I was travelling, the mate of a cargo boat showed me an apparatus that, he informed me, had belonged to his father who had been cured of a very severe and obstinate "rheumatism of the spine" by its use. It consisted of a metal piston working in a cylinder in which it could be withdrawn or released by means of a spring. On the "business end" of the piston were set concentric rings of needles projecting about % of an inch. The instrument was used by applying it over the affected part, releasing the spring sharply; by this means the skin was scarified in the same sort of way as, I believe, is employed in some modern tattooing. In this process, however, the ink was replaced by a dark brown somewhat viscous solution that I was assured was prepared from the stings of the bees. My informant's father obtained it many years ago from a German chemist and was said to have derived the greatest benefit from the use of this certainly heroic remedy.

It was a condition of the success that the remedy should be rubbed in very vigorously and it was said to produce a smart inflammatory reaction, which is hardly surprising. My informant only had a little of the fluid left and he did not know whether it could still be obtained anywhere. His father had applied it all down his spine and I imagine it was a case of osteo-arthritis and that the benefit was produced simply by counter-irritation. It is possible, however, that it may have had some specific effect as the patient supposed.

I am, Sirs,
Faithfully,
(Signed) TATTOO.
Another letter, dated October, 1907, was the following:

TO THE EDITORS OF THE *LANCET*:
SIRS:

In reply to E. W. Ainley-Walker's letter in The *Lancet*, June 22d Page 1737, an interesting review of the history and literature of formic acid will be found in Dr. Heinrich Stern's paper *Sixteen Years' Experience with Formic Acid as a Therapeutic Agent, in the Journal of the American Medical Association*, April 28, 1906, Page 1258. Dr. Stern states that when formic acid is applied to a paralyzed limb or to a rheumatic joint its beneficial influence is solely due to its power of exciting circulation and setting up a somewhat enduring counterirritation.

Several cases of arthritis deformans are described by Dr. L. B. Couch in the *Medical Record*, N. Y., June 24, 1905, Page 972, full details being given as to the symptoms, treatment, and results as regards bee stings. Dr. Couch heard of a bee farmer in Long Island who had been speedily cured of chronic rheumatism, being stung by honey-bees. He wrote to the farmer for corroboration and was informed that the story was true.

Dr. Ainley-Walker will probably have no difficulty in collecting clinical evidence from medical literature as to the value of formic acid in rheumatism, though authentic records of the efficacy of bees' stings are less easily obtained.

(Signed) HESPERUS.
Baltimore

It is rather curious that both "Tattoo" and "Hesperus" (the resplendent "Evening Star" of the Cimmerian darkness) were reluctant to give their names. I certainly fail to discover any reason for it because both letters are not only interesting, but perfectly professional and ethical.

One answer to *The Lancet*, in August, 1907, was the following:

TO THE EDITORS OF THE *LANCET*:
SIRS:

In connection with the correspondence which has appeared in your columns upon the subject of bees' stings and rheumatism, it is interesting to recall that several years ago a patient wrote me asking whether physicians of today continued to use bees for stinging the inflamed joints in rheumatism, as a curative measure, stating that he had read in an ancient classic that such treatments were practiced along the eastern shores of the Adriatic, I believe some time prior to the Christian Era. I am, Sirs,

> Yours faithfully,
> (Signed) EDWARD F. WELLS, M.D.
> Chicago, July 17, 1907.

The *British Medical Journal* received another letter from Dr. Joseph William Gill, mentioning that he had written to "The Journal" on February 8, 1906, relating the case of a patient suffering from rheumatic gout who was stung on the forehead by a bee. A severe swelling resulted, he became very ill for a few hours, after which he improved rapidly, the rheumatic gout left him, and for six months he had good health. The patient had since died from rheumatic fever. Dr. Gill added the suggestion that, if an active principle of the poison ejected by the bees could be isolated for medicinal injections, it would prove a most valuable remedy for those conditions.

In the past fifty years, a comparatively larger number of physicians have undertaken the unthankful task of administering the treatments. Terc, of Marburg, was without doubt one of the most persevering among them. Keiter, of Graz, his pupil and collaborator, swore to the miraculous healing power of bee stings. Langer, Professor of Pediatrics of the University of Prague, also an untiring and lifelong worker in this field, encountered even more difficulties in treating children, who have a natural horror of bees. Langer later produced an injectable bee venom, but the results obtained. from its use were not satisfactory.

Other workers with live bees were: Maberly, of London (report published in 1910); in France: Lamarche (1908), Bouquet (1924), Jubleau (1925), Molinery (1925), Prof. Boinet, Drs. Vigne, and Bougala (the last three from Marseilles); and some others.

Only in 1928, Herbert Pollack, of Munich, succeeded in producing an injectable bee venom, called "*Apicosan*," which was free from albumin and could be injected without anaphylactic danger of proteotoxic shock.

Contemporaneously, Franz Kretschy, of Vienna, after many years of experiments, also succeeded in producing an injectable bee venom, which he named "*Immenin*" (Imme in Old German means bee). Immenin is a sterile, abiuretic substance free from anaphylactogen elements, and can be used without any danger. The injections are almost painless.

These two preparations are very extensively employed in all parts of Europe, and the number of successfully treated cases increases daily. Kretschy introduced Immenin to the medical profession in 1928, during the 43d Balneologic Congress in Baden, near Vienna. He administered the preparation to cure himself of a very obstinate case of rheumatism, which had tortured him for years, not yielding to any other treatment. Later Pollack became Kretschy's collaborator in Vienna.

The Weleda Company, Ltd., of Arlesheim, Switzerland, also put an injectable bee venom on the market, called "*Apisin*." It is, likewise, distributed in ampoules of various concentrations, to be administered subcutaneously or intramuscularly, for the treatment of rheumatoid ailments.

Just before this volume went to the press, the British Medical Journal mentioned a new injectable bee venom preparation which appeared on the market. It is called British Bee Venom, and is prepared by the Antibody Products Ltd., Watford, Hertfordshire, England. It is dispensed in I c.c. ampoules, in progressively stronger doses, each vial being marked with the number of units it contains. In one box, called one course, there are twelve vials, ranging from 5 to 60 units. Ten units are supposed to be equivalent to one bee sting. It is administered intradermally or subcutaneously for the treatment of rheumatoid disorders.

Since the introduction of the injectable venom, many hospitals and clinics in Europe have made special studies in this field. I enumerate chronologically the fellow-workers who published reports:

1927   Prof. Passow, of Munich.

1928   H. Pollack, of Vienna.
F. Kretschy, of Vienna.
K. Wasserbrenner, of the Vienna Polyclinic (Prof. Strasser).
W. Krebs, of Bad-Aachen.

1929   J. Kroner, of the Friedrich Wilhelm Hospital, Berlin.

1930   R. Loebel, of Hofgastein.
A. Simo, of Schallebach.

1931   S. Becker, First Med. University Clinic of Vienna (Prof. Porges).

1932   H. Nowotny, of the Orthopedic Hospital in Vienna (Prof. Spitzy).
W. Fehlow, Berlin University (Prof. Aug. Bier).
G. Koehler, of Berlin (Prof. H. Zondek).
M. Grünsfeld, of Vienna.

1933-   M. Roch, Professor of the Faculty of Geneva.
M. Perrin and A. Cuènot, of the Faculty of Nancy, France (Perrin and Cuènot still use live bees (1933) during the summer months; but in winter, a special preparation of their own, described in Chapter III section "The production of Injectable Bee Venom").

All the inconveniences and difficulties of the old tedious treatments do not exist today and there are no obstacles which would prevent the medical man from giving this remedy a fair and deserving trial.

Lately, an ointment which contains bee venom has been produced in Germany. It is called "*Forapin.*" The preparation was perfected under the direction of Forster, for many years assistant of the Pharmacological Institute of Würzburg. The ointment is rubbed in over the painful nerves, muscles, and joints, and is supposed to possess rubefacient and vesicant action in addition to an absorptive effect. It is attested by a number of physicians and hospitals.

R. Schwab, in a recent article in the *Münch. Med. Wchnschr.*, reported 40 cases of acute and chronic arthritis, muscular rheumatism, and sciatic neuritis which had been favorably treated with the ointment. He stated that it contains no formic acid but salicylates, which were in too small an amount to be effective but sufficient to soften the skin. He did not notice any idiosyncrasy or unusually strong reactions from the use of Forapin, but did observe that a real rheumatic reacted less than a normal person.

Forapin is dispensed in graduated tubes, each containing the venom of 80 bees. To promote absorption, one-half percent sinapis oil, and for preservative effect, eight percent salicylic acid are added. A cork "rubbing pad" is furnished with each tube.

The Weleda Company, also, introduced recently a two percent Apis ointment.

CHAPTER REFERENCES

ALTSCHUL. Real-Lexicon für homöopath. Arzneimittellehre, Therapie und Arzneibe reitungskunde, Sonderhausen, 1864.

AMERICAN BEE J. Bees and Medicine, Febr. 1925.

BECKER, S. Behandlung rheumatischer Erkrankungen mit injizierbaren Bienengift präparat Immenin, Therap. d. Gegenw. Berl. u. Wien, 6, 1931.

BOINET, E. Deux cas de guérison du lupus par les piqûres d'abeille, Marseille Med., 60, 1923.

BRANDT, u. RATZEBURG. Die Honigbiene, Mediz. Zoologie, I, 1829.

DALE, SAMUEL. Pharmacologia seu manuductio ad materiam medicam. Lond. 1737.

DAVIS, F. P. Medical Summary, 1908.

EDWARDES, TICKNER. The Bee-Master of Warrilow, London, 1920.

FEHLOW, W. Die Bienengiftbehandlung rheumatischer Erkrankungen, Deutsche Med. Wchnschr. Berl. u. Leipz., 9 Febr. 1932.

"FORAPIN," Neue eingeführte Arzneimittel und Pharmaceut. Specialität., Deutsche Med. Wchnschr. Berl. u. Leipz., 2, 1934.

GALEN. Kühn, Leipz., 1820.

GOULLON, H. Das Bienengift im Dienste der Homeopathie, Leipz., 1880.

GRÜNSFELD, M. Das injizierbare Bienengiftpräparat Immenin von Standpunkte des praktischen Arztes, Wien. Med. Wchnschr. 8, 1932.

HERING, C. American Provings, 1853.
Condensed Materia Medica, Apis mellifica, 1877.
The guiding symptoms of our Materia Medica. Phila. 1879.
Kurzgefasste Arzneimittellehre, 3d Ed. Berl. 1889.

JÜHLING, J. Die Tierre in deutscher Volksmedizin, Alter und Neuer Zeit.

KAFKA, J. Therapeutische Erfahrungen über das Bienengift, Berl. 1858.

KEITER, A. Rheumatismus und Bienenstichbehandlung, 1914.
Bienenstichkur, Umschau & Therap. Mon. Bericht, 1913.

KOEHLER, G. Über die Behandlung chron. Gelenksaffectionen mit Apicosan, Med. Welt, 43, Oct. 1932.

KRETSCHY, F. Die moderne Bienengifttherapie, Ztschr. f. Wissensch. Bäderkunde, 2, 1928.

KRONER, J. Die Behandlung der chron. Polyarthritis im Spätstadium, München. Med. Wchnschr., 39-40, 1930.
—Spätstadien rheumatischer Erkrankungen und ihre Behandlung, RheumaJahrbuch, 1929.

LOEBEL, R. u. SIMO, A. Uber ambulatorische Behandlung chron. Gelenkskrankheiten, Neuralgien, Myalgien mit unspecif. Reiztherapie, Med. Klin. Berl. u. Wien, 10, 1930.

MABERLY, F. H. Brief Notes on the Treatment of Rheumatism with Bee Stings, Lancet, Lond. July 23, 1910.

NOWOTNY, H. Immeninbehandlung chron. entzündlich. Processe, München. Med. Wchnschr., 29, 1932.

PASSOW, PR. Über Apicosanbehandlung bei Iritis rheumatica, Klin. Monatsbl. f. Augenh., 79, 1927.

PERRIN, M. ET CUÈNOT, A. Rheumatisme et Venin d'Abeilles, Rev. Med. de l'Est, Apr. 1933.

PLINY. C. Plinius secundi naturalis historia, Teubner, 1870.

POLLACK, H. Über Apicosanbehandlung bei Iritis rheumatica, Klin. Monatsbl. f. Augenh., 81, Nov. 1928.

QUINCY, JOHN. Pharmacopoeia officinalis, extemporanea or complete English Dispensatory, Lond. 1733.

RICHET, CH. Diction. de Physiolog, Abeille, 1895.

ROCH, M. Le venin d'abeille dans le traitment des sciatiques. Rev. Med. de la Suisse Rom. Genève, Febr. 1933.

SALMON, WM. Pharmacopoeia Londoniensis or New London Dispensatory, Lond., 1716.

SCHWAB, R. Eine neue Applikations methode des Bienengiftes bei rheumatischen Erkrankungen (Forapin), München. Med. Wchnschr., 81, 1934.

SOZINSKEY, TII. S. Medical Symbolism, 1891.

STRASSER, PR., 1928.

VIGNE ET BOUGALA. Soc. de méd. Col. Hyg. D'Marseille, Dec. 12, 1923.

WASSERBRENNER, K. Über Behandlung von rheumatischen Erkrankungen mit Bienengift, Wien. Klin. Wchnschr., 35, 1928.

WOLF, C. W. Apis Mellifica, or The Poison of the Honey Bee considered as a Therapeutic Agent, Berlin, 1858.

Chapter III Animal Venom

If we reflect upon the general utility of animals to mankind, we find that certain of them are useful to man, supplying him with food, like meat and milk; some furnish clothing necessities, like leather and furs; others again supply domestic and industrial needs, feathers, horns, horsehair, and even luxuries, such as pearls, ivory, and hundreds of other different materials. Many animals render vital commercial and agricultural services. Last but not least, they also produce important medicinal substances.

On the other hand, there are animals harmful and dangerous to man, even damaging his property. Some beasts attack man and devour him; to them he is a source of food. Again, various animals imperil the human race by inflicting grave, even mortal injuries. They kill man but leave the corpse. Apparently, this is done with no definite object, but on closer investigation we usually discover it to be simply an act of self-defense in their struggle for self-preservation. In the latter class, serpents and venomous insects predominate.

Now, if we try to classify the animal kingdom according to harmful characteristics, we have to assign a place to the bees. Here, once again, we are confronted with their paradoxical and complex character. No doubt, the bees are venomous insects, but still we cannot call them harmful in the strict sense of the word. As Muffet said, "Bees are neither wilde nor tame creatures, but a middle kinde of nature between both." Man has domesticated the bees, and made them house pets, cultivating the species with great interest, diligence, and care. Bees are utilitarian and profitable, producing honey and wax; they have great commercial and economic value, and, from the viewpoint of their horticultural and agricultural benefits, they are simply indispensable. We have to place the bees in the class of useful insects, considering that their beneficial services (pro bono publico) predominate, and that they are productive of far more good than harm. In consideration of the fact that their venom is credited with important healing power, we certainly ought to accord them a still higher rank.

Bees unquestionably produce and secrete a substance of poisonous quality. If we intend to utilize their venom as a therapeutic agent, it is expedient not only to know the anatomy, morphology, histology, physiology, and biology of the bees, but also the chemical, toxicological properties and clinical effects of their venom. (My intention was to include in this treatise the first mentioned subjects which afford not only an absorbing and captivating field for research but also have considerable scientific interest for all real students of medicine. On the advice of the

34

publishers, I withdrew these with the prospect of inserting them in another volume, to be published shortly.)

Before all, we had better discuss first the respective position of the bee among venomous insects, and settle also the much debated question of what constitutes a poison. It is hard to say which of the two problems is more difficult to solve.

What is the definition of poison? The lay conception of poison is an organic or inorganic substance having a temporary or permanent harmful effect on the human or animal system. The scientific, toxicological definition is quite different. From a scientific viewpoint, there are no absolute universal poisons. All toxicity is only relative, depending on quality, quantity, and on the media of their action. The quantity, of course, is a most important and essential factor. Strychnine, arsenic, and morphine are called poisonous and still are well known curative agents. Vice versa, sodium chloride, sugar, and alcohol are not considered poisonous, but in large quantities or in the blood stream they are injurious and even fatal. For instance, there is recorded a death which was caused by half a pint of concentrated solution of common table salt.

It is evident that the definition of a poison is arbitrary. Any harmless substance in large quantity will answer all the requirements of the term "poison." Water is not a poison; still in large quantities, it can be destructive. Heat is necessary to the body, but high temperature will destroy life. Powdered glass cannot be classified as a poison; but if introduced into the gastro-intestinal tract, even in small quantity, it will mechanically destroy the tissues and may cause death.

From a comparative physiological viewpoint, cadaveric poison and snake venom are fatal in the blood, but if they enter the system through the digestive tract they are harmless. Many poisonous reptiles and insects are eaten by other animals (even men) without ill effects. For example, the Spanish fly is eaten by birds. Socrates died from the poison of the hemlock, and yet the aphis anthrisci (leaf louse) thrives on its juices. The hog, crane, and mongoose are bitten by serpents, and also eat them with impunity, though even the snake's blood is decidedly poisonous.

Individual sensitivity, idiosyncrasy, and likewise lack of detoxicating power, all play important parts in poisoning. We know of Baermann's published case, the death of a grown-up person, as the result of taking half a gram of quinine sulphate. Habitat, also, is an important factor. Fresh water fish will die in the ocean and deep sea fish, as a rule, will perish in a lake or river. And how many other relational, often contributory causes influence the effect of poisons! The experiment with phosphin is only one example. A solution of phosphin has no effect on infusoria at night, but in the daytime the same concentration will kill them, the accumulative effect of sunlight influencing the efficiency of the substance.

The production of venom by animals and insects, and their method of administering it, differ greatly. Some animals and insects discharge their venom in the medium in which they live, like toads and salamanders; others first inflict mechanical injuries, and through these avenues inoculate, convey, and transmit their venom. The organs which they employ in inflicting wounds are located in different parts of their bodies: in certain instances, they are in the front; in others, in the rear. The organs located in the front are usually an integral part of the digestive tract, like teeth. Snakes, spiders, ants, utilize their bite to accomplish the injury. When the "retributive" organ is located in the rear of the body, as in the case of bees, wasps, and hornets, the insects possess a special apparatus, usually a sharp-pointed instrument, and with the aid and employment of this so-called weapon, perform an act called stinging, thrusting this instrument into the victim, and through the resulting channel inject their venom.

After these preliminaries, we might discuss animal venoms in general. There is no other branch of medicine where fear, fiction, legend, and superstition are more intermingled with truth and real facts than in the chapter on venomous animals and insects; there is plenty of thrill, adventure, and even serious danger in store for the scientist and medical man. First, we have to extract the venom for scientific research or therapeutic use. Collecting and handling this material derived from living animals is not, by any means, a simple task, but a rather intricate and complicated procedure. In addition, it often involves considerable time, labor, and expense. The work is not like that of handling mineral or vegetable matter. The extracted substances are very perishable, they rapidly deteriorate, and are not infrequently subjected to chemical changes, viz., autolytic ferments, bacterial invasion, etc.

ANIMAL VENOM

In classifying animal poisons, we divide them into three classes:

1) Active poisons: supplied by special glands and introduced or injected by a more or less complicated apparatus into the organism of the victim.

2) Passive poisons: administered without the aforementioned contrivances but also limited to a certain confined part of the body, like toad venom, cantharidin, etc.

3) Cryptotoxic substances: those in which the toxic material under normal conditions is not active but must first be produced in an experimental way, like adrenalin, thyroid, bile acids, etc.

The treatise on animal poisons, outside of its general human interest, is, also, an essential and significant chapter of chemistry and toxicology. In medical sciences, in pharmacology and in the study of immunity and serology, animal venoms have fundamental importance. Through their occult and mystic attributes they supply a wealth of material for myths, folklore, literature, drama, poetry, and law.

ACTIVE POISONS

Though by logical inference, the process of administering active poisons implies aggression, the use of the weapon, in the majority of instances, is strictly a defensive performance. Of course, there are some snakes, wasps, and hornets which kill their prey to consume them afterwards, but even these are given the benefit of the doubt by some scientists, who, in spite of it, claim that primarily they acted in self-defense.

PASSIVE POISONS

Toad poison and cantharidin are typical examples of this class. The poison of the toads is not only found in the glands of the animals but is contained in their blood, just as in snakes. Cantharidin, as we know, has an old and renowned history. It not only has a general constitutional effect, but also is a strong local vesicant-the Spanish fly stings when alive, and blisters when dead. Hippocrates, Aristotle, Pliny all mention its aphrodisiac effects.

CRYPTOTOXIC POISONS

These represent the largest group of animal poisons. Extracts of the ductless glands and biliary toxins are numberless. Bilirubin is very toxic, even in small quantities. We may include our human body as a great potential poison producer. Urinary toxins are very powerful poisons, especially under certain specific pathological conditions. We cannot go into detail in the enumeration of the various ptomaines and leukomaines.

If we now thoroughly investigate and examine for facts and principles the relationship among mineral and vegetable (also synthetic) poisons, animal venoms, and bacteria, with the purpose of recording, from a comparative viewpoint, their similarities and divergencies, we are certainly confronted with an all-absorbing, momentous problem. Comparing from a chemical, physiological, clinical viewpoint the individual characteristics of these four principal groups-mineral, vegetable, animal, and bacterial—we cannot fail to notice that there is no sharp boundary, nor a fixed line of demarcation between them.

For instance, if we investigate the characteristics of the animal venoms, we note that:

1) They have no, or slight toxicity when administered perorally, being easily destroyed by digestive ferments.

2) Heat, chemicals, antiseptics, oxidizing substances will attenuate or destroy their efficiency.

3) Through habituation to their use, they confer immunity.

4) They are capable of being transmitted into vaccines.

5) After vaccinating animals with increasing doses of animal venoms, their sera possess immunizing properties which are effective for a certain limited time. This serum acts like an antivirus. Injected into a nonimmunized animal, it will confer a so-called passive immunity against the venom.

6) The immunity is passed on by heredity, both through the transmission of the blood, in placental circulation, and through the milk, during the lactation period.

Now if we consider all these enumerated phenomena as characteristic attributes of animal poisons, we cannot fail to notice that they are almost identical with those of the bacteria. Bacterial toxins, viewed as proteins, are colloidal molecules, and are affected also by proteolytic enzymes. They are so powerful that they are efficient even in such diluted states as will not react to any analytical tests. Bacterial toxins have great antigenic characteristics. Detoxicated with formalin, they lose their toxicity (toxoid), but still retain their antigenic action. Toxins and enzymes have striking similarities: both are colloids.

The most important difference between the two groups is that, while the full effect of the bacterial toxins is preceded by a state of incubation, the animal venoms have instantaneous effect. The difference is apparently a radical one, but upon closer scrutiny it will only prove to be rather superficial. The bacteria have the faculty of multiplying in the invaded host (a requisite for the attainment of their full potency), while the animal venoms possess their maximum strength and have an almost immediate and violent effect. In a word, animal venoms are formed, complete toxins; bacterial toxins are unformed and incomplete at the time of their entrance into the body, but the time which they require for their development really corresponds with the period of incubation. Many hemolytic poisons also have a latent state in the organism.

If we continue our line of investigation and compare the animal venoms with some of the vegetable poisons, we find that both these groups show not only a similar chemical composition but also analogous physiological action. The chemical structure and physiological effect of the vegetable glucosides are almost parallel to those of the animal venoms. Toad venom, a mixture of carbylamine substances and phrynin, has a physiological action similar to digitalis. Quillaja acid, according to Faust, greatly resembles, physiologically and chemically, ophiotoxin (compound of cobra venom) the whole chemical difference is that one atom of hydrogen is missing in the latter. Quillaja acid and sapotoxins, in gradually increased doses, will immunize the organism in the same manner as animal venoms. But it is much beyond the limit of our dissertation to discuss further the defensive factor in the system, whether it is the increase of cholesterin in the plasma, or something else.

Our last point, to compare the similar physiological effects of mineral with those of the vegetable poisons-the alkaloids, for instance-is the least difficult, as the modus operandi of the two classes is very much alike.

In addition to the statement that there is no sharp boundary between these four groups of poisons, if we now survey the field of bacteria, it is not surprising to find that Besredka, of the Pasteur Institute, made the statement, "I believe there can no longer be any doubt that the effect produced by antivirus is a nonspecific one."

Sera of animals immunized against anthrax and tetanus have antitoxic effect on the venom of serpents; likewise have the sera of dogs highly immunized against rabies and erysipelas. Rabbits vaccinated against snake venom become resistant to poisoning by abrine; on the other hand, those vaccinated against abrine acquire a certain immunity to snake venom, diphtheria, ricine, occasionally even to anthrax.

THE THERAPEUTIC USES OF ANIMAL VENOMS

In conjunction with the subject of this treatise, namely, the treatment of arthritis and rheumatism with bee venom, I wish to mention the fact that many attempts have been made to use other animal venoms for curative purposes.

Quite some time ago, Alphonse LeRoy suggested viper venom for hydrophobia and yellow fever; rattlesnake venom for leprosy, diphtheria, and febrile conditions; and cobra venom for cancer. Levin, in 1900, treated leprosy with rattlesnake venom. It is very peculiar that an otherwise fatal dose of the venom was well tolerated by lepers; they possess a certain immunity to it, a fact having remarkable analogy to the action of bee venom, which is endowed with a powerful curative effect on rheumatoid patients and, at the same time, is well tolerated by them.

Calmette and Mezie, in 1914, treated epilepsy with snake venom. They made the observation that attacks become lighter and less frequent. Mays reported a case in 1909. A male epileptic, 35, who had had epileptic fits for 15 years, was bitten by a snake two years previous and since that time had been free from attacks. Ralph H. Spangler treated a great number of cases with crotalus venom, and found the character of convulsions modified, the intervals between the attacks lengthened, and the mental and physical condition of the patients noticeably improved.

F. W. Fitzsimons, Director of the Port Elizabeth Museum and Snake Park, South Africa, published many cases of epilepsy cured with "Venene," a combination of various snake venoms. Innumerable instances are reported where epileptics, bitten by venomous reptiles, have greatly improved of never suffered further attacks. Snake venoms are powerful antispasmodic and anticonvulsive agents. Fitzsimons also successfully cured, with injections of Venene, many dogs of chorea, an after-effect of distemper, which so far had been considered incurable. In a lecture to a gathering of scientists at the American Museum of Natural History a short time ago, Dr. Fitzsimons said that the nontoxic serum derived from puff-adder venom had cured 20 percent of 500 cases of epilepsy. Only 6 percent of the epileptic patients failed to respond to the serum; the rest improved in varying degrees. Fitzsimons stressed the effectiveness of the treatment for St. Vitus dance and readily accessible cancerous tumors. The puff-adder is a South African snake which resembles the American rattlesnake. Fitzsimons explained that the puff-adder toxoid causes intense blood congestion, which, in turn, attracts the white blood corpuscles to attack the normal cell area.

ANIMAL VENOM

Chopra and Chowhan, of Calcutta, India, gave a detailed account of the extensive use of snake venoms by Hindu physicians. Pills containing cobra venom are used for collapse and cholera. The medical use of cobra venom as a heart stimulant was, they thought, on the increase. It is also highly valued as a hepatic stimulant. The Mohammedan physicians in India use the venom for leukoderma. In some parts of Burma, the natives eat snake flesh as a food. Crotalus is used for epilepsy, *hemophilia*, and chorea. It is supposed to have a depressive effect on the nerves, increasing also the fibrin content of the blood. In blackwater fever, profuse and painful menstruation, viperine venoms are used with great success.

Cobra venom is used in the *Farmachidis* test for cancer diagnosis. This test depends upon the activation by cobra venom of the hemolytic action of the serum in the complement deviation test, and it is asserted that the test is positive only with the serum of persons suffering from a malignant disease. Recently, André Gosset read a paper before the Academy of Medicine in Paris, reporting 115 so-called incurable cancer cases treated by our New York colleague, Monae-Lesser, with the serum of black cobras. (His first experiments were made with rattlesnake venom, and only later, on Calmette's advice, with the venom of the cobra.) Patients obtained considerable relief and in some instances, even, the disease was checked, producing retrograde metamorphosis and a marked healing tendency. On the same occasion, Calmette spoke of the neurotoxic qualities of cobra venom and advocated its use in the treatment of other diseases. Laignel-Lavastine and Koressios found that cobra venom is an effective substitute for morphine as an analgesic in inoperable cancers, the effect being more durable. One injection was sufficient to keep the patient painless sometimes for 8 to 10 days. Phisalix, in 1914, was not so optimistic about the therapeutic effects of snake venom and made the statement that according to his opinion it had very little future or importance in therapeutics.

Yoannovitch and Chahovitch wrote an interesting article which appeared in the June, 1932, number of the *Bull. Acad. de Médicine*. The subject was the treatment of experimental cancerous tumors with bee venom. They based their research on the fact that erysipelas complicating cancer not only arrested the growth of the tumor, but greatly favored the cure of the disease, and successful results, even complete cures, were reported. The favorable action of erysipelas is the inflammatory phenomenon. Naturally, it would be dangerous to employ such a method, infecting patients with streptococci; the septicemia might be fatal before the tumor had a chance to recede. For this reason, they never attempted such experiments.

The fact that inflammation had such pronounced effect on neoplasms induced them to try a substance which, when injected, would provoke inflammatory phenomena without any serious danger. Yoannovitch and Chahovitch knew that bee venom would produce such an inflammatory state, which was supposed to increase with its amount and strength. But after repeated injections, the inflammation was not so noticeable, in accordance with the laws of immunity. Cancer statistics show that people occupied in the bee industry are rarely affected by malignant growths.

Yoannovitch and Chahovitch first produced experimental cancers on the ears of a rabbit and then treated them with bee venom. Both ears presented numerous tumors, some the size of a hazelnut. The tumors were dry. Injections were given daily, later on alternate days, at first with a weak solution of venom, gradually increasing the concentration. The injections were administered subcutaneously around the largest tumor. Several hours later, the inflammatory symptoms appeared and their intensity gradually increased, but next day subsided. The tumors became soft and succulent, their bases diminished and parts fell off, followed by cicatrization. The most noteworthy fact was that bee venom had an effect even on the tumors of the other ear, proving that it had not only local but remote action. After the cessation of the injections, the tumors did not continue to regress, but commenced to grow again.

These authors had the same experience with another rabbit. They also treated an orbital cancer of a goat, and noticed the development of granulating tissues on the surface of the tumor. Unluckily, the goat perished as the result of an accident. The experiments were not completed, but they proved two facts: (1) under the influence of bee venom, which provoked inflammatory phenomena, the size of the tumor and its growth were arrested; (2) after the discontinuance of the injections, the tumors did not disappear but commenced to grow.

Their summary was: The inflammatory process produced by bee venom was not sufficient to effect the complete disappearance of the tumors, which would require a combination of the inflammatory action of the venom and injections of some other substance, capable of digesting the tissues of the malignant growth.

The venoms of reptiles and insects have a wide usage, especially in the tropics. In Guyana it is a common practice among the natives, if one of them becomes paralyzed by drink, just to put a big ant on the victim, and he will immediately regain consciousness. Stanley, in his African travels, told us that the natives pulverize dry ants, mix them with olive oil and dip their arrows into the substance, which accounts for their deadly effect. Many savage tribes poison their arrows with snake venom.

In South America, certain ants are used as an aphrodisiac, like cantharidin. In the 17th Century, in all European courts Hoffman's "Vinegar of Magnanimity," made with formic acid, was very popular. It was extensively used as a general tonic, stomachic, diuretic and aphrodisiac remedy.

Bufagin (buffaline), obtained from the secretion of the poison glands of the tropical toad (bufo agua), a substance which is probably also present in the skin glands of other species of toads, proved to have cardiotonic properties, very much like digitalis.

THE THERAPEUTIC USES OF FORMIC ACID

I do not wish to omit here the mention of the use of formic acid in the treatment of rheumatoid conditions. For centuries, there has been a generally accepted belief that the potent part of bee venom was formic acid. Even Langer, one of the first scientists to make an exhaustive research with bee venom, mentioned formic acid as one of its important components. Theodor Merl, in 1921, by very carefully conducted chemical experiments, positively proved that bee venom does not contain even a small trace of formic acid. All the distinctive tests for it proved negative. In spite of this, many authors, even today, erroneously refer to formic acid as the effective component of bee venom. The domestic ants' venom contains a considerable amount of formic acid, which never was, and never will be doubted, having in certain respects an effect similar to that of bee venom, but it is not nearly as powerful.

Formic acid was introduced into therapeutics at the end of the last century and extensively used as a rheumatic remedy. Its reputed efficacy was based on the belief that bee venom was supposed to contain formic acid and on the observation that persons suffering from arthritis and rheumatism, when stung by bees, noticed considerable amelioration of the symptoms and were often cured. Formic acid, on the other hand, when concentrated, produces a stronger local effect on the uninjured skin than bee venom. It may cause inflammation, severe pain, and even blistering-in a word, a real vesicant effect.

The pharmacopoeia lists several preparations of formic acid: a 25% aqueous solution, spiritus acidi formici, sodii formas, elixir formati comp. It is given internally and, to imitate the action of bee stings, in diluted solutions, intradermally injected. It causes local inflammation and, besides,

43

has an absorptive effect. The preparation is extensively used in homeopathic practice. It is put up in ampoules and used intracutaneously, intramuscularly, and intravenously.

Louis Bradford Couch, in 1905, related three years' experiments with formic acid and the therapeutic results obtained. He used a five percent aqueous solution in subcutaneous injections of five drops each, and found the remedy of greatest value in all rheumatic affections, such as lumbago, sciatica, and muscular rheumatism. In acute inflammatory rheumatism and arthritis, the fever and pain ceased in 48 hours. Couch also reported several successful cures of arthritis deformans, and made up his mind never to use anything else for the treatment of these ailments.

Heinrich Stern, in 1906, reported his results, after experimenting for 16 years with formic acid, likewise obtaining excellent cures.

H. M. Sylvester, of Philadelphia, published an article in 1929 reporting 93 cases of gout and various rheumatic and arthritic disorders treated with injections of formic acid. He injected one cubic centimeter, usually about three doses, at three-week intervals, intravenously or hypodermically. Sylvester thought that it changed metabolism in a hitherto unknown way, possibly by assisting in the removal of waste, also rendering living conditions unsuitable for bacteria. Albert E. Hinsdale stated that Apis contained formic acid and protein, and that there was more to any medicine than its active principle; he believed the poor results so far, in the treatment of arthritis and rheumatism with formic acid, were due to the fact that no Apis was administered. The substitution of an active principle for the whole drug is a cardinal mistake and it should be discouraged.

CHAPTER REFERENCES

BACHMETJEW, P. Experimentelle entomologische Studien, 1901.

BESREDKA, A. Are antivirus specific? J. Immunol. Balt. & Cambridge Eng., X, 1932-33.

BOLLINGER. Infektionen durch Tiergifte, Ziemssen Handbuch der spec. Pathol., 652, 1876.

BROWN, TH. R. On the Chemistry, Toxicology and Therapy of Snake Poisoning, Johns Hopkins Hosp. Bull., Balt., 105, 1899.

CALMETTE, A. Le venin des serpents, Par., 1896.
Les venins, les animaux venimeux et la serotherapie antivenimeuse, Par., 1907.

ANIMAL VENOM

CARLET, M. G. Sur le venin d'Hymenoptères et organ. excreteurs, Comt. rend. Ac. d. Sc., Par., 98, 1884.

CHOPRA, R. N., and CHOWAN, J. S. Snake Venoms in Medicine, Indian M. Gas., Calcutta, 67, 1932.

COUCH, L. B. Formic Acid in Rheumatic Conditions, Med. Rec. N. Y., June, 1905.

FARNSTEINER, K. Der Ameisensäuregehalt des Honigs, Ztschr. f. Untersuch. d. Nahrungs u. Genussmittel, Berl., 1908.

FAUST, E. S. Die tierischen Gifte, 1906.
Vergiftungen durch tierische Gifte, Handbuch der Inner. Mediz. (Mohr u. Staehlin), Bd. 4, Th. II, Aufl. II.
Über Ophiotoxin aus dem Gifte d. Cobra di Capello, 1907.
Darstellung und Nachweis tierischer Gifte, Handbuch biolog. Arbeitsmethoden, IV, 7, 1923.
Handbuch d. experiment. Pharmakolog., Bd. II, 2, 1924.

FITZSIMONS, F. W. Snake Venoms, their therapeutic uses and possibilities, Cape-town, 1929.

FLURY, F. Über die Bedeutung der Ameisensäure als naturl. vorkommen, Gift, Bericht. deutsch. pharmazeut. Ges., 1919.
Lehrbuch der Toxicologie, 1928.

FONTANA, F. Abhandlung über das Viperngift, Berl., 1787.

FORCHHEIMER. Therapeusis of Int. Diseases (Billings a. Irons), II, 150, 1917.

GAUTIER, A. Les Toxines microbiennes et animales, 1896.

GUNN, J. A. Snake Venoms, Cambridge Univ. Med. Soc. Mag., 1, 1929.

HINSDALE, A. E. The writings of A. E. Hinsdale, J. Am. Inst. Homeop., N. Y., 22, 1929.

HUSEMANN, F. Handbuch der Toxicologie, I, 273, 1862.

KOBERT, R. Practical Toxicology, 1910.
Beiträge zur Kenntniss der Saponinsubstanzen, 1904.

LAIGNEL-LAVASTINE et KORESSIOS. Traitment des Algies cancereuses par le venin de Cobra, J. de Méd. de Par., 30, July 27, 1933.

MATHESON, R. Medical Entomology, 1933.

MERL, TH. Bienenkörper als Ameisensäureträger, Ztschr. f. Untersuch. d. Nahrungs u. Genussmittel, Berl., 42, 1921.

MITCHELL, S. WEIR. Research upon the venom of the rattlesnake, etc., Wash., 1861.

MONAELESSER, A. Effets du venin de Cobra modifié sur les tumeurs cancereuses, Par., 1933.

NOGUCHI, H. Snake Venoms, 1909.

NOTHNAGEL. Speciel. Pathol. u. Therap. Bienengift, Bd. I, 1910.

PATTON, W. S., AND EVANS, A. M. Insects, Ticks, Mites and Venomous Animals, I, II.

PAWLOWSKY, E. N. Gifttiere und Ihre Giftigkeit, 1927.

PHISALIX, M. Animaux Venimeux et Venins, 1922.

POZZI-ESCOT, E. The Toxins and Venoms and Their Antibodies, 1906.

RILEY, W., and JOHANNSEN, O. A. Handbook of Medical Entomology, Ithaca, 1915.

SOLIS-COHEN, S., and GITHENS, TH. S. Pharmacotherapeutics, Mat. Med. and Drug Action, 1928.

SPANGLER, R. H. The Treatment of Epilepsy with hypoderm. inject. of rattlesnake venom, Crotalin, N. York M. J. (etc.), Sept. 1910, 1911, 1912.

STANLEY, H. M. In Darkest Africa, 1890.

STERN, H. Sixteen years' experience with formic acid as a therapeutic agent, J. Am. M. Ass., Chicago, Apr. 1906.

STUMPER, C. R. Venins des fournis, Comt. rend. Acad. d. Sc., Par., 174, 1922.

SYLVESTER, H. M. Formic acid in its therap. relation to joint diseases, J. Am. Inst. Homeop., 222, 1929.

TAGUET, CH. La cure des Algies et des tumeurs malignes, Jour. de Méd. de Par., 3 Août, 1933.

TASCHENBERG, O. Die Giftige Tiere, 1909.

VAN HASSELT, L. Handbuch der Giftlehre, II.

YOANNOVITCH, G., and CHAHOVITCH, X. Le traitment des tumeurs par le venin des abeilles. Bull. Acad. de Méd. Par., Juin, 1932.

Chapter IV Bee Venom
THE CHEMISTRY OF BEE VENOM

Bee venom is a substance secreted by special active glands and ejected with the aid of the sting apparatus. It is a water-clear liquid with a sharp, bitter taste and aromatic odor (comparable to ripe bananas), having a distinctly acid reaction. Its specific gravity is 1.1313. It is easily soluble in water and acids, almost insoluble in alcohol. It contains 30 percent solid matter. The weight of an average drop of venom is about 0.2 to 0.3 mg., that is, about 1/500th part of the bee's body weight. Flury succeeded in extracting from 1,000 bees approximately 50 to 75 mg. of venom and even this small amount was mixed with a certain percentage of honey.

The venom dries quickly in ordinary room temperature. Drying will convert it into a gum-like substance, without any loss of potency. It thermostabile, withstanding 100° C. temperature for ten days without losing any of its power. Boiling will make clear bee venom cloudy, but if boiled in a sealed glass tube even for two hours its appearance will not be affected. Cold, even freezing, does not destroy its effect. Yeast does not change the venom, even when exposed to its influence for several hours. It cannot be dialyzed through a membrane, which signifies that it belongs to the colloidal group. By various manipulations the venom gives a sediment rich in albumin.

Bee venom is easily destroyed by oxidizing substances: potassium permanganate, potassium sulphate; halogen elements-chlorine and bromine destroy it very quickly; the effect of iodine is much slower. Alcohol possesses a strong and quick destructive effect on the venom. In contact with tincture of iodine, the alcohol is more destructive than the dissolved iodine.

Digestive ferments-ptyalin, pepsin, pancreatin, rennet, likewise vegetable ferments—papayin, papayotoxin, rapidly weaken the venom and, *vice versa*, bee venom quickly impairs their effectiveness-in a word, they are destructive to each other. This action is, also, a common characteristic quality of both groups of ferments toward other animal venoms, for instance, snake venom.

The neutralizing effect of alkalies on bee venom is likewise very rapid and strong. For instance, ammonia will speedily neutralize it. Powerful acids -picric, chromic, carbolic-and also strong antiseptics, of course, will rapidly destroy the venom but all these substances themselves have poisonous and caustic effects. Fouling, autolytic ferments and bacteria are destructive to the venom.

It has no effect on uninjured skin. Still there are references to the fact that in certain sensitive people eczematous rash develops on parts of the body, whenever there is any contact with bee-materials, such as gloves, veil, frames, etc., which had been previously used. It is a kind of skin-allergy, produced by prior sensitization. The best proof that bee venom affects the skin is that absorption takes place. The recent introduction of a bee venom ointment for arthritic joints and rheumatic muscles, about which there have been many reports of very favorable results, confirms the supposition. This ointment must be vigorously rubbed in. It is possible that the consequent injury to the skin assists in the absorption.

On the other hand, its action is powerful on the mucous membranes, except, as mentioned, on those of the alimentary tract; the salivary, gastric, and intestinal ferments will quickly destroy it. On account of this fact bee venom (like snake venom), if taken internally, is usually ineffective. It is a generally accepted belief, based on past experience that, if another person sucks the wound of a victim bitten by snakes, he may swallow the venom with impunity. Innumerable statements have been made that this is not the case with bee venom. Many a good Samaritan, performing such an act for a victim stung by a bee, to prevent an anticipated violent intoxication, has become violently ill, suffering distressing headache, circulatory disturbances, even indigestion. There is no better proof than this of the high potency of bee venom, which would likewise explain the homeopathic successes in the administration of Apis.

On the conjunctiva and nasal surfaces, it produces an especially strong effect. A 1 to 1000 solution, tested on the conjunctiva of a rabbit, will at once produce a distinct reaction.

The venom dries quickly. If preserved from moisture, it will keep for years. In glycerin, it keeps indefinitely without losing toxicity. Snake venom has the same characteristics. According to Weir-Mitchell, dried snake venom kept for 22 years without losing potency.

Bee venom is an efficient, active poison, producing not only a strong local reaction when injected under the epidermis, but at the same time a very powerful, absorptive, remote, systemic effect.

According to Langer, 0.1 percent bee venom solution retards the growth of the streptococci which are supposed to be important antecedents of arthritis. The streptococci, removed to another indifferent solution, regained their former virulence. Bee venom, as a rule, is free from bacteria and, to a certain degree, it will prevent their growth. On the other hand, bacteria weaken the efficacy of the venom. They are mutually destructive, but the venom is the more potent of the two. While bee venom is normally bacteria free, it is not considered by any means a powerful antiseptic.

The venom, in addition to albumin (which can be easily detected by various tests), contains inorganic salts, sodium, and calcium (none of them very toxic organic base-a nitrogen-free compound-which is the effective poisonous), besides hydrochloric acid, phosphoric acid, volatile oils and a part. The volatile oils evaporate while the venom is drying. The smarting and painful effect of the venom and also its rapid absorptive action are ascribed to these volatile oils. When the venom is dried and redissolved, the pain produced is considerably less and, likewise, the absorption, slower. This is one of the advantages in the administration of injectable bee venom (the volatile oils) have been removed.

So far, science has been successful only in the study of the biological, physiological, and clinical effects of the venom, but plenty of uncertainty still surrounds its complex chemical composition. All we know is that it contains a substance of protein-like toxicity which can be only partially separated and isolated. It was not so long ago that every animal venom was called and considered a toxalbumin. Langer, with fairly extensive knowledge not only of the clinical but also of the chemical phase of bee venom, succeeded in producing its effective component in an albumin-free state, which is known to-day as Langer's base. The efficiency and toxic quality of the venom are attributed to this base.

Flury, in 1920, through hydrolysis of Langer's base with hydrochloric acid, found in it the following elements: Tryptophan, choline, glycerin, phosphoric acid, palmitic acid, fatty acid (non-crystallizable), a volatile acid, likely butyric, and a non-nitrogenous substance.

Flury was convinced that the last named substance is the pharmacologically active and physiologically effective component of the venom. According to the way it was isolated, it produced a neutral compound which was slightly soluble, or an acid compound, easily soluble in water. The slightly soluble neutral compound was very probably a cyclic acid-anhydride, much like cantharidin, having an inflammatory, and, in oil, a vesicant effect; the freely water-soluble acid compound, with strong hemolytic effect, was a saponin substance.

Flury felt justified in concluding that bee venom was a complex substance, a combination between an albumin-free sapotoxin of animal origin, like crotalotoxin and ophiotoxin of snake venoms, and a poison similar to the cantharidin group. The active element was always in combination with lecithin.

Langer made a good start in examining the chemical qualities of bee venom. He thought that, in a pure state, it was an organic base, which when precipitated with alkalies, especially ammonia, gave a general alkaloidal reaction, and could not be destroyed by a temperature of 100° C. Flury, the other hand, believed it was improbable that the effect of the venom was due to a base. Most compounds, in a toxocological sense, which possess inflammatory or hemolytic action, are nitrogen-free. Of course, there are some alkaloids which have strong local, irritant effect, like veratrin and colchicin. Doubtless, the substance isolated by Langer had a basic character, but still it is inadmissible-in spite of the fact that bee venom gives a general alkaloidal reaction-to consider it an alkaloid. Against its alkaloidal nature is the fact that it does not form any definite salts. Even in other characteristics, *viz.*, solubility, it differs from alkaloids. Flury, one of the most productive workers in the field, extracted, according to Langer's procedure, this base from 200,000 bees, and from that number he gained only one gram of venom for chemical experiments. This preparation had to be cleaned six times, by dissolving it in acetic acid, and then had to be precipitated with ammonia, to rid it entirely of the albumin. As a result the substance further shrank to half a gram which still did not represent the pure active principle (in the Production of Injectables Bee Venom section).

Scientists, for many years, were greatly interested in the chemical composition of bee venom and also in its physiological action. Many animal experiments were made to study and determine its toxic qualities and also the post mortem organic changes after fatal doses. Langer, Flury, Arthus, Phisalix, Lyssy, Bert, Gautier, Philouze, Calmette and many other leading scientists made innumerable animal experiments and extensive chemical research in the thorough study of bee venom.

THE PRODUCTION OF INJECTABLE BEE VENOM

Bee venom can be procured in many ways. In the cleanest form, we can obtain it by pressing carefully with thumb and index finger the lower part of the bee's abdomen. In this procedure the sting protrudes, and a clear drop of venom becomes visible on its end. This can be collected in capillary tubes, absorbed by a blotter, or flushed off in a normal saline solution. If we quickly dip this minute amount of poison into water, it will form a solution, as it is extremely water-soluble. By this method, the bees, with careful handling, can be used repeatedly as they will remain alive if the sting is not injured. A more complicated way, after pressing the bee's abdomen, is to grasp the protruding sting with fine forceps, and then with slight effort the whole sting apparatus (the sting and adnexa, poison sac, glands, etc.) can be pulled out easily. If we collect a large number of these stings and immerse them in water, a cloudy fluid will result. This must be repeatedly filtered. If the stings are extracted and dropped into 96 percent alcohol, the alcohol must be filtered and the remaining substance dried at 40° C. This substance can be rubbed into a fine powder, extracted with water, and refiltered. We thus obtain a clear, brownish-yellow liquid which, after proper concentration, will give all characteristic toxic reactions.

It required about 25,000 bees for Langer to produce one milligram of pure venom. The venom, when evaporated, forms regular crystals; with ammonia, a whitish substance; with tannin, a sediment. All these properties show that the venom has an organic base.

Flury succeeded in producing the material in several ways. In the beginning of his experiments, he used dead bees. He tore out the stings and adnexa, dried them, extracted the venom with water, and precipitated it with alcohol. With three successive precipitations, he obtained from 1,000 bees approximately 20 milligrams of dry venom, which, however, contained albumin. Later on, he continued his research with live bees. He put a swarm of about 25,000 bees, in several sections, into a large glass vessel, covered the opening with a blotter, on which he poured ether. The ether fumes irritated the bees; they discharged their venom, some of which remained on the glass and a certain quantity on their bodies. When the bees were in deep narcosis, the glass and the bees were washed off with water, which brought the venom into a solution. After evaporation of the water, the remaining substance had all the toxic qualities of the venom and could be kept for several months. Flury, by this method, obtained from a thousand bees about 50 to 75 milligrams of venom, mixed with a certain amount of honey. Later he let the bees dry in the sun; many of them recuperated and flew away. (Flury obtained valuable assistance in his experiments from Dr. Enoch Zander, Professor of Apiculture in Erlangen.)

The rinsing liquid was of varying quality and purity, yellow, cloudy, but always of acid reaction. The sugar which it contained could be easily separated. By various manipulations, Flury gained a sediment rich in albumin which completely precipitated in alcohol. Mixed with a little sodium or ammonia, a very effective albuminous substance was obtained, wholly or partly soluble in water. The watery solution of this precipitate had a strong hemolytic action and caused, on the conjunctiva of a rabbit, according to its strength, a more or less severe inflammation.

BEE VENOM

Subcutaneously injected into the rabbit's ear, it produced edema with a consecutive necrosis. The wet precipitate, after exposure to the air, turned gray, brownish, and finally black. In a dry state, it retained its effect for years. Out of this filtratum with alcohol, sodium, and ammonium sulphate, Flury obtained other effective parts of the venom. The precipitate, in acid, was more complete than in alkaline solution. In the former, he gained a colorless, in the latter a colored filtratum. The ammonium sulphate precipitate was very soluble in water, of acid reaction, and could be precipitated either with ammonia or acetic acid. The albuminous bee venom, isolated through ammonium sulphate, very powerful even seven years later. Five or ten milligrams in a rabbit intravenously caused death in several minutes. With metaphosphoric acid in the original rinsing fluid, or in alcohol, ammonia or sodium, the filtratum ammonia and retained its effect for years. The filtratum with ammonium gave a very powerful precipitate. This last precipitate was easily soluble in sulphate and metaphosphoric acid was not so efficacious. All fractions which were effective in animal experiments gave biuretic reaction and a positive Millon test. The substances obtained through fermentative reduction or hydrolytic splitting had all the qualities of the lipoid group.

In another important experiment, Flury obtained pure venom in "native" state, without impurities. He put the bees on a heavy, wet blotter. They stung it immediately and the poison was absorbed. This method was very simple and, on a sunny day, very successful. With a little experience, in one day the venom from several thousand bees could be collected. The venom soaked paper was then dried and placed in a well-closed jar. This way he obtained an albuminous venom which kept for years. The watery extract, especially when 1/3 or 1/2 volume of glycerin was added, gave a good stock solution for animal and immunizing experiments. The stings, caught in the blotter (from which the greatest amount of poison had already been extracted), could be collected and from them some additional venom obtained. Out of 10,000 of these stings, which, when dried, weighed about 32 grams, about 0.08 to 0.12 gram of venom was still extractable.

LANGER'S METHOD

Langer's method, rather his directions for producing bee venom, are as follows:

1) Kill the bees with chloroform. In the rear of the abdomen, the protruding sting is visible.

2) With fine forceps, pull out the sting (actually the whole apparatus) to which the glands, poison sac, muscles, and chitin parts will be attached. Place them in 96 percent alcohol and let the mass coagulate.

3) Strain the alcohol through a funnel. Dry the stings at 50° C.

4) Rub the dried stings into a fine powder. Make an extract in several c.c. of distilled water and let it stand for 24 hours.

5) Drop this watery extract through a filter funnel into 96 percent alcohol, which will produce, first, a cloudiness, and finally, a sediment.

6) The sediment which gradually settles on the bottom consists of venom and albuminous substances.

7) Change the alcohol repeatedly; add some ether, and let it evaporate.

8) The pure venom represented by an organic base is produced from this final sediment.

Perrin and Cuènot still (1933) use live bees during the summer months in the administration of their treatments. For winter they prepared a special venom product. They extracted the stings and their adnexa (which always remain attached) with forceps. Placing about a thousand stings in 5 c.c. of alcohol, all microbes were destroyed, and the albumin fixed. After the alcohol was evaporated, by drying the extract in a vacuum, placed over calcium chloride, the dry venom remained. This was later diluted in normal saline solution and standardized.

Personally, I consider the simplest and most practical procedure to extract the venom of the bees is the following:

Take a wide-mouthed glass jar, approximately two to four inches in diameter, and opening in the rear of the hive, just large enough for a worker bee to pass through; animal membrane (a ram's dried scrotal sac is most appropriate). Make a small place several drops of honey at this exit; the emerging bee will delight herself in consuming it, and there is no difficulty in catching her with two fingers. (Of course a beekeeper will not require all these preparations, as he has no difficulty in catching them, with the greatest ease, at the entrance of the hive.)

Place the bee over the membrane of the jar, which she will sting with great eagerness. The sting penetrates the membrane, and the venom will be ejected, in a pure state, into the water, where it will form a solution. The stings will be caught and remain in the membrane. The final concentration of the solution will, of course. depend on the quantity of water contained in the jar, and the number of bees which were used. This is a very simple procedure to obtain a supply of venom for experimental purposes-its toxicity must be subsequently standardized.

Though we obtain the venom in a fairly pure state, it is not yet fit for therapeutic purposes; the *protein must be entirely removed, which is a rather intricate task.*

The foreign manufacturers *carefully guard the secret* of the method by which they eliminate the protein. The writer, so far, has not been successful, even with the assistance of chemical experts, in producing a protein-free solution suitable for injections, and failed to gain the coöperation of the foreign manufacturers.

In toxicological studies, animal experiments have rendered a great service. Success in the administration of all toxic substances for therapeutic purposes has been facilitated by them. The effect of bee venom on the animal kingdom is interesting and instructive.

The lower types, e.g., molluscae, rain worm, are extremely sensitive to bee venom. One-twentieth milligram at first paralyzes, then kills them. The venom is effective even without an act of stinging; just a surface contact will produce full toxicity.

Calmette took the venom of two bees in one c.c. of water and this solution, when injected, was sufficient to kill a mouse or a sparrow in several minutes. The animals died from respiratory paralysis (just as they do after the administration of cobra venom) which is manifestly a neurotoxic symptom. The blood in the heart was liquid and black on account of hemolysis. A fly stung by a bee died in ten or twenty seconds, but a sting of a hornet or wasp was sufficient to kill it instantaneously-a proof that their venom is more violent than that of the bee.

One and one-half percent solution of clear bee venom injected into a four and one-half kilogram dog caused a low pulse rate and a lowered blood pressure, in 15 minutes after the first injection. The next produced an increased blood pressure, clonic trembling, trismus, nystagmus, emprosthotonus, and the dog soon died from respiratory paralysis. The autopsy findings were hyperemia of the kidneys, liver, pancreas, in fact of the whole intestinal tract, not infrequently hemorrhage of the bowels; the pericardium blood showed methemoglobin. Intravenously injected into an animal, the was tense and filled with bloody fluid. Spectroscopic examination of the venom produced quicker and greater destruction of the blood cells, a distinct erythrolytic effect. The most characteristic postmortem changes were hyperemia, hemorrhage and hemolysis.

The erythrolytic effect of bee venom on the blood varied considerably in different animals, *in vivo* as well as *in vitro*. Dog's blood was very sensitive to its action; on the other hand, the blood of a rabbit or rat, only slightly. When in a test tube, some rabbit's blood was added to canine blood, the former increased considerably the latter's resistance to the erythrolytic influence of bee venom. Even serum from the blood of a rabbit had a pronounced destructive effect on the hemolytic power of the venom, an evident antihemolytic action. The local inflammatory effect on the animal conjunctiva was ameliorated also by the addition of some blood serum of a rabbit. Cholesterin had the same effect.

The erythrolytic power of bee venom, on the contrary, was markedly augmented by the addition of lecithin. When lecithin was added to bee venom, it formed a combination, "toxolecithid," of a surprisingly increased toxicity; in fact, the erythrolytic power of the combination was 200 to 500 times greater than that of the original venom itself.

Small fish quickly perished when stung by bees. A small quantity of bee venom added to the water in which they lived soon killed them. Frogs were not so sensitive when stung, but a slight touch of 1/100th milligram of venom stopped the frog's heart.

Birds are rather sensitive. Let us give here Marie Phisalix's vivid description of some of her experiments. A sparrow stung by two bees will very soon show all signs of general weakness and lack of motor power; the bird sinks down to its feet, tries to fly, but falls. The paresis gradually increases, the victim just scrapes the ground with incoördinated movements. General tremor and regular chorea will soon follow. Respiration fails; the victim gasps for air. Intellect is not affected; the bird defends itself with beak and claws. Death is finally caused by respiratory paralysis. The heart beats for several minutes after the respiration has stopped.

There are innumerable instances mentioned where geese and chickens have died from a few stings. Flury disagreed with the statement that birds are very sensitive to bee venom. His experience was that they were not extremely so.

Professor Phillips reported an interesting case, proving the great variability in birds as to their response to bee stings. A correspondent in Australia sent him a bird's stomach which was punctured by over ninety stings. Some of them extended through the outer wall, and yet the bird had appeared normal when shot. The bird was of the type which is a real pest in apiaries similar to the bee-martin in this country.

Accidents where horses, goats, dogs and sheep have been killed by bees are many. Horses are unusually sensitive. They become ill and die. Even Aristotle mentioned that horses were killed by bees. Many lawsuits for damages have been filed. Delpech reported eight, and Conradi five instances where a large number of horses were killed by bee sting injuries. Eugene Clichy, a French veterinary, was called by a farmer to attend to five of his horses. They had gone into the garden where the hives were placed. All were overrun by bees. The stings were found around the eyes, mouth, ears, neck and rectum of the animals-a proof of how skillfully bees select the most vulnerable places. The horses all died and autopsies were performed. Their abdomens were bloated like a drum; severe hemorrhagia of the internal organs, especially of the kidneys, were the main findings.

Cats are rather resistant to the action of bee venom (likewise to snake venom); whether there are antibodies present or it is just a lack of susceptibility is another point still awaiting solution.

While bee venom has no effect on the intact skin of higher animals, their mucous membranes, except those of the digestive tract, are very sensitive. A small quantity of the venom instilled in the eye of a rabbit will soon cause hyperemia, chemosis, purulent and croupous conjunctivitis, ulcerations of the cornea, and iritis-even cataracts have been observed. This effect is of very important service in the production of injectable bee venom. The produced effects on the animal conjunctiva increase correspondingly with the concentration of the solution; in fact, they are so characteristic and dependable that, when the substance is dropped into the eye of a rabbit, the time of development of the inflammatory symptoms and the degree of other manifestations are reliable tests of its strength and they are accepted as true standards. The pupils of the animal dilate; it tries to rub the venom from the eyes with its forelegs. When a medium concentration of the venom is applied, this will usually happen in about half an hour. If the rubbing act starts earlier or later, the difference in time will approximately indicate the respective strength of the concentration, which also will correspond with the inflammatory changes of the conjunctiva. One usually starts with a weak solution, gradually increasing its strength with careful control of the consecutive changes, of which an exact score must be kept.

It is a rather remarkable fact that bee venom is effective even on the bees themselves. One would assume that they were immune to their own venom. The killing of the rival queens, the massacre of the drones, and the battles with hostile groups are proof of how quickly they succumb to the stings of their own kind. Of course, we must not forget that the bees always use their diabolical skill by stinging their own kind and other insects (for instance, flies, spiders) in the narrow, connecting bridge between the thorax and abdomen, or in some abdominal segments through which the nerve ganglia pass; and the insects quickly expire.

CHAPTER REFERENCES

ARISTOTLE. Historia Animalium, IV (Bekker, J. 1837).

ARTHUS, M. Réchérches experimentales sur le venin des abeilles, Compt. rend. de Soc. de Biol. Par., 182, 1919.

BERT, P. Gaz. Méd. de Par., 771, 1865.

BERT ET CLOEZ. Venin des Hymenoptères, Compt. rend. de Soc. de Biol. Par., Juillet, 1865.

BERTARELLI, E., U. TEDESCHI, A. Experimentelle Untersuchungen über das Gift der Hornisse, Centralbl. f. Bakteriol., Jena, Bd. 68, 1913.

CARLET, M. Memoirs sur le venin et l'aiguillon de l'abeille, Ann. Sc. Nat. Zool., 9, 1890.

COHN, S. Beiträge zur Kenntniss des Bienengiftes, Inaug. Dissert. Würzburg, 1922.

FENGER, H. Anatomie und Physiologie des Giftapparates bei der Hymenopteren, Arch. f. Naturgeschicht, 7.

FLURY, F. Über die chemische Natur des Bienengiftes, Arch. f. Exper. Path. u. Pharmakol. Leipz., 85, 1920.

GAUTIER, A. Les Toxines microbiennes et animales, 1896.

HOLTZ, H. Anatomische Studien des Bienenstachels, Nordl. Bienenzeit., 1883.

HYATT, J. D. The Sting of the Honeybee, Amer. Quart. Microsc. J., I, 1878.

KARSCH, F. Über eine Doppelrolle des Stachels der Honigbiene, Entomolog. Nach. richt, 1884.

KOEHLER, A. Zur Funktion des Bienenstachels, Arch. f. Bienenkund., III, 1921.

BEE VENOM

KRAEPELIN, C. Untersuchungen über den Bau, Mechanism. und Entwickelungs geschicht. des Stachels der bienenartig. Tiere, Zeitschr. f. wiss. Zool., XXIII.

LANGER, J. Über das Gift unserer Honigbiene, Arch. f. Exper. Path. u. Pharmakol., Leipz., 38, 1897.
Der Aculeatenstich, Arch. f. Dermat. u. Syph., 43, 1898.
Abschwächung und Zerstörung des Bienengiftes, Arch. internat. de Pharmacodyn. Grand et Par., 6, 1899.
Versuche zur Anwendung von Bienenstich und Bienengift als Heilmittel bei chron.-rheum. Erkrankungen des Kindesalters, Jahrb. d. Kinderh., Leipz., 81, 1915.
Uber Bienenstich, Vortrag d. deutsch. Bienenwirtschaftl. Centr. Vereins, Prag., 1895.
Bienengift u. Bienenstich, Bienenvater, Jahrg., 33, 10, 1901.
Die Entgiftung des Bienengiftes, Vortr. deutsch. bienenwirtschaftl. Centr. Ver., 1898.
Neure Ergebnisse über Bienenstich, Vortr., Stuttgart, 1930.
Zur Frage der tötlichen Bienenstiche, Vortr. Wandersammlm deutsch. Bienenwirte, 1927.
Das histolog. Bild des Aculeatenstiches, Arch. f. Derm. u. Syph. Leipz. u. Wien, 1932.
Die Fixation des Bienengiftes an der Stichstelle, Biochem. Ztschr., Berl., 1932.
Beurteilung des Bienenhoniges und seiner Verfälschung mittels biolog. Eiweissdifferenzier., Arch. f. Hyg. München u. Berl., 71, 1910.

LEDERLE, P. Über das Gift der Honigbiene., Die Biene und ihre Zucht, 56, 11-12, 1919.

LYSSY, R. Réchérches experimentales sur le venin des Abeilles, Arch. internat. de Physiolog. Liege & Par., 16, 1921.

PHILOUZE. Du venin des abeilles, Ann. Ste. linéenne de Meine et Loire, IV, 1860.

PHISALIX, C. Réchérches sur le venin d'abeilles, Compt. rend. Soc. de Biol., Par., 1904.

ROCH, M. Les piqûres d'hymenoptères au point de vue chimique et thérapeut., Rev. med. de la Suisse Rom. Genève, Nov. 1928.

SOLLMAN, A. Die Bienenstachel, Ztschr. f. Zoolog., XIII, 4.

SPALIKOURSKY. Piqûres des Abeilles, Rev. Scientif., 1899.

WEINERT, H. Über Bau und Bedeutung des Wehrstachels der Bienen u. Wespen, Wissenschaftlich. Wchnschr., 15, 1920.

ZANDER, E. Beiträge zur Morphologie des Stachelapparates der Hymenopteren, Ztschr. f. wiss. Zoolog., 56, 1899.

Chapter V Physiological Effects of Bee Venom

During the entire last century and part of the present one, a great many prominent scientists have devoted considerable time and energy to the study of the effects of bee venom, as already mentioned, but they concentrated their whole attention on chemical and physiological experiments. They were all very well aware of the fact that bee venom has therapeutic properties, but evidently few of them tried to utilize these qualities *and produce a preparation properly adapted for clinical use.* Even Langer, who did untiring research in both laboratory and clinical fields, when he started to administer treatments to his patients, used live bees.

Flury, the well known Würzburg toxicologist, recognized its curative value long ago. On account of his close contact with beekeepers, from whom he learned the remarkable healing power of bee stings, he repeatedly suggested that the medical fraternity ought to investigate the known facts more carefully, and stated that *there was undoubtedly great need of an injectable bee venom preparation fit for therapeutic use,* instead of putting up with all the inconveniences of using live bees for the treatments.

I will try to enumerate the conclusions drawn by various research workers-the laboratory animal experiments of some, as well as the clinical observations of others.

C. Phisalix, in 1904, found three characteristic toxic effects of bee venom:

(1) Flogogen (inflammatory).
(2) Convulsive.
(3) Paralyzing.

Phisalix thought the flogogen and convulsive toxins were the secretions of the acid and the paralytic poison, of the alkaline glands.

Arthus, in 1919, administered bee venom intravenously to rabbits, and noticed that the produced symptoms had exact similarity to those of a distinct anaphylactic shock. He was convinced that the active element in bee venom was a protein body. He observed many analogies between bee venom and the venoms of the scorpion and crotalus.

PHYSIOLOIGICAL EFFECTS OF BEE VENOM

Morgenroth and Carpi came to the conclusion that the hemolytic property of bee venom is analogous to that of cobra venom. Calmette held the same opinion. Lyssy likewise found a great similarity in the neurotoxic qualities of bee and snake venoms.

Felix Fontana, the personal physician of the Grand Duke of Tuscany, made the statement 150 years ago, in his well known dissertation, *Ueber das Viperngift*, that bee venom taken from the sting or expressed from the poison bag and dried had the same effect as the venom of the viper, caused the same pain, swelling and general symptoms. Brandt and Ratzeburg, over a hundred years ago, in 1829, also called attention to the fact that *bee and snake venoms are alike.*

Lyssy, in 1921, after extensive research, arrived at the conclusion that bee venom has typical proteotoxic qualities. These experiments proved that the venom:

1)   Lowered blood pressure.

2)   Accelerated the respiration.

3)   Diminished the coagulability of the blood.

4)   Greatly increased peristaltic movements.

Arthus also noticed the great acceleration of the peristaltic movements—a typical symptom of protein intoxication, a sero-anaphylactic phenomenon. Roch, in experimental animals, counted as the effect of bee venom intoxication 78 fecal boli in 18 minutes, a characteristic sero-anaphylactic symptom. Murakami ascertained, after injection of bee venom into rabbits:

1)   The nitrogen elements in the urine increased.

2)   Urates increased.

3)   Hyperglycemia.

4)   Decrease of cholesterin.

5)   Hemolytic, leukolytic, and plasmolytic action.

Perrin and Cuènot noticed two special clinical manifestations after bee stings: hypotension and leukopenia, symptoms of proteotoxicity. With regard to types, they made the following classifications:

PHYSIOLOIGICAL EFFECTS OF BEE VENOM

1) Cases in which a larger amount of venom (multiple stings) caused a proteotoxic condition.

2) Cases in which a strong reaction was formerly never manifested and suddenly a violent one was experienced. This must have been due to anaphylactic sensibility or to a higher seasonal virulence of the venom.

3) Congenital hypersensitivity or hereditary idiosyncrasy.

Essex, Markowitz, and Mann, of the Mayo Foundation in Rochester, Minn., also noticed *a similarity in the physiological action of bee venom and the venom of the rattlesnake* (crotalus). The depressor action seemed to be more peripherical, judging from the local reaction. It proved to be a distinct capillary, i.e., an endothelial poison, a marked stimulant of the smooth muscles, comparable only to histamine. The mechanism of the depressor action enhanced the splanchnic dilatation. The womb of a rabbit perfused with a solution of bee venom rapidly contracted, while the heart, with a similar perfusion, manifested a markedly feebler contraction. In their summary, they stated that they found bee venom:

1) Intravenously in dogs and rabbits induced rapid fall of blood pressure, preceded by a very short increase.

2) Produced an occlusive bronchospasm.

3) Intradermally in humans, had an effect practically identical to that produced by the venom of the rattlesnake and histamine.

4) Had a marked hemolytic action; the coloring matter of the blood dissolved.

Lacaillade, of the Rockefeller Institute for Medical Research, determined the potency of bee venom in *vitro* from a known standard solution, and noticed that the cytolytic and hemolytic action of the venom lasted much longer when injected into guinea pigs hypodermically.

We cannot fail to observe, in severe cases of bee venom intoxication, that the venom produced physiological effects similar to those of snake venom, especially crotalin. The consensus of opinion of all research workers was that bee venom, like snake venom, so far as its physiological action was concerned, had three distinguishing and characteristic toxic effects:

1) Neurotoxic.

2) Hemorrhagic.

3) Hemolytic.

NEUROTOXIC EFFECTS

An important toxic attribute of bee venom is the effect on the nervous system-its neurotoxic effect. This is produced by neurotoxin, which by neurolysis destroys the central nerve tissues. A detailed description of the histological changes of the nerve tissues produced by the lytic destructive effect of the venom would occupy too much time and space. The process is similar to the action of other neurotoxic venoms, for instance, snake venom (cobra). The literature on this subject is very extensive.

The neurotoxin of bee venom has a definite, specific, selective action on the nerve cells, especially on the convulsive center. It has an important rôle in deaths caused by bee stings, when a sufficiently large amount of venom is absorbed, e.g., in multiple stings. While the hemorrhagic and hemolytic effects (the two other toxic attributes of the venom) have more extensive, widespread, general activities, the neurotoxic effect will produce a central destructive action which is later followed by peripheral disturbances.

It is interesting to note G. Billard's discovery that animals even slightly intoxicated with alkaloids, like spa like spartein, can tolerate more than ten fatal doses of cobra venom. This effect of the alkaloids applies also to bee venom. Perrin and Cuènot called this apparent immunity "metathesis." The influence of certain alkaloids is explained by the theory that they have a greater power of displacing the neurotoxin of the venoms on account of a greater selective affinity to these cellular tissues.

Neurotoxin is much more thermostabile than hemorrhagin or hemolysin. According to Weir Mitchell, the effects of the latter ones are destroyed by a temperature of 80° C. while neurotoxin requires about 120° to 135° C. to lose its toxic effect. It is, also, much more resistant to alcohol.

Bee venom, like snake venom, has greater resistance when in a dry form than when in solution, and the same can be said of neurotoxin. The neurotoxic effect of dry bee venom will not be destroyed by 190° C. below zero temperature. Sun rays have a strong destructive effect on the venom in solution, but not on the dry venom.

For clinical illustration of the neurotoxic effects of bee venom on the organism, produced by bee stings, I quote some instructive cases:

Mme. Marie Phisalix reported the following: Woman, 24, was stung on the palmar surface of the left little finger. It occurred in July, 1918, at 10 A.M. She paid no attention to it and resumed her work. An hour later there followed malaise, general pruritus, nausea, vomiting. Soon there were clonic and tonic convulsions of both the upper and lower extremities, trismus, constriction of the pharynx and chest, and severe dyspnea. The hand which had been stung was edematous, painful. The swelling extended over the whole upper arm, even reaching the chest. The tetanic convulsions kept up until late in the afternoon, with considerable headache and stupor. Patient looked anguished, could not speak, her pulse was rapid and feeble. Camphorated oil was injected and antivenin administered. She soon came out of the stupor and responded to questioning. The phenomena gradually attenuated around 2 A.M.; next day the critical phase passed off but somnolence persisted all that night and the following morning. Took nourishment only in the afternoon. The complete detoxication required almost a week.

F. G. Cawston reported a characteristic instance where bee stings caused typical neurotoxic symptoms. A middle-aged man was stung on his hands by several bees from his neighbor's hive. The local reaction was not unusual but he broke out in very profuse perspiration and his main and conspicuous complaint was extremely severe pain in the back of his legs. The pulse was weak. Strychnine was injected, after which the general feeling improved, but he continued to complain bitterly that the severe pain in his legs did not stop. Cawston was compelled to administer some aspirin and, later, heroin to relieve his distress. He suggested that the pain in the legs was caused by spinal involvement probably due to the neurotoxic effect of the bee venom.

Dr. W., of Munster, Indiana, in answer to my questionnaire, wrote that while he had been moderately sensitive to stings at first, his sensitivity seemed to increase gradually, with marked local reactions-burning, swelling, soreness, and also slight vertigo and weakness. On September 26, 1933, he was stung on both ankles and on the right arm and hand. Two days later, incapacitated him for several days. He had to walk with the aid of two canes he felt severe pains, principally in the spine and lower extremities, which for ten days, and was partially disabled for 30 days. The symptoms were apparently of distinct neurotoxic origin. He had several stings after that time, without any marked reaction.

W. Zimmermann reported recently two cases of bee sting injuries with distinctly neurotoxic effects.

A woman, 44 years old, who never paid much attention to bee stings, while pouring water on a swarm (around 11 A.M.) for the purpose of hiving it, was stung by a bee on the left side of her neck. Disregarding it she went into the kitchen, to fetch something, with the intention to continue the watering. Suddenly, after bending, she experienced a violent headache, a feeling "that her head almost burst." Very soon she felt a pressure at the region of the heart. Her whole body, down to her toes, was paralyzed. Respiratory anguish set in; she felt that her breath gradually became shorter.

She was put to bed, her chest massaged with brandy and she was able to rise only late in the evening still feeling spasmodic contractions all over her body. Zimmermann thought that the venom may have reached the brain and produced central paralysis (perhaps of the capillaries).

A man, 31 years old, beekeeper, who, as a rule, paid no regard to stings received one on the tip of his ear. Soon like an electric shock cramp-like contraction crept through his whole body. The spasmodic pains lasted for about half an hour, which paralyzed him to such a degree that he was utterly helpless.

HEMORRHAGIC EFFECTS

The hemorrhagic effect of bee venom is one of its most distinguishing, characteristic qualities; in fact, the writer is firmly convinced that the *therapeutic value of the venom is mainly due to this hemorrhagic property*. The hemorrhagin (endotheliotoxin) which bee venom contains is a blood poison. Its primary action, as we learn from animal experiments, is upon the blood elements but it also has a strong effect on the blood vessels themselves. *Hemorrhagin causes the capillaries to become permeable to blood*. This results in hemorrhages from the nose, conjunctiva, peritoneum, rectum, etc. Blood escapes from all mucous and serous surfaces without any visible lesion. Hemorrhagin, at the same time, has a depressing effect on the various nerve centers and nerve endings, causing a rapid fall of blood pressure. This active principle has the nature of albumoses. The reaction which hemorrhagin provokes resembles that of the proteins and bacterial vaccines, greatly contributing to the anaphylactic complex. The sensitivity which it produces can be transferred by injecting the blood or serum from one subject to another (passive anaphylaxy); the sensitivity can also be inherited.

Langer performed many necropsies on animals after fatal doses of bee venom had been administered, and always noticed a considerable effusion of blood in the pericardium, kidneys, and intestines, in addition to general hyperemia. Most of these animals showed a very pronounced meningeal congestion, blood effusion in the brain ventricles, and other intracranial hemorrhages.

PHYSIOLOIGICAL EFFECTS OF BEE VENOM

The hemorrhagic action is produced by the venom proteids, globulins, which are precipitated but not destroyed by alcohol. The hemorrhagic efficiency of the venom is parallel to the amount of these globulin-like bodies.

Before Flexner and Noguchi made their successful discoveries with various snake venoms, there was great confusion; and no distinct line of demarcation was drawn between hemolytic and hemorrhagic processes. They made the statement: "We look upon hemorrhagin in the light of a cytolysin for endothelial cells of blood vessels, the destruction of which is the direct cause of the escape of blood into the surrounding structures." The extravasation takes place not by diapedesis, but through actual breaking of the walls, and the escape is not limited to red blood cells, as white blood cells, also, emigrate.

Hemorrhagin invades the central nervous system only rarely. It is the chief toxic component of crotalus venom as well as of bee venom, both having a special affinity to the endothelial cells, of which the walls of blood and lymph vessels are constituted. Cobra venom, on the other hand, has a specific affinity for the nervous system, producing hardly any general tissue changes. Is it, perhaps, an affinity for lecithin?

The experiments of Monae-Lesser, Taguet, Laignel-Lavastine and Koressios, in trying to cure cancer with cobra venom, seem to me to be based entirely on an erroneous principle. It is, of course, not surprising to note the remarkable analgesia (greatly surpassing that of morphine) which they report in even incurable cancer cases, on account of neurotoxic action of cobra venom. The selective affinity of the venom for the phosphatides of nerve cells is conclusive but *only venoms with hemorrhagic effect, like crotalin or bee venom, could accomplish a reconstructive process.*

This disparity in the action of neurotoxin and hemorrhagin has a great importance in the use of various antivenins. Antivenin, which neutralizes the neurotoxic, has no influence on the hemorrhagic effect of the venom of another species and, inversely, antivenin, which is strongly antihemorrhagic, is not antineurotoxic. In a word, *cobra antivenin has antineurotoxic but no antihemorrhagic effect and, vice versa, crotalus antivenin has antihemorrhagic but no antineurotoxic effect.* (Ricin has hemagglutinative, hemorrhagic, and also neurotoxic properties.) Crotalus antivenin was successfully used to counteract the effects of bee venom.

From a clinical viewpoint, the hemorrhagin of bee venom is extremely important. This is fully described and explained in Chapter IX.

After bee sting injuries, we often find, in the symptoms which follow, typical hemorrhagic effects. I have already expressed the opinion that many fatalities were due to cerebral hemorrhages.

Professor Roch, of Geneva, published a very instructive case, which clearly illustrated the correctness of this supposition. The patient was a farmer who, at the age of seven, had acquired chorea from a sudden fright. Was a little backward mentally but attended to farm work. On the 25th of May, 1925, during a thunderstorm, he took refuge in an apiary, where he was attacked by a great number of bees. Immediately ran home, undressed and went to bed. His parents counted about 200 stings on his face and neck.

Patient became very ill, vomited freely and soon fell into a coma, which lasted three days. He was taken to the Medical Clinic of Geneva. In addition to aphasia he was paralyzed on the entire right side. The reflexes of that side were exaggerated; Babinski reflex was positive. Right leg was edematous and cyanotic. Lumbar puncture showed nothing pathological. Roch thought that cerebral hemorrhage caused by the venom resulted in a hemiplegia of central origin.

HEMOLYTIC EFFECTS

Another important characteristic physiological action of bee venom on the blood is its hemolytic, hemotoxic effect. If we add to the blood in a test tube even a small quantity of bee venom, we find under the microscope very few erythrocytes. We do find dissolved hemoglobin and, under the spectroscope, methemoglobin. Bee venom is a powerful hemolytic poison. The hemolytic effect is produced by hemolysin, which acts not only on the red blood cells (erythrocytolysin) but also on the white blood cells (leucocytolysin). Blood serum, in itself, has great antihemolytic capacity, a strictly defensive measure which is supposedly due to its cholesterin content. The whole theory of immunity seems to rest on the fact that when an organism is immunized by gradual doses of some venom or toxin an automatic increase of cholesterin in the blood plasma acts as a neutralizing defensive, antitoxic substance. Phisalix has already made the statement that cholesterin has an immunizing effect on snake venom, and is a real antidote for it. Kyes and Sachs found that there are hemolytic poisons on which cholesterin has no effect.

PHYSIOLOIGICAL EFFECTS OF BEE VENOM

Lecithin plays an important rôle in biological chemistry, especially in the study of immunology and serology. The action of lecithin is just opposite to that of cholesterin. If we add lecithin to pure bee venom, the combination will increase enormously the hemolytic action of the venom. Morgenroth and Carpi found that the lecithid of bee venom is 200 to 500 times more hemolysing than the venom by itself. Bee venom without the addition of lecithin gives a scant precipitation with ether. If we dissolve this precipitate in physiological salt solution, it possesses hemolysing power. The lecithid, on the contrary, will dissolve the red corpuscles almost instantaneously. The hemolytic action of these lecithids is very powerful, but this is not applicable also to its neurotoxic effect.

Preston Kyes mixed 1 ½ c.c. solution of venom with 1 ½ c.c. 5% solution of lecithin, in methyl alcohol. After the solution was kept for 24 hours at 37° C., 22 c.c. absolute alcohol was added. The liquid was decanted and the clear filtrate mixed with 150 c.c. of ether. There was a slowly-formed, somewhat copious flocculent deposit, which was collected in a filter, washed several times with ether, and finally dried. The lecithid which remained on the filter completely dissolved in physiological salt solution.

The researches of Kyes and Sachs have an importance of greater magnitude in the science of immunity than we realize. The discovery of the toxin -toxolecithid-a product between a chemically unknown substance of amboceptor character, the so-called prolecithid, in combination with the chemically known substance, lecithin, is of great fundamental value. The quantitative relationship of lecithin and venom corresponds to that of amboceptor and complement-the more venom present the less lecithin is needed for complete hemolysis-and the reverse.

The hemolytic effect of cobra venom depends on the lecithin content of the blood. Flexner and Noguchi found that the hemolytic substance of cobra venom has two components: one is in the venom and the other component is in the blood serum which activates it-in brief, the venom consists of a substance of amboceptor character which is greatly activated by certain complements of the serum. Calmette calls it "substance sensibilisatrice." Lecithin is an activator.

Morgenroth and Carpi thought that further study of the characteristics of toxolecithid is worth more than the study of all the rest of the toxins, including those of bacterial origin. Many questions about the theoretical knowledge of immunity lead us to toxolecithid as a bridge to the important bacterial toxins. In every difficult problem of physiology, we must select a proper experimental animal. In the science of immunity, we must, also, look for a proper substance in conducting our experimental work, though it might seem entirely unimportant from a medical viewpoint. What importance had ricin and abrin in Ehrlich's researches in the field of antitoxins? The substances had, and at present have, very little value or importance. Morgenroth and Carpi thought it very peculiar that prolecithid has similar character in animals zoologically very far apart, e.g., the venoms of the scorpion and cobra. According to Calmette, scorpion and cobra venoms have very similar effects on the central nervous system.

The thermostability of the prolecithid of bee venom is much less than that of cobra venom. In a neutral solution for two to three hours under 37° C., its hemolytic effect is weaker. On the other hand, toxolecithid shows very great thermostability.

Hemolytic poisons have a latent state in the body. With careful and gradual injections, immunity can be reached. This leads us to Ehrlich's theory that certain haptophore cells will bind the invading bacterial or other kind of poison.

I wish to mention here one fact: that syphilitics in the early stages of their disease are hypersensitive to hemolytic poisons, but later show a heightened resistance. This point may also demand some consideration in bee venom therapy.

CHAPTER REFERENCES

ARTHUS, M. Réchérches experimentales sur le venin des Abeilles, Compt. rend. Soc. de Biolog., Par., 182, 1919.

BILLARD, G. La Phylaxie, Par., 1931.

BRANDT, J. F., und RATZEBURG, J. T. C. Die Honigbiene, Med. Zoolog., I, 1829.

CARLET, M. G. Sur le venin des Hymenoptères et ses organs excreteurs, Compt. rend. Acad. d. Sc., Par., 98, 106, 1884.

CAWSTON, F. G. Acute Poisoning from Bee Stings, J. Trop. M. (etc.) Lond., Dec. 1930.

ESSEX, H. E., MARKOWITZ, J., and MANN, F. C. The Physiological Action of the Venom of the Honey Bee, Am. J. Physiol., Baltimore, 94, 1930.

FABRE, P. Le Venin des Hymenoptères, Bull. Acad. de Med., Par., 1905.

FLEXNER, S., and NOGUCHI, H. Snakevenom in Relation to Hemolysis, Bacteriolysis and Toxicity, J. Exp. M. N. Y., 6, 1902.

FLURY, F. Über den Bienenstich, Naturwissenschaft, 11, 1923.

FONTANA, F. Abhandlung über das Viperngift, Berl., 1787.

KYES, P. Über die Wirkungsweise des Cobragiftes, Berl. Klin. Wehnschr., 38-39, 1902.

KYES, P., und SACHS, H. Zur Kenntniss der Cobragiftactivierenden Substanzen, Berl. klin. Wchnschr., 2-4, 1903.

LACAILLADE, C. W., JR. The Determination of the Potency of Bee Venom, Am. J. Physiol., Baltimore, 105, Aug. 1933.

LEDERLE, P. Über das Gift der Honigbiene, Bienen Zeit., 204, 1919.

LEGIEHN, D. Eigenthümliche Wirkungen eines Bienenstiches, Berl. klin. Wchnschr., 787, 1889.

LYSSY, R. Réchérches experimentales sur le venin des Abeilles, Arch. internat. de Physiol., 16, 1921.

MITCHELL, S. WEIR. Researches upon the venom of the rattlesnake, Wash., 1861.

MORGENROTH, J., UND CARPI, W. Über ein Toxolecithid des Bienengiftes, Berl. klin. Wchnschr., 43, 1906.

MURAKAMI, K. Influence of bee's poison on blood picture, blood corpuscles and cholesterol content of blood in rabbit, Okayama Igakkai Kwai Zasshi, 40, 1928.
Influence of bee's poison on protein and carbohydrate metabolism, Okayama Igakkai Zasshi, 40, 760, 1928.

PERRIN, M. ET CUÈNOT, A. Le traitement de l'Hypersensibilité au Venin d'Abeilles, Bull. gen. Therap. (etc.), Par., 183, 1932.

PHISALIX, C. Réchérches sur le venin d'abeilles, Compt. rend. Soc. de Biol., Par., 1904.

PHISALIX, M. Symptômes graves determines chez une femme jeune par la piqûre d'une seule abeille, Bull. du Mus. d'Hist. Nat., 7, 547, 1918.

PLATEAU, F. Venins D'Abeille. Art. Dict. Physiol. de Ch. Richet, 1895.

ROCH, M. Les piqûres d'Hymenoptères au point de vue chimique et thérapeut., Rev. Med. de la Suisse Rom. Genève, Nov. 1928.

SACHS, H. Hemolysine, Ergebn. d. allg. Path. u. path. Anatom. (etc.), Wiesb., 735, 1901.

THOMPSON, F. About Bee Venom, Lancet, Lond., 2, Aug. 19, 1933.

ZIMMERMANN, W. Bienen und Wespenstich-Vergiftungen, Samml. von VergiftungsFälle, Bd. 5, June 1934.

Chapter VI Effects Produced by Bee Sting Injuries

With the purpose in mind of studying the physiological effects of bee use, I deemed it advisable to devote more time and attention to the changes in the human organism produced by bee stings. By treating the subject of bee sting injuries more thoroughly and at greater length-since as a rule they are really nothing else but intradermal applications of bee venom-we will indirectly gain a more complete knowledge of the venom's effect.

The study of the effects of bee stings has a decided medical interest, but in our field of investigation it has an added significance. Bee sting injuries are, of course, very common occurrences. Medical literature abounds in a large number of published reports, which will provide us with ample material for our proper enlightenment. It is much more practical and also more fair to patients, to acquire an accurate understanding of the effects through the study of these records than to count on experiences to be gained during the course of treatments.

Another significant aspect is that by collecting sufficient material from a large number of cases, the medical profession will also obtain a clearer view of bee sting injuries. The reports are so widely scattered among various periodicals that it is rather difficult for the average physician to collect the data himself, especially in the country, without the necessary library facilities. City physicians are only slightly interested in bee sting injuries; on the other hand, in the country this type of injury might have considerable importance. To my knowledge, so far there is no complete textbook available on the subject. That there is a demand from the profession for more knowledge is shown by a letter which appeared in *The Lancet* of Sept. 24, 1932.

TO THE EDITOR OF THE *LANCET*:
Sir:

In those stung by bees severe symptoms are not uncommon. They may include faintness, pallor, cyanosis, urticaria, diarrhea, unconsciousness, and, exceptionally, death within a few minutes; yet textbooks seem to be completely silent on the subject.

I recently had a case of a laborer, aged sixty-nine, who died five minutes after being stung by a bee on the back of his neck. A week previous he had been stung on the top of the head without ill effects; but four years before he had been unconscious for some hours and unable to work for three weeks following a sting (location unknown).

Is this idiosyncrasy a form of protein shock, or does it depend upon the entry of the poison into a superficial vein? I am told that the bee has both acid and alkali poison glands; are they both used and why and when?

I am, Sir,
Yours faithfully,
(Signed) NEVILLE M. GOODMAN.

This letter speaks for itself, demonstrating the exigency for more enlightenment on this topic. May I add confidentially-because I was looking forward to the elucidating replies with almost as much avidity as Dr. Goodman-that I am convinced the doctor was just as much in the dark about the subject afterwards as he was when he inserted his appeal for the coveted information?

The present chapter, in which we intend to discuss the effects of bee stings, *is one of the most important parts of this work.* To make it more intelligible, it was expedient to subdivide the vast material.

First, in classifying the effects of bee stings, we have to divide them into two main groups, which at the same time designate the field of their action, namely: I, Local Effects; II, General Effects.

I. The *Local Effects* are produced on or around the spot where the injury was inflicted and where the sting penetrated the dermal or epithelial covering of the body.

II. The General Effects are the systemic, organic changes produced by the absorption of the toxic venom into the circulatory stream.

What is the physiological definition of "effect"? Effects are subjective, functional changes produced by physicochemically efficient substances. They are: (a) Beneficial; (b) Injurious.

The body is provided and invested with abundant, almost unlimited, inherent and constructive power to: (1) Utilize beneficial effects; (2) Protect itself against physical and chemical injuries, to preserve its safety, often its real existence.

The forces for the utilization of beneficial effects are, of course, predominant. They are continuously active and serve to maintain the normal body functions. The organism depends entirely on these beneficial effects and they are familiar to the system.

The injurious effects are innumerable and multiform. As a rule, the body s not accustomed to being harmed. Injuries, mechanical or chemical, are abnormal effects and are usually unexpected. The defensive power of the system is ready for all emergencies but, first, this defensive force must be organized and mobilized, to check, withstand, and counteract any harmful invasion. When the two rival (the systemic and the invading) forces face each other in the encounter, the systemic always represent a reverse action, counter-tendency, against the attacking forces.

In the aggression by these invading physical or chemical agencies, the natural defensive power of the body will be aroused to neutralize and annihilate these harmful influences-in a word, the two opposite, hostile, antagonistic energies conflict and clash. When the attacking contender is rather feeble, the conflict is hardly noticeable, as there is plenty of reserve power it the system to dispose of it with the greatest ease. If it is of considerable strength and, in addition, sudden and violent, the conflict will be noticeable and we shall see a manifestation of the mutual, reciprocal action. We call this a "reaction."

Possibly, the defensive powers were even inert-in a state of lethargy, just in repose-and had to be aroused first, to respond to the unexpected and unfamiliar attack. The defensive forces will be more prepared for the next similar or identical aggression, which would mean a state of increased defense, preparedness. If there is a repetition of the attack, it becomes familiar, expected, and the system grows accustomed and habituated to it, which means that a tolerance has been acquired, attributable to certain neutralizing substances. This defense reaction is really an immunological reaction.

As already mentioned, the invasion can be mechanical or chemical. The external, injurious mechanical forces, in the great majority of cases, will meet the relatively impervious skin-the greatest defensive medium of the organism against external harm. If the mechanical attacks are frequent, the preparedness of the skin will manifest itself in hyperplasia, callous formation. The skin, besides, has a vast defensive power against chemical attacks. This protective response against chemical injury is called metaplasia, which is explained by the theory of mobilized phagocytes, a very important digestive function of the mesodermal cells.

According to Frederick P. Gay, the immediate response manifesting itself in reactive inflammation is the outpouring of the polymorphonuclear cells which, here, play the major rôle. Nobody questions the rapidity of the response of the polymorphonuclear cells, their ubiquity and their phagocytic capabilities. When they fail, the inflammation is ineffective. In delayed phagocytosis, the recovery depends on the mononuclear cells, macrophages (Metchnikoff).

The chemical invader can be a simple or a more complex chemical compound, like bacterial toxin, foreign protein, animal venom, etc. Bee venom belongs to this latter class. We may call the invading substances antigens; the defensive ones, antibodies. The antigens are colloidal bodies which may be chemically different but immunologically identical. According to our present knowledge, only protein bodies can act, almost exclusively, as antigens. "Sometimes an infinitesimal amount of protein is concealed in mixtures of great complexity" (Wells). Proteins are colloidal aggregates of amino acids. So far, about 20 of them are known. According to Abderhalden, they are able to form at least 2,432,902,008,176,640,000 different compounds.

There is no theoretical reason why complex carbohydrates should not exhibit antigenic functions.

LOCAL EFFECTS OF BEE STINGS

The extent of the local effects of bee stings, just like the general effects, depends on the bee and its victim. The intensity of the mechanical act, its depth, the quantity and quality of venom, the region of the body where the sting was applied, the constitutional state of the victim, eventual pathological conditions, etc., will all influence the degree of the development of the local effects.

As a rule, in bee stings the local and general effects are not only not correlated but, often, there is a great contrast between the two. A person can be stung on the eyelid or even in the eye or ear, with very violent local but with hardly any general effects. Another time, a sting may be administered intravenously and may cause very violent constitutional effects without any noticeable local reaction. Anaphylactic states and extreme idiosyncrasy may also produce no local but serious systemic reactions.

The sting of the bee is nothing else but a poisoned wound, a combination of a physical and a chemical injury. Accordingly, we must consider and distinguish between, first, the more or less painful mechanical injury caused by a barbed sting gradually penetrating the epidermis, and second a burning, extremely excruciating sensation which accompanies the injury and is produced by the chemical action of a caustic venom progressively irritating new nerve filaments of the skin. It is a characteristic, interrupted, lancinating pain.

The local physiological effect of the bee sting is generally violent inflammation, hyperemia, edema, caused by the escape of blood plasma, and a leukocytic circulatory hardening, in the center of which is often a local necrosis.

At first, a pale papule forms. We call it the "wheal," and this gradually extends in circumference with more or less rapidity, depending, of course, on the strength and quantity of the venom and on the individual sensitivity of the victim. In the center, a little red spot and sometimes a minute drop of blood are visible as the direct result of the mechanical injury. Around the wheal the hyperemic and edematous tissues become harder, increase both in size and elevation. The area is painful on pressure but not very sensitive to superficial touch. There is always a certain numbness in the center on account of the anesthetizing effect of the local infiltration.

The best proof of the efficiency of this formed phagocytic defensive ring is that Langer, even two weeks after an injury, found some virulent venom in the central necrotic tissue.

Soon the skin takes on a "goose-flesh" appearance, followed by a pruritus of various intensity, frequently accompanied by more or less extended urticaria, which is not always confined only to the immediate proximity of the sting but sometimes spreads all over the body. Quite often, especially in a sensitive person, a distinct erysipelatous inflammation sets in. In the center of the wheal, we usually find a small brownish-black substance. This is the sting and its adnexa. In the case of a normal sting injury, the local symptoms gradually disappear, corresponding to their development: first the pain, then the itch attenuates, later the inflammation, and finally the edema recedes. In other cases, the inflammation keeps up for several days. We can distinguish three phases in the formation and disappearance of the local effects: 1, State of development; 2, Stationary period; and 3, Retrogressive stage.

These three states have a great significance. Often they go hand in hand, corresponding to the constitutional symptoms.

The skin is an important visible, reactive organ when toxic or pathologic substances enter the body through its medium. The obviousness and visibility of the reaction have great value-in immunology, for instance, they are simply indispensable.

The local reaction in bee stings, however, cannot always be utilized as a safe, exact indicator or a correct dependable gage to measure the simultaneous or later-developed general effects. In the course of treatments with injectable bee venom, the visible local signs have much more value; they are helpful and dependable. We administer a proper dosage, with proper technic, in the intradermal tissues and avoid many complications produced by the unskilled and inconsiderate surgical technic of the bee. But we may overlook and condone it-this is the only act for which she deserves censure and reprimand. She still remains our friend!

GENERAL EFFECTS OF BEE STINGS

In discussing the general effects of bee stings, I wish to emphasize right here the important fact that bee venom is not only a local irritant, but a substance with powerful, remote, and far-reaching constitutional effect.

The organism makes many efforts to check, destroy, or dispose of any introduced poison. The heart, circulatory system, especially the portal circulation, the liver, the kidneys, all play important parts in arresting its course. Theophrastus von Hohenheim (Paracelsus) has already said: "If there is any disease in the body, the healthy organs, not one, but all, must fight against it. Any disease may bring death to them all. Nature knows it and fights with all its might."

The general systemic effects of bee venom on the organism are extremely variable and complex. They demand careful consideration. There is no possible way to judge, still less to put up a standard from which we could foretell, the consequences from the stings, or *vice versa*. Some cases end fatally as the result of only one sting, while others, where hundreds of stings were inflicted, might not show any ill effects. The modifying circumstances are so manifold that it is almost impossible even to attempt explanation of certain phenomena. We continually meet new, unexpected, and strange incidents. The effects of the majority of bee sting injuries are unquestionably normal, but then again we are often confronted with plenty of surprises-even miracles.

A person *sensitive* to bee stings is likely to exhibit the following symptoms within several minutes: Chills, high temperature, diffuse perspiration, headache, vertigo, dizziness, nausea, vomiting, diarrhea, great thirst, laryngeal and thoracic constriction, extreme weakness, and unconsciousness. The pulse is rapid. Later a general itching, urticaria, in

75

places edematous swelling may develop all over the body. Lips may be cyanotic and swollen; face, especially eyes, congested; sometimes epileptiform convulsions manifest themselves; patient is often greatly agitated, feels expressed anguish or lassitude. After a day or two, the symptoms may gradually disappear, but persistent fatigue frequently lasts much longer.

This is about the average case of a sensitive individual. The syndrome is not always complete. Sometimes certain symptoms are missing; other times, the intoxication progresses with such rapidity that it gives plenty of cause for anxiety, or may even terminate fatally.

In homeopathy, the bee is considered a valuable remedy and is very extensively used. Constantine Hering, one of the outstanding homeopaths, introduced it into their practice and it is still one of their favorite remedies. The homeopaths have most practical experience in intoxications with bee venom. On account of the frequent administration of the substance, they are bound to confront repeated toxic complications, and, likewise, they have gained knowledge in the control and treatment of such cases. Hering, in his condensed *Materia Medica*, furnishes a complete list of all the general toxic symptoms of bee venom, which are similar to those caused by bee stings. This might be very useful in controlling the eventual toxic symptoms likely to be produced during the treatments with injectable bee venom. I cannot do better than to enumerate the list of toxic syndromes compiled by Hering:

Mind: Feeling of faintness, general weakness, stupor, apathy, anxiety neurosis, fear of death, sometimes delirium, and loss of consciousness.

Sensorium: Great prostration, trembling, restlessness, confusion and vertigo. Vertigo is worse with closed eyes or sitting, and still worse lying down; while walking it is less severe.

Sleep: Tired, but restless sleep; incessant dreaming.

Skin: Cold perspiration; burning, prickling, itching eruptions, scattered local edema, occasionally small pustules.

Head: Dizziness; dull, throbbing, sensitive headache; fullness in occiput. Face: Pale, sallow, waxy, and swollen.

Eye: Nystagmus; burning, stinging pain; congestion, corneal ulcers. Mouth: Bitter taste, fetid breath, frothy saliva; lips bluish and swollen; gums bleed easily.

Ear: Difficulty in hearing.

Neck: Stiff.

Throat: Considerable swelling, internally and externally.

Chest: Great dyspnea, constriction of the chest, severe cough.

Heart: Pulse accelerated, increased palpitation, full, strong, often intermittent; in a later state, feeble, almost imperceptible.

Appetite: Very poor, no desire for food, great thirst, craving for milk and sour substances.

Stomach: Bilious vomiting; bitter, acrid belching; heartburn; dry, frequent gagging.

Intestines: Considerable griping; greenish-yellow, watery, foul-smelling diarrhea.

Kidneys: Renal pains; irritation of the bladder; burning, frequent urination; strangury; urine scanty and fetid.

Sex: Male: Frequent, long-lasting erection; testicles swollen; itching and redness of the scrotum. Female: Sharp ovarian pains, extending to the thighs; burning, swelling, and hardness of the breasts, often complicated with suppuration. Abortions rather frequent, especially in the early stages of pregnancy.

Extremities: Violent, rheumatoid pain in the shoulders; hands edematous; fingers numb; sometimes complicated with paronychia.

We cannot fail to recognize in the above enumerated symptoms, which frequently manifest themselves in cases of bee venomization, the typical syndrome of anaphylaxy, that is the introduction of a foreign protein into an organism, previously sensitized by the supposedly same, or similar substance. We know that chemically entirely different substances will produce similar, even identical anaphylactic reactions. Accordingly, when we deal with a severe case of bee venom intoxication, the degree of sensitivity must not be, necessarily, a consequence of former stings-*it might have been produced by some other vegetable protein, a different animal venom, even a cryptotoxic body poison.* The individual is simply in an anaphylactoid state.

It is an old saying that the soil is just as important as the seed, but in our case the subjective conditions-the soil-seem to play an incomparably more important part in the development of symptoms than the objective one-the venom-respectively, the seed; so we had better change the phrase and say that the soil is more important than the seed. The *proper resistance and the defensive strength of the body are of cardinal importance.* The organism is subjected to many and multiform altered functions, which are sometimes difficult to trace and explain. This often requires a circumspect and thoughtful study.

EFFECTS PRODUCED BY BEE STING INJURIES

To have a clear and complete understanding of the variform effects of bee stings, I believe it is the best plan to cite a comparatively fair number of cases reported by different authors in various medical books and periodicals. Some are more or less typical examples of normal bee stings, others are more unusual, even seldom met with, but all are rather instructive and illustrative.

Normal bee stings are at least in the majority of instances-benign, and on account of this fact come only very seldom under clinical observation. The victims of the injuries rarely ask or require medical intervention. They usually apply some house remedy, if such is at hand, knowing the effects will wear off anyhow and the wisest thing, under the circumstances, is "to forget it," the old slogan of veteran beekeepers.

On the other hand, we frequently have to deal with cases of serious nature, not always as a consequence of multiple stings (which, naturally, are more dangerous on account of the larger quantity of venom injected) but, as we will see, not infrequently a single bee sting injury has terminated fatally.

No individual physician, even though his observations have extended over many years, not even a large hospital, has sufficient material to be able to form an intelligent and concrete conception of the multiform and erratic effects of bee stings. Only collective teamwork can accomplish this difficult task. For this reason, I was compelled to search the widely-scattered world literature for records with characteristic, instructive, and rare manifestations of the effects of this rather occult, mystic substance, *to gain abundant material for the study*. The classification and perusal of this assembled mass experience, the intellectual survey of similar, sometimes diverging symptoms of bee sting effects, the conclusions and observations of other co-workers, their therapeutic methods of treating the injuries and results they obtained will greatly assist us to acquire a clear, comprehensive, and thorough understanding of this rather chaotic problem.

The great majority of bee stings occurs in the country and very often on account of the distance it is rather inconvenient, even difficult, to provide medical aid. Invariably when the country physician takes charge of the injury, he has no time or still less inclination to publish his experience, no matter how instructive or interesting it may be. In consequence, without any doubt, we lose much valuable information.

It was imperative to collect sufficient material to acquire an understanding of the effects of bee venom because it is a prerequisite for the successful administration of the treatments. The produced symptoms of a natural bee sting are not any different from those of an artificial inoculation. The whole conduct of a *successful treatment with injectable bee venom depends entirely and absolutely on the clinical symptoms of past administrations*; therefore, the toxic effects of the venom must be well understood before we undertake these treatments, where we must follow a carefully projected plan to secure good results. Keen observation, great solicitude, cautious concern, and discriminating judgment are required to manage obstinate and chronic cases of the type we are bound to confront if we expect to treat maladies which so far have been so refractory to most therapeutical measures.

The clinical management of the different bee sting injuries, and the therapeutic suggestions made by various authors have great medical interest and importance. I mention here, while we are discussing the effects of bee stings, that the initial shock and occasional collapse of the patient are not always due to the chemical influence of the venom. The sudden excruciating pain, in a sensitive person, may produce a mental, or rather reflex action, like swooning when a finger is crushed.

In general, the study of the effects of bee stings and their consequences is very intricate. *We encounter fewer difficulties in the treatments with injectable bee venom*, because we follow certain principles, rules, and standards; by their guidance we are able to control both the quantity and strength of our solution, inject it on the dorsal surface of the body, avoid arteries, veins, lymphatic and glandular tissues-in brief, we follow strictly certain technical rules and are not exposed to so many surprises, unexplainable complications, as when we are dealing with bee stings.

The surgical technic of the bee is very poor, even careless. All she has in view is to hurt you as much as possible. She will sting you on the tongue, palate, ear, cheek, penetrate your eyelid, inject the venom into your arteries, veins, not even attempting to test your tolerance. With bee stings, we can never figure on the consequences; the effects are uncertain, often even puzzling. Occasionally a person is stung by quite a number of bees without an important reaction; another time the same person is stung by one bee with serious consequences. Flury quoted a case where a two and a half year old child was stung by about 50 bees, without any ill effects while another child, stung by one bee, died.

The effectiveness of the sting depends on many incalculable circumstances and conditions, and this is the reason why often we cannot explain certain manifestations. There is no standard, rule, or principle, not even a seemingly logical connection, between the cause and effect. I wish to lay stress on this particular fact, and save ourselves surprises which we may encounter when looking over the case records.

The study of the general effects of bee sting injuries is very broad and important. To facilitate the classification of their systemic effects, and enable us to treat such a wide field in an appropriate manner, we have to subdivide it again into two groups. The influences which cause, ameliorate, or aggravate the general effects are: A, *Objective*; B, *Subjective*.

OBJECTIVE INFLUENCES

Objective, that is, external influences depend mainly on the bee and its venom. They are modified by:

1) Quantity of venom: multiple stings, aggressiveness of the bee, depth, direction of the sting.
2) Virulence of venom: species of bee, type of pollen, temperature and seasonal changes.
3) Septic and other complications.

The Quantity of Venom -The quantity of venom, i.e., the contents of the poison bag, contributes considerably to the effectiveness of a sting. It is only rational to include under the same heading the multiple bee stings. In single stings the variations are less pronounced.

The quantity of venom depends on many circumstances. The species of bee, the season of the year, the eagerness of the bee to empty the entire contents of its poison bag, the quality of pollens on which the bee feeds, and, also, the fact of whether it is well fed or hungry-all these contingencies will influence greatly the amount of venom which the bee will inject. Weak, very young, or aged bees have less venom.

To go into detail, the species of bee is very important. The Egyptian or Italian bee will produce a larger quantity of venom.

In spring, when the bees first start to collect their pollen, the quantity of venom, respectively the contents of the poison bag, is very low. In midsummer, the quantity is largest.

Bees are very peculiar and capricious. Sometimes when they are angry, infuriated, or in a stinging-mood, they will discharge the entire contents of the sac into the wound. The direction of the sting is, also, important, as the only way the bee can eject the contents of the bag is by applying her sting vertically. An oblique sting is never effective. As a rule, bees can sting only once; therefore, they always have the full contents of the sac at their disposal, the venom not having been used up by previous stings. In the case of wasps, which use their stings repeatedly, every subsequent sting is weaker. As early as 1719, Reaumur mentioned that the second sting of the wasp is not so painful, and the third, less than the second.

The type of flowers from which the bees collect their nectar and pollen is also an essential factor. Certain pollens produce a large quantity of venom. Bees fed on sugar syrup never produce as large an amount as those fed on pollen because in the former instance the vitality of the insect is lower, the sting is not so deep, and the venom is four or five times less potent.

It is only natural that the quantity and quality of venom are more or less correlated, interdependent. When we speak of a larger quantity of venom, it ordinarily applies to multiple bee stings. It stands to reason that in multiple stings a larger amount of venom is involved.

The effects of multiple bee stings are variable. The individual sensitivity, the body resistance, respectively any pathological state or predisposing constitutional cause, even sex, weight, age, color, all play important parts in the produced effects.

As illustrations, I quote the following cases:

J. O. Beven, of Ceylon, reported that he attended simultaneously a medical man and two ladies, stung by numerous bees at the same time.

Dr. S. was stung in about 120 places on his head, neck and shoulders. Beven abdominal cramps, profuse diarrhea, air hunger; rapid, weak pulse; sweating profound him in a collapsed state. Incessant vomiting of a greenish-yellow fluid, severe fusely.

Mrs. B. had been stung in about 80 places. The action of the venom in her case was slower but later she became clammy and almost pulseless. Continuous vomiting but no diarrhea. Very comatose.

Mrs. S. escaped very lightly though she received an equal number of stings. Developed a general erythema, urticaria, and most intense pruritus, which disappeared in about five days, followed by general furunculosis.

Beven thought we must always make allowance for weight and sex.

Virulence of Venom. The virulence of the venom, that is, the degree of its intensity, also varies considerably, even if we ignore entirely the subjective condition of the victim, which will, of course, greatly modify its effectiveness. The species, the seasonal differences, the weather conditions, the various pollens on which the bees feed, all will change the strength of the venom. Sometimes the same kind of bee may sting with unlike effects. In various species of bees, the venom differs. In tropical countries the stings have violent effect. Even there, the changes of temperature will alter their efficiency. On hot days, the stings will also become very "hot." One would think that the bees impart the fiery, glowing rays of the sun to their victims. Stings on a hot midsummer day are most powerful. (Snake bites are likewise influenced by changes of temperature. Tropical snakes are most dangerous, but even the toxicity of their venom increases in warmer seasons and depends on the changing heat of the day. Hungry, poorly-fed snakes are less dangerous.)

Cold and humidity attenuate the virulence of bee venom. The stings of young, old, hungry, weak, poorly-fed bees, or those fed on sugar syrup instead of pollen, lack intensity. At the beginning of spring, when the bees start to collect their pollen, the sting is very mild. It increases in strength during the summer; decreases again during autumn days, and will have but slight effect in winter. All these conditions influence not only the quality but also the quantity of the venom.

The flowers from which the bees collect their pollen will determine to some extent the strength of the venom. Buckwheat flowers and bass-wood blooms produce powerful venom. Even the health of the bee is a contributory factor, e.g., the sting of a dysenteric bee is severe.

Langer experimented with new-born bees which had just emerged from their larvae; they were note capable of stinging, but the poison bag already contained a minimum amount of venom. On the first day of their lives, with care and gentleness one could provoke a sting, but it would leave hardly any mark. On the third day, a wheal would form, but without any inflammation. On the fifth day, inflammation and edema already accompanied the wheal. A five-day old bee, though capable of stinging, would show no special inclination, and still less the usual eagerness to sting. Langer thought it would be a practical idea to let ourselves be stung by three to fiveday old bees, become accustomed to it, and be gradually immunized.

Septic and Other Complications. The sting of a bee is not only aseptic, but reputedly antiseptic, on account of the chemical composition of the venom. Langer proved that the venom has destructive effect on various microbes, particularly on staphylococci. There is no need to disinfect a sting injury. The bees feed on the clean nectar and pollen of flowers and never come in contact with decayed animal matter, like wasps or hornets, which are scavengers-carnivorous insects, killing their prey with the intention of eating it. There are plenty of other insects which feed on decayed, in fact, any putrid matter. Such stings are simultaneously septic inoculations.

If secondary septic complications follow a bee sting, they are always due to some extraneous contributory cause-never to the direct consequence of the sting injury. We will sometimes encounter a septic infection after a bee sting, e.g., an erysipelatous inflammation or plain suppuration, like furunculosis. This is generally attributable to the fact that an extremely intense pruritis accompanies stings and, of course, there is an abundant scratching. A microbial infection is inoculated possibly by the finger nails or, later, through the denuded skin by soiled underwear, clothing, or any other infective matter. Legal, of France, suggested that septic complications are often due to very energetic local treatments, producing extensive lesions of the skin, which open the gate for later infections.

There is a possibility that the necrotic slough, which often forms on the top and center of the inflammatory wheals, may cause septic complications, though this seems rather improbable on account of the firm leukocytic dam which surrounds it. The best proof of the obstructive and phagocytic protection of the inflammatory wheals is that, even several weeks after the stings have been inflicted, we find in the necrotic tissues some virulent venom (a similar occurrence is found in tetanic infections).

There have been cases reported with complications of lymph-adenitis, cellulitis, gangrene, even erysipelas. Dupuytren mentioned the case of Follin, who had a tetanus complication after a bee sting; and Penada, of Padua, in 1793, an instance where hydrophobia followed a bee-sting injury. Without any doubt, these were not direct but subsequent contaminations.

Nietlispach, of Switzerland, related a rather unusual and instructive casualty. A man, 42, was stung by about ten bees. He became unconscious, was cyanotic, with dilated pupils, pulse and heartbeats imperceptible, eyes turning backwards. Massage, artificial respiration, and stimulants revived the patient and he was able to resume his work two weeks later, but never recovered entirely. A year later, he acquired pulmonary tuberculosis. La Suval (a Swiss accident company of Lucerne) recognized the liability and paid the claim. Half an hour of apnea, intense passive congestion of the lungs, were considered sufficiently conducive to the acquisition of tuberculosis, as a consequence of the impaired resistance of the organism.

SUBJECTIVE INFLUENCES

Subjective influences, relating to inherent or acquired attributes of the individual who suffered the injury, are mainly dependent on:

1) *Predisposing constitutional conditions:* distinctive characteristics of the recipient-age, sex, weight, etc., an eventual pathological state, lessened resistance, idiosyncrasy, anaphylaxy, or just the reverse, an immunity of varying degree.

2) *Topographical conditions:* the particular location of the injury, e.g., face, especially eyes, nose, mouth; injection of the venom into arteries, veins, lymph ducts, producing rapid absorption, etc.

Predisposing Constitutional Conditions. Constitutional causes, pathological conditions, unusual sensitivity, idiosyncratic and anaphylactoid states, will greatly influence the effects of the stings.

Cardiac, arterial, and renal conditions predominate as important factors in increasing the gravity of the stings. When we speak of cardiac conditions, we mean myocardial, sclerotic, or valvular affections, not rheumatoid inflammations, because, as we shall see later, of all arthritic and rheumatoid involvements, the rheumatic inflammations of the heart respond so favorably to bee venom that it might be considered a specific.

Persons suffering from arteriosclerosis, nephritis, and albuminuria are very poor subjects for bee stings. Those with unstable, defective circulatory equilibrium, on account of their lessened resistance, are great sufferers and are always in danger when stung by bees. On diabetics, for instance, the effect of the venom is very pronounced. A neuropathic disposition may considerably aggravate the symptoms.

Children, even adults, of the catarrhal, lymphatic, and glandular types are generally poor subjects. Every kind of diathesis and dyscrasia is an important contributory factor, not only in producing severe general effects but also intensified local reactions. In women and children, the reactions are usually more severe, which is probably due not only to the fine texture and sensitivity of the skin but to their circulation. Keiter differed in this respect; he thought that children are less affected than older people.

Menstruation makes women sensitive to stings and the injury itself has a great effect on the menstruation. Bees are much attracted to women during their periods; it seems to provoke in the bees a certain eagerness to sting. The venom has a strong hemorrhagic and circulatory effect. Aisch, a German priest, reported in one of the bee journals that a woman aborted after a single sting, experiencing a repetition of the mishap during her next successive pregnancy. Keiter, Terc's collaborator, noticed, in treating women with bee stings, that their periods always commenced earlier. This also proves the hemorrhagic effect of the venom.

Even the weight of a person has influence on the effectiveness of the venom. The same quantity in a smaller person means higher concentration. When we use antivenin in children, we have to give a much larger dose because we must counteract higher concentration. In adults, the poison is distributed over a larger area.

Dold's experiments have shown that in albino rabbits the reaction to bee venom was stronger than in dark ones. The same principle applies to the human race-blondes suffer more than brunettes.

As an illustration of what an important part individual resistance plays in the development of the symptoms, I will cite Langer's personal experience. In 1904, he took a vacation just after he had recovered from an appendicitis operation. While convalescing on his parents' farm, he was stung on the neck by a bee. In a few minutes, he reported, all over his face and body a general and very annoying urticaria developed. He had been stung many times before by a large number of bees and wasps without showing any reaction, and was convinced that since he was in a state of convalescence the low alkalinity of the blood failed to neutralize the acid effect of the venom.

The old are quite resistant to bee venom. The more advanced the age, the less the reaction. This is consistent with the theory, or rather, the fact, that rheumatics and arthritics react slightly or not at all to bee venom, as elderly people are subject to these infirmities. Then again, we are more likely to find various, even advanced pathological conditions.

Alcoholics possess strong resistance to bee venom, yet it is a curious fact that bees have a passion for attacking them. The odor of liquor arouses their fury. Nothnagel mentioned this exceptional resistance of drunkards to bee stings. Hermann cited (*ibid.*) the case of a 74-year-old peasant who was stung by approximately 600 bees. The victim recovered quickly, without any of the serious complications which might have been expected. Of course, he had three facts in his favor: his age, his occupation as a beekeeper, and also that he was a strong alcoholic. *Alcohol* taken internally *is one of the most helpful remedies* in the treatment of the general effects, especially in severe bee venom intoxication.

EFFECTS PRODUCED BY BEE STING INJURIES

L. Bouchacourt, in a recent article about the therapeutic value of bee venom, made the interesting statement, that bee venom in certain subjects acts like a habit-forming drug, comparable only to toxicomania-an insane longing for toxic substances, like morphine, alcohol, etc.

He reported an interesting observation communicated to him personally by Mr. Mamelle, professor of the apicultural school of Grignon. A young student occasionally got drunk and incorrigible. The next day, after such a drinking spree, he was unable to attend to his work. His teacher once punished him for his intemperance by applying a number of bee stings. Since then every time the young man became intoxicated, he applied the stings himself the "morning-after." Mamelle thought that he did this, not so much to punish himself, but probably because he found that one poison counteracted the other and restored his equilibrium and this later developed into a real toxicomaniac craving.

Extreme heat will aggravate the effects, because the absorption of the venom is accelerated. On a very hot day, the heart may also be weakened and the resistance of the organism lowered. I am firmly convinced that pre disposing causes due to lessened resistance often play a more important part in grave complications than anaphylactic states. We frequently find cases with the semblance of a typical anaphylactic shock which, however, are really attributable to low body resistance.

As a very illustrative example, I quote the personal experience of G. M. D. Bartholomew, of Nebraska. He was stung by one bee in March, 1929, which produced all the symptoms of an anaphylactic shock, lasting for 24 hours. In May of that year, he was stung by three bees with still stronger effect. Unconscious for eight hours. Two weeks later, he was stung again by about half a dozen bees, in 10 minutes became unconscious, and remained so for nearly 12 hours. Aromatic spirits of ammonia gave him most relief. Bartholomew thought that, judging from the intense effects of his previous experiences, if he had been stung by three or four bees the first time it surely would have ended disastrously. He felt certain that each year there are more deaths caused by bee stings than by snake bites.

I strongly suspected that Dr. Bartholomew's unusually severe symptoms were due more to other pathological conditions than to just plain anaphylaxy. I wrote to him asking him to be kind enough to inform me about his general physical state, which might have accounted for the extraordinary reactions he suffered. The letter was returned, marked "Deceased." I then wrote to the Nebraska State Medical Association, requesting information about his death. The reply stated that he had died in 1930 from a gastric hemorrhage produced by ulcers.

Undoubtedly, Dr. Bartholomew's physical condition in 1929, a year before his death, was already quite weakened, which induced or intensified the symptoms.

The following report of Edwin L. Goss, of North Dakota, is also very instructive.

A beekeeper, for years immune to stings, after a *hearty dinner* and otherwise in a generally rundown condition, suffered serious effects from a single sting. The incident happened on a hot August day. He was dressed as usual for attending to the bees-veil, gloves, overalls, rubber boots. Bees have consummate skill in clambering into any small opening of the clothing. The beekeeper and a friend were examining some hives when a bee got under one of his gloves and stung him on the wrist. There was no swelling, but this was usual with him. He continued to work for a while but suddenly noticed that he was becoming, he said, "sick all over." He started for the house, which was nearby, hurriedly removed his clothing, and got into a tub of soda water. After this bath, his face commenced to swell and became quite puffed. There was pruritus all over the body, especially on the scalp, abdomen, and groin. Suddenly he became unconscious, fell on his face, broke his eyeglasses and suffered a cut around an. eye. Recovering from the shock, he started for the bathroom again. There supervened vomiting and diarrhea, which completely cleaned him out. In the meantime he perspired profusely, and suffered extreme itching and burning. He tried to get back to his bedroom, but fell unconscious in the hallway once more, remaining there for he did not know how long. After he had recovered, he went to bed and fell asleep for about three or four hours. Barring all the bruises, he felt only an extreme exhaustion.

The patient, at the time of the experience, was physically in a state much below par, his resistance was low, blood pressure only 100, had had a hearty dinner, besides it was a very hot day-all these conditions (possibly even the bath after a meal) contributed to the severity of the attack. Later, he was stung again, with no reaction. (Goss knew of several deaths in his practice, which we will mention later in this same chapter under FATAL INJURIES CAUSED BY BEE STINGS.)

This cited instance is unusually interesting and instructive. Let us analyze it. A beekeeper, considered immune to the effect of stings-and justly so having been often stung previously, even by a large number of bees at the same time, without the slightest reaction-is suddenly stung by a single bee and becomes violently, almost critically ill. Logically, we might exclude anaphylaxy, as he was again stung soon after the related experience without ill effect. The sudden metamorphosis therefore must be attributed to some temporarily superinduced constitutional complications. The search for these often hidden causes demands a careful scrutiny.

I have frequently noticed serious consequences from a single sting injury during (1) *a postprandial* or (2) a *menstrual period*. We have to ascribe this "revolutionary" state to a limitation or lack of defensive or responsive power in the organism, due probably to insufficiency or possibly to incapacity of the blood supply, *restrained, monopolized or altered* by (1) the digestive or (2) the reproductive organs.

To make this contention more convincing, I quote another supporting case, reported by L. Cornil:

A young woman apiarist was stung many times before, when she developed only ordinary minor reactions. In June, 1916, she was stung by a bee on the dorsal surface of the left hand. Her menstrual period had just started. She had little pain from the sting and the effects seemed to take a normal course. An hour later, she was seized with a general itching sensation which spread very rapidly. Soon diffuse urticaria and erythema developed. Her face was red and congested; the conjunctiva injected; her eyelids and lips, edematous. Nausea, vomiting, respiratory anguish, and dyspnea supervened. Two hours after the sting there was syncope, with the pulse rapid and small. Several hours later, only the hand showed edema. The symptoms, 13 hours later, gradually disappeared, first the erythema, then the urticaria, the edema of the face, and finally, the dyspnea. Only a light headache persisted.

In this case the victim was a woman apiarist, likewise stung many times before—without ill effects. The symptoms developed slowly, an hour after the injury, and disappeared only gradually 13 hours later. Unquestionably, the phenomena somewhat suggest anaphylaxy, but the time is rather against this diagnosis, as anaphylactic symptoms manifest themselves sooner and vanish more rapidly. We might exclude (with certain limitations) intravenous inoculation, as the sting was inflicted on the dorsal surface of the hand. An ovarian and uterine congestion, especially at the beginning of menstruation, the vicarious anemia of other parts of the body (cerebral, cardiac and pulmonary), and a certain circulatory restraint, seem to be the most plausible explanation. A *splanchnic congestion*-particularly after a hearty or heavy meal is an almost parallel instance.

EFFECTS PRODUCED BY BEE STING INJURIES

The fatal case of Mrs. Gertrude Mason a woman of 47, in the "best of health," "stung many times before without bad effects," occurred at six o'clock, also *after supper*, which in this case was the main meal of the day.

If we carefully study the fatal case of Henry Stizel who "did not pay much attention to the sting, had his dinner and later attended to some household duties," the fact that the sting had no immediate effect though inflicted on a region rich in vascular and lymphatic tissues, and that fatal symptoms developed only *after dinner*, deserves some consideration.

The case reported by L. Franck is somewhat similar; there the patient apparently recovered from the sting injuries, but next day, after dinner, collapsed and died.

Most of the reports seem to mention only incidentally-rather, accidentally-that a sting with serious or fatal consequences was inflicted after a meal or during menstruation, apparently considering the facts just as nonessential concurrences. To my knowledge, so far no one has paid the particular attention to these circumstances which they deserve. I hope *in future reports these "coincidences" will not be disregarded.*

Topographical Conditions. The topographical conditions, that is, the regions of the body where the stings are inflicted often greatly influence their efficiency. The facility of absorption will both quicken and aggravate the symptoms. The venom is more effective when introduced into the intradermal tissues. Subcutaneously, in the fatty tissues, where there is less circulation, it travels more slowly. On the other hand, when the venom is injected into parts of the body, rich in arterial, varicose, and lymphatic vessels, this will considerably increase the effects; fineness of the skin, as

in women and children, will also favor a rapid absorption. Stings inflicted on the face: lips, nose, eyes, ears, and on the neck or scrotum are usually serious, and are followed by severe local and general reactions. Stings in the mouth, on the tongue, palate, uvula and esophagus are always fraught with danger. In such cases, it is not always the direct toxic effect of the venom which causes the trouble, but more often the mechanical obstruction of the air passages; the consecutive edema is the danger because the patient is exposed to the hazard of suffocation. Only an early, opportunely performed tracheotomy may save such victims. In the medical and lay press there are published numberless accidents of this type caused by insects lodged on or in food material. Wasps and hornets predominate in such casualties. Bees, as a rule, restrict themselves to flowers.

Dupuytren related an instance when a farmer bit into an apple in which a wasp was hidden. He was stung in the mouth and died a short time later from asphyxia, produced by pharyngeal edema. Legal described a similar case of a young girl who, while eating grapes, was stung in the throat and died soon afterward, suffocating in the arms of her friends. Legal also gave an account of the accident of an English physician, Dr. Powel, who died in a like manner from glottis edema after three hours of "atrocious" suffering.

The eyes are supposed to be fairly well protected by the eyelids. It was thought for a time that the sting of the bee was not long enough to penetrate them. It is different with wasps; they have longer and stronger stings with more powerful muscular action.

Very often, we hardly notice any important local reaction and still the general effects are very violent. In such instances, we are usually dealing with intravenous "medication."

I quote some characteristic cases to demonstrate the importance of topographical influences:

Bee Sting Injuries in the Mouth.-Geiger and Roth reported the following:

M. J., 26, male, was riding on a motorcycle, when an insect flew into his mouth and stung him on impact. The dislodged insect proved to be an ordinary honey bee. Violent gagging and vomiting followed before he was able to reach the doctor's office. He was given a gargle. Several hours later he had difficulty in speaking, likewise in swallowing, with considerable edema in the mouth, which was inflamed and tense. The uvula was the size of a man's thumb. Palate and pillars were as edematous as the uvula. Locally, cocaine was applied. At the junction of the uvula and anterior pillar, there was a circumscribed pale area, a wheal, 5 millimeters in diameter, with a black foreign body in the center, which, after it was extracted, proved to be the sting. A 10 percent solution of silver nitrate was applied locally and a concentrated solution of bicarbonate of soda was given as a gargle. The patient was soon relieved. Without quick medical attention, this injury might have ended fatally. In the parallel case of Henry Stizel, described under fatal injuries, even a tracheotomy, possibly performed rather late, was of no avail.

W. Scholz, of Germany, related a unique accident:

A 16-year-old boy, while playing, suddenly felt a sharp pain in his cheek. He went to the doctor's office with a swollen face, especially under the angle of the mandibula. The pharynx was edematous and had all the appearance of a peritonsillar abscess-redness, swelling and considerable sensitiveness on pressure. The patient had great difficulty in breathing. On the height of the swelling, in the mouth, there was an aptha like, yellow erosion, and in its center a black speck. The doctor extracted the foreign body, which, under the microscope, proved to be a bee sting. The boy did not even have any idea that he had been injured inside the mouth. Under usual local and antiphlogistic treatments, the inflammation subsided in several days.

Only recently, April 1, 1934, The San Francisco Chronicle carried the following:

Stung internally by a bee that flew into her mouth, Lindelle Martin, 2 year old daughter of Mr. and Mrs. William Martin of Lansdale, Marin County, is fighting death at Stanford Hospital, while science marshals its forces to save her.

After a week of struggle physicians yesterday held out a ray of hope. The child's life still hung on a slender thread.

The girl's condition resulted from an accident unique in the experience of medical men. She was in a swing at her home when suddenly her rippling laugh became a scream. Her frantic parents ran to her side. Her screams of agony continued. The cause of her pain, of course, was a mystery.

Physicians were summoned and the child was removed to the hospital, where Dr. Annie Lyle, well known local physician, discovered that an insect, probably a bee or wasp, had flown into the baby's mouth, had stung the esophagus and produced a swelling extending to the child's bronchial area.

Dr. J. A. Bacher, of Stanford, with Dr. Lyle, performed a bronchoscopy. It revealed an immense swelling by the baby's trachea. For days the patient's breathing had been labored and her temperature mounted rapidly. Tanks of oxygen have been used to give her relief.

Yesterday, while still in a critical condition, the child was resting easier.

Bee Sting Injury on the Cheek. Legiehn, of Germany, reported the following:

EFFECTS PRODUCED BY BEE STING INJURIES

A woman of 40 was stung by a bee on the left cheek. The *Lancet* was immediately extracted. In three minutes, a burning feeling spread from the place of injury all over the face, head, and, in fact, the whole upper part of the body. There was distinct oppression in her head and constriction of the neck. She tried to speak but there was perfect aphonia. On the place of the sting, just a red point, no infiltration or redness around the wound, but her whole face, neck, chest, and upper part of the back were red, with many urticarial wheals and violent itching over the whole body. Pharynx was intensely red. In two hours, all symptoms suddenly disappeared. Former stings on same person on other parts of the body showed only the usual normal reactions.

Bee Sting Injuries of the Eye. Charles A. Young, of Virginia, related a very instructive case. So far, it had been thought that a bee sting was not long enough to penetrate the cartilage of the eyelid. In this instance, the sting not only penetrated the eyelid but was so deeply wedged in the cornea that it was a source of great pain and irritation. Patient, to obtain relief, even requested an enucleation of the eye. Four operations were necessary to remove the sting and save the eye.

J. H. Strebel, of Switzerland, reported several eye injuries caused by bee stings. He invariably observed severe panophthalmitis, great swelling, and considerable pain. The discharge from the eye was bacterium-free, just as though it were caused by some caustic chemical substance.

Vormann, surgeon-general of the German Army, published a report of a bee sting injury of the eye which he thought was the only one ever printed in medical literature. The sting penetrated the cartilage of the eyelid. (See cases reported by Young and Huwald.) The patient was stung on the eyelid by a bee and three days later came to Vormann's office. The eye was extremely painful, edematous, and there was a general panophthalmitis. Corresponding to the injury on the eyelid, there was a 0.75 millimeter long, fine, brown, foreign substance in the cornea which proved to be a part of the sting (the usual length of a sting is 3 millimeters). Patient very distinctly remembered that when he was stung it felt as though the eyelid were glued to the eyeball.

Huwald, of the University Clinic in Heidelberg, also, reported an injury to the cornea:

A carpenter of 35 came to the clinic a day after he had been stung by a bee on the cornea through the eyelid. The eye was considerably swollen and there was a severe conjunctivitis with muco-purulent discharge. It took fully two weeks before the inflammation subsided.

Bee Sting Injury on the Head. Edward Derrick, of Australia, described the following incident:

A boy of 19 was stung by one bee behind the left mastoid process. Sting was promptly removed. In several minutes his scalp and face became very itchy. His face was flushed, his eyes bloodshot. Shoulders first goose-fleshed; later, arms, shoulders, chest, abdomen, legs, in fact the whole body, became red and patient felt warm all over. The itch passed off as soon as the flush developed. About 10 minutes later, patient shivered, trembled, and felt very anxious. There was a brilliant generalized erythema. At the site of the sting there was a swelling the size of half a dollar, but no urticaria. Half an hour later the flush began to fade and soon entirely disappeared, likewise the local reaction.

Derrick suggested that we have to assume the bee administered the venom intravenously.

Bee Sting Injuries to the Male Genitalia.-This is a case reported by Perrin and Cuènot:

A young man of 18 was an apiarist. Had been stung many times before without ill effects. One day he was stung on the scrotum by a bee which had penetrated his clothing. Five minutes later he developed general pruritus, urticaria, chills, and a temperature of 105° F. There was an enormous scrotal edema. The urticaria disappeared next day, but the fever lasted two days longer, and the edema for four days.

Nietlispach reported a bee sting on the penis, producing retention of urine. Rapid absorption of the venom by tissues, rich in arterial and lymphatic vessels, invariably produces severe reactions.

FATAL INJURIES CAUSED BY BEE STINGS

If we try to apply the law of cause and effect to bee sting injuries and expect a logical sequence, we soon shall discover that this principle is utterly inapplicable. The symptoms which are the consequences of these injuries are produced and influenced by so many incalculable contingencies that to prognosticate an eventual outcome of the injuries, is an impossibility. Vice versa, we are often at a loss to explain certain phenomena by reasonably supporting facts. Therefore, we may just as well desist from trying to make even an approximate guess as to what constitutes *a fatal dose*.

Constitutional pathological conditions will, of course, greatly contribute to a fatal outcome; topographical influences are often instrumental. The injection of the poison into arteries, veins and lymphatic vessels will produce rapid absorption and full toxic effects. The multiplicity of stings, which literally means a larger quantity of venom, is, likewise, an important contributory factor.

Undoubtedly, we all have had our sad experiences with various septic infections of the face above the line of the upper lip. Seemingly insignificant injuries have frequently resulted in fatal complications, producing, for instance fulgurant meningitis through rapid absorption. Below the lips, it is different; the abundance of nearby lymphatic glands often checks or frustrates the progress of an infection. In over forty years of practice I have come across many unfortunate accidents caused by minor injuries on the upper part of the face, which defied all surgical skill and have ended fatally. I vividly remember two identical cases, both originating from a slight cut on the upper lip produced by licking a postage stamp. Numerous lamentable complications resulted from boils on the face which were considered trivial. When we read our case records, we shall repeatedly find that single bee sting injuries, inflicted on these regions, have caused deaths.

The oldest annals relate such untimely fatal endings. Both Bianor and Antipater, of Thessalonica, lamented the fate of baby Hermonax, who innocently crawled near the hives and was massacred by their inmates, "driving into him their wretched stings, more savage than those of vipers" (Norman Douglas). In the archives of the ancient town of Worms, one of the chief cities of Germany in the Middle Ages (with its famous 11th Century cathedral and Nibelungen fame), we read the account of a complaint, lodged before the "Diet," that bees had killed a child. The Great Council ordered the hives and bees burned in the public square. Innumerable other fatalities are reported in ancient and modern medical literature and lay press.

Van Hasselt described a case of a three-year-old child in Dreuthe, Holland, and Caffe, of France, a parallel case of a six-year-old child, stung on the temporal region by a single bee. Both died in a short time. A. Delpech, of the Paris Board of Health, who was commissioned to investigate the numerous complaints about the bee hives in Paris, in an interesting and long report cited 16 fatal cases, all rather instructive, several with autopsy findings. Most fatalities were caused by stings on the face, ear, nose, eye, temporal region and neck.

EFFECTS PRODUCED BY BEE STING INJURIES

The experience of Henry Stizel, a rich landowner, is illustrative of how serious injuries can be if inflicted on tissues rich in lymphatic vessels. He had just arrived home and was anxious to have some cider. He could not find a glass, so poured it into a funnel. While drinking it, a bee, which was in the cider, stung him in the throat. He did not pay much attention to the injury, had dinner, and even attended later to some household duties. Soon his neck started to swell and his breathing and swallowing became difficult. A physician applied ammonia compresses, performed three venesections, and finally a tracheotomy-but all were of no avail.

Conradi and Fabre collected reports of 47 serious and 17 mortal bee sting injuries. Delpech, also, told of a six-year-old child stung by one bee on the left temporal region. The child ran to her father, who extracted the sting. Her lips became blue, she had respiratory difficulties, and was covered with cold sweats. Death followed within half an hour. The child was of a very nervous type and had had repeated collapses after previous stings. Autopsy showed a diffuse congestion of the nasal sinuses and cerebral membranes; the brain ventricles were filled with two teaspoonfuls of coffee colored liquid blood.

Desbret published a similar accident of a farmer, around 30, who was stung below the eyebrow by a bee, fell to the ground, and died in a few minutes.

In "Schmidt's Jahrbücher der Medizin," we find the report of a death following a bee sting. An autopsy was performed. The most important findings were pronounced hyperemia of the meninges and sinuses, and blood exudates in the brain ventricles.

In *Büchner's Repetitorium für Pharmacie*, mention is made of a peasant woman, Marie Stimpfl, of Landshut, who was stung in the face by a single bee, was seized with nausea and cramps, and in a quarter of an hour was dead.

The *Lancet* of June 16, 1883, quoted from the Sheffield and Rotherham Independent a case of a farmer, 59, in good health, who, while working in his garden, was stung on the eyelid by a bee. Rapid collapse followed, and he died in half an hour. His daughter stated that he had been stung twice previously, and was very ill on each occasion. The editor wondered whether in such cases it was the virus of the bee, or the consequence of some disordered physiological state which led to disaster.

In a Swiss bee journal, Howald, in 1895, reported a fatality. A beekeeper was stung by one bee on the right lower eyelid. Considerable vertigo immediately followed; 15 minutes later he jumped up with a loud shriek, and dropped dead. A year before, he had also suffered quite a prolonged collapse after one sting. Autopsy showed fatty degeneration of the heart, with extensive pleural adhesions of both lungs.

Another injury was described in the *Frankfurter Zeitung* on August 21, 1905. A mill owner named Weinhold, of Thaubenheim, was stung by one bee on his left ear and died in ten minutes. Langer was interested in this accident. An autopsy was performed and it disclosed fatty degeneration of the heart and myocarditis. In addition, the family volunteered the information that the victim was a distinct neurasthenic and had a decided idiosyncrasy for bees.

Germain Legal quoted two instances published in the *Progrès Médical*. A priest named Notelet, while collecting honey, was stung by bees. Several hours later, was found unconscious and next day he died. A Mr. Bordeau, stung under identical circumstances, died before medical help could be procured.

W. A. Hunter, of Australia, gave a detailed report of a fatal casualty.

An imbecile, 24 years old (not deaf or dumb), an inmate of a home, was found by the superintendent, his head and face covered with bees. The superintendent brushed off the bees and called Dr. Hunter. On arrival, the doctor found the head, face, eyelids, lips, neck, thickly studded with stings. He added: "I never saw anything like it. Passing a hand over his face, it felt like a three days' stubble of an unshaved face." Hunter removed the stings and applied ammonia. The face was very much swollen, extending even to part of the tongue. The patient could not open his eyes. Swallowing was difficult, but he was able to curse the bees in rather voluble language. It was rather odd, but he didn't complain very much about pain, possibly due to his imbecility. He vomited a green substance containing three bees; and next day, passed a number of bees by rectum. This happened on Friday, October 29, 1926. He was conscious all of the time after that, not much complaint, was able to take nourishment. Lived until Monday, when he died suddenly.

Possibly it was due to the shock or to the absorptive effect of the large amount of venom.

Parisius and Heimberger submitted two interesting cases of acute myelosis caused by bee stings:

A man, age 68, had been in the clinic a year before with chronic nephritis. He was attacked by some dysenteric bees in April, when he suffered about 40 stings on the face. Patient was admitted to the hospital in May. The clinical findings were anemia, hemorrhagic, ulcerative gingivitis, stomatitis, enlarged spleen. Hemoglobin, 49 percent. Red blood cells, 2,400,000. Myeloblasts, 2 percent. There was a bloody diarrhea, bleeding from the bladder, hemoglobin down to 35 percent. He died two weeks after admission.

A woman of 43, who was always well, was stung by about 15 to 20 bees on the face and head two weeks before admission. The findings were fever, vomiting, dysentery, swollen glands and stomatitis. She died two weeks later. Spleen was six times its original size.

W. Ray Jones, of Seattle, stated he had knowledge of three deaths caused by bee stings in the State of Washington alone, and felt certain that there must have been many others in the United States.

The writer tried to obtain data from the Department of Commerce about the mortality statistics of bee stings, but was unsuccessful, as they are not specifically classified.

W. Scholz also reported, not from his own observation but through personal communication, a case of a woman who, while eating, swallowed a bee, which stung her in the throat. She died very shortly from suffocation. L. Franck described a fatal case with autopsy findings. A 56-year-old farmer was stung by about a dozen bees. The local reaction was not unusual, neither had he any other symptoms worth mentioning. Next day he resumed his usual work, but shortly after dinner, while talking to a friend, suddenly complained of pain in the heart. He was put to bed and a physician was called, who administered a centigram of morphine, after which the patient expired. The autopsy showed a fatty heart. The case seems to have been myocarditis and acute indigestion aggravated by morphine, whereas what was required was a stimulant. Dr. Ditten, who performed the autopsy, stated that death was not the direct result of the bee stings. In his opinion, the effects of the stings are always violent and quick and if the crisis is passed, they gradually wear off. If stings are followed by serious symptoms, it will always happen within a short time.

Edwin Goss related that several times in his practice patients stung by one bee had died a few minutes after the injury. He also learned, through personal communication, of an occurrence on a bee farm near Montreal, Canada. A girl, stung on the lip, died 20 minutes later, though she had been stung many times before without any serious consequences. Another case was communicated to him. A boy, while riding a bicycle, was stung by a bee which flew into his mouth. The boy died soon afterward. Dupuytren mentioned, in his *Leçons orales de clinique chirurgicale*, more as an anecdote, that a postillon, while passing a bee hive, upset it with a lash of his whip. A large number of bees stung him "cruelly," and he died several days later.

Flury referred to a man 84 years old, who was overrun by bees. At the autopsy, they counted 1200 sting injuries.

In the *Journal de Médicine et de Chirurgie pratiques* (XXX, 1859), there is a report of a young Hungarian who was stung on the neck by a bee. The sting was extracted. He was seized with nausea, tried to walk but could only wobble; threw himself on the couch, stammered some words, and died, not longer than 15 minutes after he had been stung. It is very hard to say, in such cases, whether it is the influx of the venom into the blood circulation, hypersensitivity, emotional shock, or other contributory conditions which produce death.

A similar incident was published by Gelpke and Schlatter. An English society lady was stung over an artery in the neck and dropped dead. Possibly, some pathologic vascular or cardiac condition may change an otherwise normal sting into a fatal one.

F. X. Dube, of St. Bruno (Quebec), wrote to the editor of The American Bee Journal in September, 1926, that beekeeping may prolong life, as some people believe, but he could not say so. His daughter, aged 13, was stung by a single bee and 20 minutes later was dead. The editor suggested that the child must have suffered from heart trouble or the sting penetrated an artery. L. Burr advised the same editor, in the November, 1926, issue, that his child, 22 years old, was stung on the thumb by a bee and in 10 minutes was barely conscious. The November, 1932, issue of this Journal mentioned that Andrew Rossi, of Renton, Washington, while at work on September 27, 1932, was stung by a bee on the back of his neck, and died in half an hour, before medical aid arrived.

A. Hansen reported a lethal case in a Copenhagen medical journal. A woman, who had been stung two or three times, presented more severe reactions on each successive occasion. In September, 1921, was stung by a bee on the left leg, and in 20 minutes exhibited symptoms of respiratory paralysis. Artificial respiration and heart massage revived her but she fell into a profound coma and died on the fourth day. There was no sign of sepsis.

EFFECTS PRODUCED BY BEE STING INJURIES

There was an item in the April 27, 1922, issue of the *New York Times* that a farmer, Harry Collerd, of Caldwell, New Jersey, was stung by a bee on the right temple. His neck began to swell; he became unconscious and I died before a physician arrived. The coroner thought death was due to apoplexy or weak heart.

Dr. C. F. Rife, of Naperville, Illinois, wrote to me, in answer to my questionnaire, on November 7, 1933:

"There was a fatality in our vicinity. I made a trip to get the facts. The man was 46 years old, unmarried, robust, Armand Tissot by name, and lived near Downers Grove, Illinois. He acquired a colony of bees but had a friend to manipulate them. In July, a year ago, his friend was working with the bees when Tissot, who was about twenty yards away, was stung by a bee on his hand. He was in great pain, threw himself face down on the grass, arm swelled to the shoulder, tongue swollen and protruding from his mouth, frothing and unable to speak. His aunt said that his face was quite purple. No doctor was called. About a half hour later, was able to speak. Later stated that he was conscious all of the time.

"Tissot received the *fatal sting* on November 5th of last year, under similar circumstances. His friend had the hive open and Tissot was at approximately the same distance from the hive as on the previous occasion. A single bee stung him on his chin. He ran to the house immediately, removed the sting, and sat down in a chair. His aunt got some baking soda, wet it and was ready to apply it on the site of the sting when she noticed his precarious condition and sent for a doctor. The physician arrived in eight minutes, and found him dead. The aunt said that his appearance and symptoms were very similar to those caused by the previous sting, only more pronounced. There was a spasmodic contraction of the abdominal muscles, as though he was trying to vomit, which might have been caused, also, by the effort to get his breath, due to the swollen condition of his tongue. Was dead within ten minutes after receiving the sting."

A. W. Mason, of Batavia, New York, under date of November 6, 1933, sent me the following communication:

"I lost my wife on the fourth of August, 1932, from just one sting. My wife went with me and my two boys to the home yard after supper, about six o'clock. The yard is about two minutes' drive from the house. She had gone there often and had been stung many times without any bad effects. I left her and the two boys in the car and went to put some combs into the hives. I saw her get out of the car and walk toward the yard. Shortly afterwards, one of the boys called me to come quickly, as she had been stung. I rushed over to where she was. She had sat down, her head was on her knees, breathing her last. We got her to the hospital in about ten minutes, but the doctor said she had been dead at least ten or twelve minutes. From the time I saw her get out of the car until I picked her up it must have been about seven minutes. She was forty-seven years old, and was always in the best of health."

This was another case where a sting injury inflicted after a meal had mortal effect.

Clayton S. Baker, of LaFayette, N. Y., informed me on January 22, 1934, that when his father, Alexander S. Baker, a farmer, was a young man he was stung by a bee, became unconscious for several hours, and the gave him up as dead. His hands and feet turned black under the nails. He revived, but the attack left him in a very weak condition. Received the fatal sting, inflicted on the bridge of his nose by a single bee, at the age of 58 years. He just managed to reach the house and his bed, where he died within half an hour. During the period between the first incident which produced such serious consequences, and the fatal injury, he was stung repeatedly without abnormal effects.

A. E. Clayton of Peaston, East Tuluse, South Africa, sent me two records of fatal casualties caused by bee sting injuries. One, an accident to a policeman, quoted on page 202, led to legal action instituted by his widow against the government. The other was that of a Mr. and Mrs. Lange, an elderly couple, who were stung by bees which hived near their "stoep." Both became very ill. Mr. Lange eventually collapsed and died. Mr. Clayton had heard of many other fatal accidents, but had kept no record. He heard of a man who was stung, while traveling in Pretoria in a tram car which was "invaded" by bees, and who suffocated as the result of the swelling of his tongue.

Other fatal cases were reported to me, one from Centralia, Kansas, of a ten-year-old girl, who was stung by one bee on the top of her head. Death resulted within two hours (name given but omitted by request). Another was from Callicoon, Sullivan County, New York. A young man suffered only one sting, ran to the house, and dropped dead.

In fatalities caused by bee stings, as a general rule, we lack accurate and detailed autopsy findings. Prof. C. Wegelin, of Berne, Switzerland, recently described a very instructive and illustrative instance, giving a most minute description of the pathological and histological changes. It is a worthy prototype of a thorough report.

Albert A., a road builder, 40 years old, while at work on September 19, 1932, was stung on the neck by a bee. The sting was removed by a fellow-worker. There was no swelling on the place of injury, only slight edema. The victim complained of constriction of the chest, became cyanotic and had great difficulty in reaching a nearby house. He stretched out on the floor, had a couple drinks of whiskey, and rubbed some of it on his neck. He died 20 minutes from the time of the injury, after having exhibited increasing air hunger and great anxiety. There was very distinct protrusion of the eyes. The physician who was immediately called found him dead. The corpse showed extensive mottled cyanotic and red spots. According to friends, A. was always in perfect health, and was an efficient worker.

The autopsy was performed 17 hours later. Body well built. Face and neck dark blue. Eyes somewhat protruding. On the right side of the neck at the height of the larynx, on the anterior edge of the sternocleidomastoid muscle, a minute puncture was visible to the naked eye. Pharyngeal aperture was strongly edematous and cyanotic, especially around the right tonsil; considerable swelling of the soft palate diminished; mucous membranes of the pharynx, larynx and trachea dark red. Heart and uvula; the epiglottic folds were particularly edematous; laryngeal opening considerably enlarged, the lobes grayish red. Spleen normal in size, of solid consistency dark red, hyperemic. Kidneys greatly congested. Liver normal in size, dark red. Stomach inflamed, hemorrhages on the mucous surfaces. Scrotal sac tense, filled with clear yellow fluid. Lymph glands and ducts swollen only on the right side. Blood liquid and dark amount of blood. Brain, meninges and hypophysis contained a large amount of blood.

Anatomical diagnosis: Bee injury on the right side of the neck; edema of the right tonsil, soft palate, uvula; all mucous membranes, especially the epiglottic folds congested; edema of the lungs; hyperemia of all organs of the neck, brain, spleen, liver and kidneys; hemorrhages of the gastric and duodenal mucous surfaces; slight sclerosis of the margins of the cardiac valves; colloidal and parenchymatous goiter; testicular hydrocele.

Microscopic findings on the place of injury showed a defect of the epidermis of 0.1 millimeter in diameter, which contained a brownish-yellow broken-off part of the sting. Below the surface of the skin, at about two millimeters depth, another small retrorse part of the sting was found, which had perforated the capillary vessels. Some red blood cells in the tissues.

Epidermis and papillae somewhat raised, with blood effusions. Several subcutaneous necrotic places encircled by abundant and diffuse bluish coloring. Slight edema of the cutis. Hyperemia in the proximity of the perforation, very marked. Capillaries and venules noticeably enlarged, and densely filled with blood. The erythrocytes well preserved, with normal hemoglobin content. Arterioles less dilated. In the necrotic zones, strong hyperemia and intravasal leukocytes, *a distinct inflammatory reaction.*

Judging from the clinical symptoms, autopsy and microscopical findings, it is beyond any doubt that the 40-year-old, powerfully built man died from a sting injury on the neck. The clinical symptoms were so severe that he died, 20 minutes after the injury had been inflicted, from asphyxia, accompanied by cyanosis, great protrusion of the eyes and marbled exanthema.

Austopsy plainly proved the cause of death; the excessive cyanosis, edema and hyperemia of the lungs and liquid state of the blood, clearly indicated asphyxia.

Chemical examination of the whiskey did not disclose any harmful elements. The extravasation of the red blood cells and neutrophil leukocytes showed the *decided hemorrhagic effects of the venom.* There was no sign of hemolysis. Macroscopically, the blood did not have any lacquerlike appearance and in all organs the red blood cells were properly colored and well preserved.

The jugular vein was microscopically examined; a slight canal had been formed by the sting but the vein had not been entered. Wegelin doubted whether, considering the thickness of the epidermis, this could ever happen, as the depth of the sting is usually between two and two and a half millimeters. He thought the sting could penetrate only a vein, for instance on the dorsal surface of the hand through a fine skin.

Whether there was a special hypersensitivity to bee venom in this case is hard to say. The autopsy findings could not disclose any unusual lack of resistance of the constitution toward the venom, the heart was normal, and most of the other organs, even microscopically, showed very little deviation from normalcy. Even the histological examination of all the endocrines and lymphatic system did not prove any abnormality.

During treatments of rheumatic, arthritic, neuralgic and gouty conditions with bee venom, very probably advanced pathological states are frequently present, and still patients tolerate the treatments fairly well. Of course, injectable bee venom is protein-free and does not possess the proteotoxic properties of the normal venom.

Wegelin, in his article, cited another fatal case communicated to him in 1929 by Dr. Kloss, of Lucerne. A 36-year-old blacksmith, while hiving a swarm, was attacked and stung by the bees. About a dozen stings were extracted from his arms, the nape of his neck, and around his ears. The victim walked home, complained of headache, became bluish-black, and collapsed. The physician who was called found him pulseless, breathing his last, without stridor. Death occurred 10 minutes from the time of injury. Autopsy revealed 25 sting injuries, some on the dorsal surfaces of the hands, forearms, etc. Other findings were: bilateral dilatation of the heart, hydrocele, scoliosis, pigeon-breast, *considerable hyperemia and hemorrhages*, perivascular lympho- and leukocytic infiltrations and occasional necrosis around the wounds. In some of the channels, fragments of the stings could be found.

CHAPTER REFERENCES

ABDERHALDEN, E. Allgemeine Technik u. Isolierung d. monoamidosäuren, Berlin, 1922.

BARTHOLOMEW, G. M. D. Bee Stings, Journal-Lancet, July, 1929.

BAYLEY DE CASTRO, A. The Effects of Bee Venom, Indian M. Gas., Calcutta, 62, 1927.

BEHRENS, D. Erkrankungen und Todesfälle durch Insectenstiche, Inaug. Diss. Würzb., 1920.

BEVEN, J. O. Acidosis Following Bee Stings, Lancet, Lond., II, 850, 1920.

BIBLIOTEQUE MÉDIC. Des accidents produits par la piqûre l'Hymenoptères, 66, 1819.

BOUCHACOURT, L. Sur la valeur thérapeutique du venin des abeilles, et sur l'apithérapie. La Méd. Internat. Illustr., Mai, 1934.

BROWN, G. Med. J. Australia, Sidney, Dec. 1931 (quoted by Cleland).

BUCHNER. Repetitorium für Pharmacie, 1857.

CAFFE. Schmidt's Jahrbücher, 12, 1852.

CATOLA. Crises vasomotrices céphalique et menièreformes par venin d'abeille, Rev. neurolog., Par., 35, 1928.

CLELAND, J. B. Insects in their relationship to injury and disease in man in Australia, Med. J. Australia, Sydney, Dec. 1931.

CONRADI, A. F. Osservationi di puncture di api sussequita da fenomen. extraordinari, Animal. Univers. di Medicina, 257, 1822.

EFFECTS PRODUCED BY BEE STING INJURIES

CORNIL, L. A propos d'un cas d'accidents toxiques graves consecutifs à une d'abeille et rapellant les phenomènes d'anaphylaxie, Bull. Soc. Pathol. comp. Mars, 1917.

D'ABREU, A. R. Effects of Bee Venom, Ind. M. Gaz., Calcutta, Nov. 1926.

DELPECH, A. Les dépots de ruches d'abeille existant sur differents points de la ville de Paris, Ann. d'Hyg., Par., III, Janvier, 1880.

DERRICK, E. A striking general reaction to a Bee Sting, Med. J. Australia, June, 1932.

DITTON, D. Bienenstichvergiftungen, Aerstl. Sachverst. Ztg., Berl., 22, 1930.

DOLD, H. Immunisierungsversuche gegen das Bienengift, Ztschr. f. Immunitatsforsch. u. exper. Therap., Jena, 26, 1917.

DOUGLAS, N. Birds and Beasts of the Greek Mythology.

DUPUYTREN, G. Leçons orales de clinique chirurgicale, 85, 1839.

FABRE, P. L'intoxication par les piqûre d'Hymenoptères, J. des Pract., 802, 1903.
Sur les phenomènes d'intoxication dus aux piqûres d'Hymenopt., Paris, 1906.

FRANCK, E. Bienenstich Vergiftung oder Herzleiden als Ursache plötzlich. Todes. Aerztl. Sachverst. Ztg., 18, 1930.

GAY, F. P. Tissue Resistance and Immunity. J. Am. M. Ass., Oct. 1931.

GEIGER, C. W., and ROTH, J. H. Bee Stings of the Uvula. J. Am. M. Ass., Aug. 1923.

GELPKE, L., und SCHLATTER, C. Unfallkunde, 82, 1917.

GOODMAN, N. M. Anaphylaxis from Bee Stings, Lancet, Lond., Sept. 24, 1932.

GOSS, E. L. A Bee Sting, Journal-Lancet, 46, 1926.

HANSEN, A. A. Fatal Bee Sting on Leg, Ugesk. f. Laeger Kjobenk, 83, 1921.

HELD, F. Beiträge zur medizinischer Bedeutung des Bienengiftes, Inaug. Diss. Würzb., 1922.

HERING, C. Condensed Materia Medica, Apis Mellifica, 1877.

HOWALD, S. Tod eines Bienenzüchters nicht infolge eines Bienenstiches, Schweiz. Bienen Ztg., 31, 1895.

HUNTER, W. A. Med. J. Australia, Sidney, Dec. 1931. (Quoted by Cleland.)

HUWALD, G. Klinisch-biologisch, Befunde bei Verletzung der Cornea durch Bienenstiche, Graefe's Arch. f. Ophthalmol., 50, 1904.

JONES, W. R. Bee Sting Treatment, Northwest Med., Seattle, 25, 1926.

LEGAL, G. Contribution a l'étude des Conditions des Gravité des Piqûres d'Hymenopt., Thèse Méd., 1922.

LEGIEHN, D. Eigenthümliche Wirkung eines Bienenstiches, Berl. klin. Wchnschr., 787, 1889.

MABARET DU BASTY, P. G. Des accidents produits par la piqûre des Hymenopt. port aigullon, Thèse de Par., 2875, 1875.

MEASE, D. Grave accidents produced by the sting of bees and other insects, Am. J. M. Sc., Phila., 1836.

NETOLITKY, F. Insekten als Heilmittel, Pharmazeut. Post, Wien, 1, 1916.

NIETLISPACH, W. Insektenstich und Unfall, Zürich.

NOTHNAGEL. Spec. Pathol. und Therapie, Bd. I, 1911.

PARISIUS, W., und HEIMBERGER, H. Acute Myelosen nach Bienenstichen, Deutsch. Arch. f. klin. Med., 143, 1924.

PERRIN, M., et CUÈNOT, A. A propos de 13 observations nouvelles d'hypersensibilité au venin d'abeilles, Rev. Méd. de l'Est, 60, 1932.

PHISALIX, M. Symptômes graves determines chez une femme jeune par la piqûre d'une seule abeille, Bull. du Mus. d'Hist. Nat., 7, 547, 1918.

SAJO, K. Örtliche Empfänglichkeit für Bienengift, II, Kosmos, Stuttg., 1914.

SCHMIDT. Jahrbücher der Medizin, 76, 1852.

SCHOLZ, W. Bienenstich in den weichen Gaumen, Deutsch. Med. Wchnschr., Berl u. Leipz., 51, 1926.

SPALIKOURSKY. Piqûres des abeilles. Rev. Scient., Par., 504, 1899.

STREBEL, J. Binnen und Wespenstichverletzungen des Auges, Klin. Monatsbl. f Augenh., 86, 657, 1931.

VAN HASSELT, L. Handbuch der Giftlehre, II.

VORMANN. Perforation des Augenliedknorpels mit Verletzungen des Augenapfe bindehaut durch einen Bienenstich, München. Med. Wchnschr., 71, 1924.

WEGELIN, C. Tod durch Bienenstich, Schweiz. Med. Wchnschr., 32, Aug. 12, 193.

WELLS, G. H. Chemical Pathology, 1925.

YOUNG, C. A. Bee Sting of the Cornea, Am. J. Ophth., 208, 1931.

Chapter VII Decreased and Increased Sensitivity

IMMUNITY

The study of the immunity of cells is a very broad subject which has an invaluable interest for us: in fact, our main object, the treatment of arthritis and rheumatism with bee venom, is founded on immunology-or, perhaps, just the reverse. If we give credit to the bee as the performer of the first hypodermic injection, we really ought to give her credit, also, as one of the originators of immunity. It is a long-established fact that beekeepers, stung repeatedly by bees, usually react less and less to their virus and finally do not react at all-they become immune. This ought to be the oldest, most common, illustrative example of immunity. The whole theory could have been developed from this principle.

The fundamental explanation of immunity has already been expressed by Metchnikoff: "The cells of the host are actively concerned in its defense against invading substances." It is a defensive act of Nature against chemical aggression-a struggle between the host and the invaders. While this process is taking place, a chemical and physical rearrangement, a new equilibrium, is created by the introduction of foreign elements into the organism. Fundamentally, it is a physicochemical reaction. As Wells says: "We attribute this altered re-activity to the presence of 'antibodies,' despite the fact that we have absolutely no knowledge of what these antibodies may be or even that they exist as material objects. We recognize them by what they do, without knowing just what they are."

I do not wish to enter into the details of this almost unlimited field, but certain facts and principles must be briefly discussed to make our main subject clear and intelligible.

Bee venom is not by any means a bacterial toxin but, as propounded before, the action and nature of animal venoms and microbial toxins are so intimately correlated that there is no sharp line of demarcation between them. Their characteristics are so analogous, often even homologous, that we are able to utilize the laws of immunity and serology which are supposed to be applicable to bacterial toxins. I treated the subject under the chapter of animal venoms and enumerated their mutual characteristics: both are destroyed by digestive ferments; heat, chemicals, antiseptics, and I oxidizing substances attenuate or destroy them; they are capable of being transmitted in vaccines; through habituation to their use they confer munity; the serum of vaccinated animals possesses immunizing properties; their sera confer passive immunity, and the immunity is passed on by heredity.

The laws and principles of immunity which are so well known and generally accepted will be of great assistance in the administration of bee venom treatments.

If an organism is systematically vaccinated with any special, properly attenuated venom, it becomes immunized. It will be endowed with antitoxic properties, and will be capable of counteracting the toxic effects of that venom. The venom, with its selective affinity, will try to form a close combination with certain tissue-cells, which the antitoxin will prevent. A very important point, taken again from serology, is *if the antitoxin is introduced late into the system the toxin has already formed a close union with the tissue-cells, and the antitoxin will be powerless to break up and destroy this combination.* The longer the time which has elapsed from the introduction of the toxin, the less effective the antitoxin will be, and it may prove even useless.

Another essential law of immunity is, it wears off, *as it is very seldom absolute.* It is an interesting phase of this retrogression that the longer the time required for acquisition of immunity, the more permanent it is; rapid immunization is quickly lost. We know that if beekeepers who have acquired immunity are not stung for a certain period they will find that it has partly or considerably diminished or has been entirely lost. Of course, this depends on the degree acquired and on the length of time which has elapsed. Beekeepers are aware of the fact that, while during the summer they acquire immunity, they will lose part of it in the winter and the next spring the stings will produce more severe reactions than at the end of the previous fall. The longer they continue their occupation, the more permanent the immunity will become and they will lose less of it each winter. In a certain number of years they will eventually become definitely immune. This condition, however, varies greatly in different individuals.

DECREASED AND INCREASED SENSITIVITY

Langer sent out a questionnaire to apiarists. He received from 126 beekeepers the following answers to his question about the period of time necessary to acquire a fairly permanent state of immunity:

71 beekeepers:	from	1 – 5 years	56%
19 " "	"	6 -10 years	15%
16 " "	"	10 – 20 years	13%
3 " "	"	10 -30 years	2%
17 " "	"	A longer period	14%

On the other hand, abnormal susceptibility was frequently observed. We must not forget that by immunity to bee stings we literally mean that a person loses his sensitivity toward the toxic effects of bee venom.

We refer to the chemical action and not to the mechanical sensation of having a barbed *Lancet* penetrate the skin, especially on a very sensitive of the body, for instance the lips, nose, eyelids, ears, although even these parts become more or less accustomed to it.

It is very peculiar that when the immunity of a person to bee venom wears off, he loses first, that is, more quickly, his general systemic, and only later his local skin immunity.

The length of time necessary to reach this relative state of immunity varies according to the individual. Darin mentioned in *La Gazette des Hôpi taux* that a man, out of curiosity, exposed himself daily to bee stings just to study their effects. On the twentieth day, he found that he had become immune. M. G. Walker gave his experiments in the *British Bee Journal*. He at first let himself be stung by one bee, increasing the number of stings, three, five, etc., and by the end of the week was receiving 18 stings. On the last day of the second week, 32 stings were inflicted. He noticed hardly any change in the reactions: the more stings he received, the less he felt their effects. Apparently, as already mentioned, a person not only grows immune to the chemical effect of the stings but also becomes accustomed to the mechanical injury.

DECREASED AND INCREASED SENSITIVITY

Flury questioned a large number of apiarists with regard to their immunity. He found:

Absolutely immune	10%
Relatively immune	66%
Acquired immunity	83%
Permanently sensitive	13%

On his questionnaire to 600 beekeepers, Langer, also, received 164 answers relative to sensitivity to bee stings:

Not sensitive from the beginning	11	7%
Sensitive from the beginning	153	93%
During their occupation, slightly sensitive	21	14%
Continued sensitivity	27	17%
Considerable decrease in sensitivity	91	60
No reaction at all (poison fast)	14	9%
(See chart derived from my questionnaire)		

According to the above statistics, 7 percent were not sensitive to bee stings from the start. It is now a question of whether we are dealing here with inherited immunity. According to the laws of immunity, it could be inherited by the children from an immune father, or rather, mother. It would be of enormous interest to substantiate this hypothesis. Possibly one day an apiarist mother will surprise us with an interesting revelation. They say that the snake charmers in India possess immunity to snake bites. Whether this is an inherent or acquired state is doubtful. Vaccinated animals not only gain protection for themselves but are also capable of giving successive sera of antitoxic power. Their sera have preventive and curative value. They can transmit this protective power through their blood to the fetuses and through the milk to their nurslings. Why would this not apply to human beings? Female rabbits are able to transmit immunity, if gestation takes place at the height of the immunization period, their young retaining it for several months; immunized male rabbits, on the other hand, are unable to transmit immunity to their offspring.

Absolute immunity in the human race is rather rare. Some animals, however, have a natural, absolute immunity to certain venoms, e.g., the immunity of the hog, hedgehog, mongoose, and some herons to snake venom. Their blood possesses antitoxic qualities. Whether this is acquired or is congenital is still disputed. It is possible that part of the immunity is acquired, as the young animals are not so resistant. H. E. Coffey, of Honolulu, Hawaii, wrote me that he thinks skunks are not affected by bee stings. He stated that in his former Texas home the skunks chewed his bees by the mouthfuls, and afterwards spat them out near the entrance of the hive. Professor Phillips thinks that skunks are bad pests of the apiary. "They visit the hive at night, the same hive night after night, scratch the front until the bees boil out and then eat them. The face and head of the skunk are covered with bees, and these are raked off with the claws and eaten. They must get thousands of stings."

Frogs and several kinds of birds eat bees and wasps with impunity. The tropical birds, merops apiaster and pernis apivorus, as their names imply, live on bees and wasps and feed them to their young. They are frequently overrun by swarms but are not afraid as they are never harmed. Their eyes are protected by stiff feathers. There is the possibility that these birds or their young ones are often stung in the mouth, on the tongue, and, although bee venom has a very violent effect on lymphatic tissues, they do not suffer any ill effects. There is nothing unusual in the fact that they eat bees without any harm, as the gastric ferments destroy the venom with great rapidity. Before we progress any further, let us divide immunity to bee venom into four classes, which will greatly facilitate future arguments:

1) Congenital or absolute immunity. Very rare in humans. Could be best explained by a theory that they are born of immune parents.

2) Active or acquired immunity (beekeepers).

3) Passive immunity through inoculation with the blood or serum of an immunized human or animal.

4) Pathological immunity (rheumatics).

We really ought to call acquired immunity artificial in contrast with the natural immunity which we know the body already possesses in various degrees. In cases where immunity wears off, sometimes it is due to the decrease of the natural body immunity (lessened resistance), and not so much to the impairment of the acquired immunity. Both contribute their share to the immune state. However, it is difficult to ascertain in what proportion, but it seems reasonable to assume that the natural body immunity contributes the larger share. Its decline is not always due to a lack of quantitative defensive capacity in the system but rather to the fact that the response of the body is not sufficiently prompt and rapid to form a defensive, neutralizing substance with qualities opposite to those of the toxin. Any antitoxin is supposed to have only an accelerating influence on the normal blood serum.

Frequently, we notice that beekeepers who have been stung many times without ill effects, suddenly react very violently to a single sting as the result of some unfavorable contributory circumstances, like run-down condition, convalescence, indigestion, heavy meal, etc.

The duration and degree of active immunity is much more lasting than that of the passive, which is relatively shorter. When passive immunity is created through the media of antitoxic sera (which are sometimes 500 to 1,000 times more powerful than the active venoms), the resulting state is incomparably more effective but not as permanent. This is a very essential point of vaccine therapy. When the system acquires active immunity through gradually increased doses of some venom, it may last for years and even for a lifetime. The fact that passive immunity is not so permanent may be due, also, to another serological law of the high specificity of antibodies, namely that when an alien serum, that is, serum from an animal of a different species (heterologous serum), is introduced into an organism it disappears more quickly than homologous serum.

In discussing the subject of immunity and anaphylaxy we are again confronted by two entirely opposite manifestations of the system. The same process, the introduction of a foreign substance into an organism, will produce in one person a state of tolerance, decreased sensitivity, or even a relative state of immunity, and in another person just the opposite, abnormal susceptibility. I almost hesitate to continue here the chain of reasoning by referring to the state of anti-anaphylaxy, which gives the impression of real immunity. What hidden forces will produce these entirely opposite and contrasting states constitutes a most complex question. In conducting our treatments with bee venom, we shall often confront this problem and it will present some difficulties.

There is another point to be solved which will give us plenty of food for thought. I previously mentioned pathological immunity. True rheumatics and arthritics seem to possess a high degree of resistance to bee venom. The degree of the apparent immunity of these subjects corresponds in direct ratio to the degree of the pathological conditions. The obstinacy of rheumatic and arthritic conditions in the response to these treatments depends mainly on their duration: the older and more resistant the pathological states, the more immune they appear to the venom. To treat and cure arthritics or rheumatics is supposed to mean that a higher immunization to the venom must be reached than the patients already seem to possess. To effect a cure is, to be exact, to establish a higher, sufficiently definite amount of immunity, or rather, an actual immunity.

DECREASED AND INCREASED SENSITIVITY

It seems rather remarkable and paradoxical that a rheumatic, because of a supposed pathological condition, shows very little or no reaction to bee venom and a cured case, which is assumed to be in a normal physiological state, is also immune. In a word, *the ill and the cured both show a similar negative reaction with an entirely heterogeneous character of the organism*. This is another very pertinent and essential question which will require careful attention during the execution of the treatments.

The writer has given this aspect of the subject special consideration. On first thought, there is almost a temptation to agree with Terc and to accept his conclusions unconditionally and without reservation. No doubt, there is an intimate relationship between bee venom and rheumatic and arthritic conditions. The inference seems plausible and logical, especially in view of the additional observation that the more advanced the ailment, the more expressed is the patient's apparent immunity to the venom. A correlation and also a certain parallelism are undeniable and beyond all dispute.

But if we are familiar with the reaction produced by bee venom in arthritis deformans and compare it with that produced in other rheumatoid conditions, we find an identical situation, namely, *both groups show a similar behavior, a diminished sensitivity toward the venom*. And yet, their respective etiologies are supposed to differ. (In spite of all the confusion which reigns over the whole field, the neurogenic origin of arthritis deformans is acknowledged, which excludes all toxic materies morbi, often suggested as the cause of arthritic and rheumatoid states.) Accordingly, if arthritis deformans and rheumatoid conditions behave and react in the same manner toward bee venom, even though their etiologies are different, the correlation between the two heterogeneous groups and the venom must be based on another, namely, a *non-toxic relationship*.

The best solution and explanation of this enigma, according to the writer's opinion, is: the absence of local reactive sensitivity toward bee venom in both rheumatoid conditions and arthritis deformans must be due to the same cause as their etiologies, namely, defective oxidation (which will be propounded later) and not to any toxic influences, as has heretofore been suspected. It seems as though the circulatory system lacks sufficient power to form a phagocytic local defensive reaction, which deficiency, at the same time, is the producing "causa morbi" of both groups. This lack of reactive response can be easily demonstrated by a simple experiment. If, after a fairly moderate constriction of the arm of a normal subject with a tourniquet, we form several wheals with bee venom, they will show a lack of reactivity, its degree absolutely depending on the amount of pressure applied. As soon as the pressure is lessened, the normal reactions will gradually and correspondingly develop. A parallel behavior, that is, a lack of reactivity toward bee venom, is found in rheumatoid conditions; here, however, it is contingent on their chronicity or degree. If we could express in units this lack of reactive response produced by pressure, we could almost compute in figures and determine, through parallelism, the state of the rheumatoid conditions; in other words, the amount of pressure causing this deficiency in a normal person ought to be equal to the degree of the pathological conditions in rheumatoid subjects.

Of course, we have to differentiate between local and general reactions. There is a possibility that even if we do not find any visible signs of sufficient local defensive power, which would normally signify that an act of toxic invasion had taken place, the venom might still have power to produce general effects. This heterogeneous or bipartite process would mean that Dr. Gay's contention (which we will soon discuss) that a local protection can be produced without a general one, might also be reversed; in brief, a generalized protection might take place without a local defense, or, at least, without any visible manifestations.

Now if we further analyze the situation: at the time when, during treatments, the first skin reaction appears, it seems that the defensive power has already been sufficiently restored through the beneficial effect of the venom so that it is able to form a reaction; conversely, when, following the postreactive phase, the organism once more does not react, only then is it literally in an immune state. In brief, the first immunity, which we called "pathological immunity" but might have called "pseudo-immunity," was due to a circulatory or oxygenic deficiency, which, at the same time, is the causative factor of rheumatoid conditions. The subsequent immunity which we secured during and as a consequence of our treatments is a true immunity, identical to that possessed by beekeepers.

We must not disregard the fact-because it will play an important part in bee venom therapy-that when we are injecting the venom into the skin for curative purposes double immunization is supposed to take place: local and general. The time of local mobilization of antibodies usually corresponds with the creation of general immunity. Reuben L. Kahn thought that the skin possesses about ten times greater power to produce immunity than the blood stream. The local defensive act is performed by the phagocytes, represented by the white blood cells: the general immunity is produced by the antitoxic power of the organic fluids, represented by the blood serum and lymph.

DECREASED AND INCREASED SENSITIVITY

Frederick P. Gay said his experiments convinced him that the locally superior mechanism for the disposal of infection can be produced without a generalized protection; for instance, the skin can be protected by skin immunization without increasing the resistance of the body as a whole. The phagocytes, in actively immunized animals, respond by specific rapid mobilization, possibly just an increased metabolism. Leukocytes of immune animals are not any different from those of nonimmunized ones, the difference is merely a superior response. The mode of action of certain protective sera of superimmune animals is supposedly due to their tropin content.

Finally, there is another question to be settled regarding passive immunity, which has an important scientific meaning; namely, that the characteristic pharmacologically active and physiologically effective chemical substance in bee venom is not an albumin body, respectively, not a toxalbumin. Can we produce an antitoxin against a substance which is not of albuminous nature?

Dold, in 1917, produced local immunity in the eye of a rabbit, but found no antibodies in the blood. He was unable to produce an experimental immunity to bee venom. Flury and Zanger, in 1928, made similar statements their attempt to produce a useful anti-bee venom serum was unsuccessful.

Muck, in the *Vienna Veterinary Monthly*, described the experiments of one of his pupils, Joseph Furch, who was anxious to find out whether bee venom was a real toxin and if it created an antitoxin, also whether it was possible to produce immunization with the antibodies of inoculated animals against the effects of the venom. He came to the conclusion that bee venom had no toxin nature; though it raises resistance, it cannot form antibodies. On the other hand, various other authors have found that rabbits, inoculated repeatedly with this venom, acquire immunity, and their sera have antitoxic and antihemolytic qualities.

As an illustration, for the purpose of comparing the immunizing effects of bee venom with those of snake venom, I would mention that Calmette, at the Pasteur Institute in Lille, prepared antivenomous sera which had both preventive and curative value in specific snake bites. A horse was inoculated with gradually increased doses of a certain snake venom, until in several months the animal subsequently yielded a vaccinal serum. This same serum has been proved to possess a very effective curative power in severe cases of bee venom intoxication, as many experiments in France have demonstrated, another proof of the chemical and physiological analogy of the two venoms.

DECREASED AND INCREASED SENSITIVITY

Why could not a horse be intensely immunized with bee venom and its serum used:

To confer immunity to bee venom?
As a curative, in severe bee venom intoxication?
As a preventive of arthritis and rheumatism?
As a curative for both?
Another fertile field for the serologist!

F. Thompson told us K. S. Thompson had shown that a precipitin reaction is obtained with a serum of those who were stung and the sting of the bee. F. Thompson received this information through unpublished communication of material demonstrated to the English Biochemical Society in 1930 by K. S. Thompson. The report follows:

"He triturated the poison sacs and glands in normal saline at a strength of ten stings per c.c., filtered through a Seitz filter into sterile flasks and refrigerated. During the process a heavy sickly odour was emitted, which caused severe frontal headache. The pH of this saline solution of bee venom was 4.2, but this was buffered to neutral by an equal volume of human serum. This saline solution, when added to a suspension of washed red cells and incubated at 65° C. (one drop of saline solution to 50 drops of suspension), caused hemolysis in 3 to 10 minutes. Similarly subcutaneous injection of the extract into the human leg caused ecchymosis in 24 hours.

"Sting extract prepared as above, extract prepared by Langer's method, extract of bee body prepared as above, the original extract boiled and filtered, original extract treated with alcohol and filtered, and the above extract fully saturated with ammonium sulphate and filtered, and Kretschy's 'Immenin bee venom,' were then tried against normal serum and sera of bee keepers who had been stung. Positive flocculation occurred in the tubes containing the saline sting solution and the sera of bee keepers.

"One drop of saline sting extract with 10 drops of a 1 in 60 saline dilution of serum to be tested, refrigerated overnight, and incubated at 65° C. caused flocculation after about 12 minutes. After injection of this extract in repeated doses into a person who previously gave a negative reaction, a positive flocculation occurred after 12 days, but not of the same degree as the bee keepers' serum tested. The bee keepers' blood was negative to the Wassermann reaction.

"The above experiments explain the facts well known among old bee keepers, that they slowly become practically immune against ill-effects from bee-stings, even in large quantities, being only slightly affected at the

115

commencement of the 'bee season' after they have been without stings for over six months."

The experience of H. Baudisch, often quoted in German medical literature, has a rather interesting immunological aspect. On June 27, 1906, a very hot day, the doctor was called to visit an eighteen-month-old girl, who had been overrun by bees near the hives. The child had been stung by about 200 bees. The doctor himself removed and counted about 150 stings. The child vomited, had diarrhea, pulse was 140, restless, with profuse perspiration. He ordered Goulard solution externally and a milk diet. Considering the child's age and the large number of sting injuries, the recovery was surprisingly favorable, almost uneventful. It was explained that the child had been very weak until she reached her tenth month, but was well after that age, because from that time on she ate unusually large quantities of honey. The doctor was convinced that the venom which the honey contained made her immune to the stings, which otherwise would have proved fatal.

The conception of anaphylaxy, in opposition to prophylaxy, is a hypersensitivity to the toxic effects of certain proteins, induced by a previous sensitization with the same or similar substance. Any part of the organism may be subjected to these anaphylactic changes: skin, gastro-intestinal canal, respiratory tract, and cardiac, or circulatory system. To-day we are able to solve and explain many puzzling questions, especially with regard to so-called idiosyncrasy. The theory is one of the most valuable and significant achievements of medical science and we have no conception of what we may yet "unriddle" with the aid of its cognizance. A thorough discussion of anaphylaxy is far beyond the scope of this work but I must mention several facts as they have very intimate connection in clearing up many points of bee venom therapy.

It is an established and fundamental biological law that foreign proteins, introduced into an organism in any other way (parenterally) than through the digestive tract (perorally), will create remarkable physiological changes. Many experiments have shown that certain protein substances, injected into an animal for the first time, will not provoke any reaction, but on the second injection-even in much smaller doses-may cause a violent one, with the possibility that the animal may succumb. While after the first (sensitizing) injection there were no visible symptoms, some profound, temporarily concealed, changes took place in the organism which evidenced themselves after the second (intoxicating) administration of the same or similar substance. The altered conditions transformed the at first perfectly harmless substance-on the second injection-into a virulent poison. The reaction to the next injection, on the other hand, may again be perfectly normal. (The law of strict specificity is a characteristic trait in all these experiments. The specificity is mainly dependent on the difference of proteins.)

A certain time must elapse (usually ten days or more) during which these functional changes take place in the organism, to develop a condition of sensitiveness. In animal experiments, this sensitivity develops gradually, reaches a maximum, diminishes again, or remains constant. G. H. Wells said: "It is a startling fact that a guinea pig, which can tolerate many cubic centimeters of such protein mixtures as horse serum in a single dose, will be almost immediately killed by as little as 0.01 c.c. of this same serum, provided a similar or even much smaller amount has been injected into it ten days or more previously. The character of the death with violent convulsions, perhaps within a minute of the time the injection is made, makes this observation all the more dramatic. I have succeeded in sensitizing guinea pigs with a single dose of crystallized egg albumin as small as one twenty-millionth of a gram. Large doses are less effective in sensitizing guinea pigs than small, e.g., one milligram of most proteins will usually be much more effective than 100 milligrams."

According to Vaughan's hypothesis, upon the first introduction of a foreign protein into the tissues, proteolytic ferments are produced (proteo and liberate by cleavage the toxic component of the protein. The freed toxic lytic zymogens), which, on reinjection of the same substance, will split up component, with rapid quantitative action, will produce the symptoms of anaphylaxy. The absence of the specific proteolytic ferments made the first injection harmless; on the second injection, the presence of the activating proteolytic zymogens produced by the previous injection, resulted in the intense reaction. At the first injection, we dealt with a nonsensitized subject; on the second occasion with a sensitized one. It is a case of protein disintegration produced by proteolytic enzymes. If the cleavage process is too drastic, it will destroy the poison entirely. The character of the changes which produce an anaphylactic reaction still have to be explained.

The mechanism of anaphylaxy is an act of protein splitting, a production of toxic substances through ferment changes, a reaction between specific antibodies of the cells and the invading antigens. The biochemical protein cleavage can be best explained by physical changes.

Richet called the substance "toxigen"-and the combination of toxigen plus antigen equals apotoxin (also called precipitin or anaphylotoxin).

DECREASED AND INCREASED SENSITIVITY

The intensity of the anaphylactic reaction or shock is proportionate, according to Scott, to the content of precipitin in the serum, this substance being consumed by the shock. We find the same antibodies in anaphylaxy as in immunity.

This sensitized state, this altered function, becomes such an inherent quality of the organism that it can be transmitted by inoculation from one subject to another. Blood serum from a sensitized animal, injected into a normal one, will transfer the sensitized state and the proteolytic zymogens (passive anaphylaxy). The antibodies are introduced through this act of transference.

Richet and Arthus were the first to prove that originally harmless proteins repeatedly injected into the same animal may produce grave toxic symptoms, even death. The animal is in a sensitized state, and the functional system is entirely changed. This sensitivity can be transmitted not only by injections but through feeding, instillation in the eye, inunction, and even inhalation. Sensitized guinea pigs will transmit this state to their young ones. If we now compare anaphylaxy with immunity, we find that:

Anaphylaxy is increased sensitivity-decreased resistance.
Immunity is decreased sensitivity-increased resistance.
Both qualities are transmittable through vaccination.

Proteins can be of vegetable or animal origin, even in the most minute quantities. The method of introducing the invading substance into the recipient host varies considerably. Intradermal or subcutaneous injections are not nearly so powerful and rapid as intravenous or intraspinal administrations.

If a sensitized animal recovers from nonfatal anaphylactic, reactive symptoms, it will be resistant (refractory) to the further introduction of the same protein. It would seem as though the substances which caused the sensitivity had lost their power. This condition is called anti-anaphylaxy. The anaphylactic state may return later, possibly as the result of the formation of new proteolytic substances. The more rapid the method used to produce an anaphylactic state, correspondingly rapid will be the development of anti-anaphylaxy. If we produce anti-anaphylaxy in a subject, we really perform an act of immunization. Sometimes varied substances, entirely different chemically, will produce similar, even identical, anaphylactic reactions, which we call "anaphylactoid" states.

Anti-anaphylaxy is explained by Vaughan as a quantitative disproportion between a small amount of specific proteolytic zymogens and foreign proteins-the anaphylactic reaction uses up most of the available ferments and the rest cannot exert any effect.

Frequently the general effects produced by bee stings are not only markedly similar to the symptoms of an anaphylactic shock, but are almost identical. If we do not know the producing causes of a certain syndrome (which occasionally we do not), we cannot even differentiate between the two. The symptoms are usually very violent, with hardly any local reaction. The introduction of a foreign substance into an extremely susceptible organism, even in small doses, may produce a very grave crisis.

The duration of the effects of anaphylaxy from a clinical viewpoint are very much like those of alkaloidal poisons; they gradually wear off. They are mainly directed toward the smooth muscles, like those of respiration, simultaneously attempting to paralyze the vasomotor endings of the blood vessels. Cardiac syncope and cutaneous irritations in human beings are very characteristic.

The whole mechanism of an anaphylactic shock sometimes almost suggests that there is a mobilization, through a defensive reflex action, of the whole available blood supply of the organism, an act of defensive transposition in an effort to counteract and combat the deleterious or destructive effects of the invading foreign toxic substances, producing thereby a corresponding vicarious ischemia and anoxemia in the cerebral and cardiac centers, with all the characteristics of a violent reactive function.

Cerebral anemia especially will produce important respiratory changes and will also greatly influence blood pressure. There is a distinct correlation and parallelism between the two. The respiratory center is most sensitive and responsive to temporary cerebral hypotension, and the same can be said of the vasomotor center, possibly on account of the harmful and noxious chemical effect of the accumulated lactic acid and CO_2.

If we try to apply the laws of anaphylaxy to bee stings, we are certainly years considered themselves immune, and were stung by numerous bees in a single day without exhibiting any reaction, sometimes, if stung by one bee, become gravely ill. How can we give an adequate explanation for such a sudden loss of immunity? One of the explanations we could offer is that such people have only a "skin immunity" and when the venom is injected into the veins and does not pass through the skin, they react very violently. This comment seems rather fantastic but still we have to give it consideration. Another explanation would be that some other temporary constitutional derangement aggravates, perhaps through negative instrumentality, the action of the venom. We note repeatedly that a veteran beekeeper's reactions are very severe after one sting, but when stung a couple of days later, he is again in the usual nonreactive state. I noticed numerous cases where the reactions were very severe after a meal, especially after a *hearty meal.*

Can it be that in such instances the power of the organism, which is supposed to be utilized for defensive purposes, is *preoccupied*, otherwise engaged, so that it is *incapable of combating an unexpected simultaneous invasion*-just an inferior response, an interfered or retarded mobilization - and the antigens and antibodies are unable to unite? Is it possible that the complement content of the blood is diminished or claimed by some priority unknown to us? *Or did the food intake constrain the oxidizing capacity of the blood?* No doubt "the emergency apparatus for parenteral digestion and consequent assimilation" is disturbed, temporarily-an untoward incident in protein digestion. Or is it a combination of other toxic proteins or the formation of some cryptotoxic body poisons? It is difficult to imagine that immunity, increased resistance, should turn into anaphylaxy, a state of hypersensitivity, *en passant.*

In severe borderline cases, it is rather difficult to decide whether the confused functional phenomena are attributable to anaphylaxy, idiosyncrasy, or to a general lowered resistance of the organism because of some other physiological or pathological state. The writer observed that in a case of typical anaphylactic sensitivity the symptoms were much more violent and disappeared more quickly than when they were the direct consequences of, or were aggravated by, other conditions. This suggestion is often helpful in the differentiation. The causes are frequently obscure, but anaphylactic phenomena and the symptoms of bee-venom intoxication are certainly very similar.

I quote some characteristic and illustrative cases. Aubry published a very interesting one:

In August, 1922, Madame B. sent for him to call immediately as the physical condition of one of the servants gave her great anxiety. When the doctor arrived at his destination, which was six miles away, he found the patient in a very desperate condition. The servant was a woman, 30 years old. He learned from the history supplied by the household that the patient had enjoyed habitual good health. She had gone to bed perfectly well but in the morning they found her prostrate, with hardly any sign of life.

Prolonged examination was out of the question. The patient was unconscious, regained consciousness only from time to time and complained of great weakness. The extremities were cold, the face cyanotic and edematous, the lips swollen and blue, with a hardly perceptible pulse. There was cold perspiration all over the body and respiratory anxiety. She was not a very reassuring sight. Heart beats were arhythmic and rapid. With all these alarming symptoms, the diagnosis was very difficult. Her surroundings did not suggest any explanation and examination of the various organs revealed nothing positive. Was it a cardiac, uremic, or a general toxic state?

Aubry remembered a bee sting injury with similar symptoms and later questioned the patient, who gave an affirmative answer. During the night it became very hot. She opened a window and in the morning when she got up to close it, while doing so felt a sting under her right knee. It all seemed to her so insignificant that she never considered it even worth while to mention. The right leg showed some edema, was thicker than the left and slightly painful on pressure. The place of the sting did not even show. The only diagnosis Aubry could make was venomization by a bee. After the usual symptomatic treatments, by the next day the patient had recovered completely.

This case, in view of the rapidity with which the small amount of venom caused such critical symptoms and the severity of the general reactions compared to the slight local reaction, is worthy of notice.

There are many similar cases reported in medical literature which can be explained only as intravenous inoculations, extreme idiosyncrasy or anaphylaxy. The paucity of local reactions and the rapid progress and intensity of the general symptoms often suggest an intravenous inoculation. In the case of anaphylaxy, the symptoms usually intimate that a colloidal substance of anaphylactizing effect was previously introduced, and, after the organism was sensitized, produced an anaphylactic shock.

Germain Legal, of France, reported several interesting cases:

A woman of 43 had, since her 18th year, worked in a sugar refinery. The last ten years she suffered from frequent migraine. There were occasional alimentary disorders and intense generalized urticarial eruptions. Examination revealed nothing else extraordinary. Her heart was normal, urine clear with no albumin. There was a slight enlargement of the liver. She often suffered from diarrhea and there was an acne rosacea on her face. While engaged in her work of packing sugar, she was stung very often by bees on her face, arms, and hands. Her symptoms were similar to those of her comrades: slight swelling, pain, and the usual consequences of a normal sting.

In July, 1919, the patient was stung on the external surface of the lower arm by a single bee. She applied the usual treatment, extracted the sting and put on a drop of tincture of iodine. In half an hour, she was seized with violent epigastric pain, disturbed respiration and spasmodic cough. Her face, especially the conjunctiva, was congested. She fell to the ground unconscious with convulsive movements. Consciousness returned rapidly. The face was edematous, the extremities cold, and there supervened bilious vomiting, intense anguish and dyspnea. The patient was soon able to sit up. The worst of the crisis passed. Her dyspnea attenuated, so did the anguish. The place of the sting was hardly noticeable except for the iodine. All symptoms gradually disappeared. Patient at first thought she had some epileptiform attack, never even thought of the sting. An hour later she had extremely profuse diarrhea; after that, just a little asthenia which lasted until the next morning. The year 1919 passed without any further accident worth mentioning.

In June, 1920, she suffered another sting injury on her left hand, immediately followed by an exact repetition of the identical symptoms described previously. In July, 1920, another sting, with a similar syndrome.

In August, 1922, she was stung on the anterior surface of the neck. This time there was a slight variation of her symptoms. Edema of the face was very intense, persisted for several days. Generalized bullous eruption appeared soon after the sting, accompanied by violent pruritus which disappeared several days later. The asthenia was more intense and obstinate. Legal thought the symptoms were suggestive of anaphylactic phenomena. The treatment consisted of desensitization not only for bee venom but for all other albuminoid substances. It seemed to him most practicable to choose for the purpose a colloidal substance, like the serum of the subject. By intravenous puncture, he aspirated from the median vein at the elbow of the patient some blood and reinjected it intramuscularly. Sulphate of soda was administered for several days for her liver. Two more autohematotherapeutic injections per week, was the established treatment. Six weeks later the patient felt better, her digestion improved, and she lost her migraine. She left her place of employment and Legal lost track of her. Legal's observations convinced him that the symptoms were attributable to previous sensitization. (Writer would suggest that the poor physical state of the patient greatly contributed to the symptoms.)

DECREASED AND INCREASED SENSITIVITY

Another case, reported by Legal, follows:

A young man of 19, and healthy, was stung on the left knee by a single bee. The pain let up gradually but the knee was very swollen. Five minutes later he developed respiratory anguish and extremely violent urticaria. The swelling even on his face was so pronounced that he could not open his eyes voluntarily. The conjunctivae were red and congested. Then there were profuse perspiration and intense general pruritus. The general symptoms rapidly regressed; only slight vertigo and headache continued. Next day he was normal.

Hugh Mackay, of Winnipeg, reported a typical case:

Mr. H. E. W., 41, a farmer, was stung in the tibial region of the right leg by a bee. The following morning, there was a generalized urticaria; the eruption was very red and itchy. Under antiphlogistic treatment, the eruption gradually disappeared but the whole right leg was painful and swollen to twice its natural size. Two days later, bullae developed, the axillary and inguinal glands became very much enlarged and tender. Fresh bullae continued to appear on different parts of the body. The temperature was 102° F. and pulse, 120. There were occasional chills and the patient was acutely ill.

Twelve days later he was stung again on the index finger of the left hand. Mackay first saw the patient in the hospital in a pitiful state; bullae on different parts of the body and a generalized exfoliating dermatitis. The skin was thrown off in huge sheets. A colloidal bath gave him some relief. Internally he was given bicarbonate of soda. He gradually improved and left the hospital five days later. The patient had been stung several times in previous years without any unusual cutaneous reaction. The diagnosis was acidosis, or the introduction of a toxic protein constituent producing anaphylaxy.

A. T. Waterhouse, of Oxford, England, published the following case:

A man of 53, had severe typhoid about 30 years previous. When taking strong aperients he was subject to fainting spells, but otherwise, enjoyed good health. He had been a beekeeper for many years and was stung often but without any other evidence except the usual local inflammation. In the month of June, while taking in a swarm, he was stung by about half a dozen bees, but was none the worse for his experience.

123

DECREASED AND INCREASED SENSITIVITY

In August, he was stung on his hand by two bees. He immediately felt constriction of the throat and intense throbbing of his head. The face was flushed, eyes congested, lips swollen; there was a distinct numbness and tingling of both hands and difficulty in breathing. Half an hour later, he lost consciousness; his breathing became stertorous and his pulse, feeble-in fact, for a few seconds, he was absolutely pulseless. He recovered consciousness in several minutes and had another milder attack in ten minutes. In 12 hours he was convalescent.

In September he was stung by a single bee on the upper margin of his right ear. Remembering his former experience, he rushed to the nearest pharmacy, feeling already a constriction of the throat and difficulty in breathing. At the chemist's he collapsed on the floor. Waterhouse saw him 10 minutes later. He was semiconscious with a sighing respiration. The right side of his face was congested and swollen, and his extremities were cold, pale, clammy and sweating profusely. Pulse could not be felt at the wrist and heart sounds were very feeble. The sting was extracted, and ammonia applied to the ear. Waterhouse administered some sal volatile by mouth and strychnine hypodermically. In a quarter of an hour the patient recovered consciousness and was removed to his home. He was listless for a couple of days, but later made a good recovery.

Waterhouse noticed nothing unusual about this case; what he considered very remarkable was the resemblance of the patient's serious symptoms to those of a typical anaphylactic shock. In a person who had been stung many times before without ill effect, the sudden onset of such grave symptoms from a minute quantity of irritant poison could be explained only by assuming that his extraordinary increase in sensitivity was due to the fact that he had been sensitized by former stings, which, at the time, appeared innocuous.

Perrin and Cuènot contributed more cases of bee sting injuries to medical literature (13 in all) than any other author. The case reports are, in general, very scattered. We usually find a single case, once in a great while two, and only rarely three or more cases reported by the same writer.

The following cases reported by Perrin and Cuènot have all the characteristics of anaphylaxy, suggesting also idiosyncrasy:

Mrs. J., 58, always showed remarkable hypersensitiveness toward bee stings. When she was 20 years old, she was stung on her little finger. She fell unconscious and was found in that state. Her face was congested; eyes, bloodshot. There were wide urticaria, profuse vomiting, diarrhea and

124

rapid pulse. Notwithstanding all precautions on account of her distinct horror of bees, she was stung repeatedly with similar grave symptoms.

A man, 44, suffered one sting on the eyelid. He was immediately seized with dyspnea, thoracic constriction and violent chills. Five minutes later he developed temporary blindness, and later, nausea, vomiting, general pruritus and urticaria. In two hours, his sight was gradually restored. In 24 hours, all symptoms disappeared.

Mrs. H., 40, was stung by one bee on her arm. In several minutes she experienced violent headache, thoracic anguish, congestion in the head and eyes; and cried violently. General urticaria and marked edema, even on the lower extremities, appeared. In about four or five hours, all symptoms disappeared. Seven months later, she was stung again, resulting in identical symptoms but the reaction in the head and eyes was even more marked.

A. L. Gregg reported a case in The *Lancet* of March, 1932. He described the experience of a medical friend of his, which is worth recording:

Dr. X had been interested in bee-keeping for the previous two years. In August, 1930, while working on his bees, though well protected with veil, gloves, etc., possibly through inexperience or poor judgment he aroused the frenzy of the insects, and was stung by approximately 20 of them. This was followed by considerable local and general reactions. He had to go to bed with headache, diarrhea, and the usual disfigurement.

He was comparatively unmolested until June, 1931, when stung by three angry bees on the chin and forearm. The stings were very painful. In ten minutes, he suffered from cramping pain over the precordial region, and felt generally sick. His surroundings-including the hive-appeared to revolve round and round in a kaleidoscopic confusion. He was conscious enough to stagger four yards from the hive, where he collapsed and remained so for some time. The attack was followed by vomiting, diarrhea, headache, and raised temperature for 12 hours. The local swelling was severe and remained for three days.

Dr. X regarded the experience as sensitization from the previous year, and was convinced that if he had fallen nearer the hive and had received more stings, it would have been disastrous.

In the July 21, 1934, issue of *The Lancet*, A. E. Mahood, of Norwich, reported several cases typical of anaphylaxy. Two sisters, instead of acquiring immunity to the venom, became highly sensitized. The younger, aged 27, who had charge of the bees at first, was often stung, but had only slight local irritation. Toward the end of the second season she had violent attacks after being stung by bees. About 15 minutes after the sting, intense urticaria started all over the body, accompanied by a feeling of serious illness, fainting, and collapse. A doctor, who was called on the second occasion, advised her to keep away from bees. Then the other sister took charge of the apiary and, apart from trivial local irritation, bee stings had no unpleasant effect on her during the first two years. About mid-season of the third year (1932), a very serious attack occurred, said to be due either to food poisoning, to a bee sting, or to both combined. She avoided the bees for the rest of the season and during 1933. She took charge of them again in 1934, had one sting in April on the leg with only slight local reaction. On May 30th several stings (two on the left hand and one on the left leg) were followed within 20 minutes by intense urticaria from head to foot. Irritation began on the scalp and spread rapidly, accompanied by a "terrible cough," much cardiac and mental distress. General condition became worse. She took two tablets of calcium sodium lactate, powdered in water, but she did not improve. After an ounce of milk of magnesia was given, marked relief was noticeable. The intolerable itching, also the cardiac and mental distress, improved. Several hours later she was quite comfortable and slept well. Mahood thought milk of magnesia is worth a further trial.

The following experience of a hardened bee keeper, described by Edwardes, is rather similar. I quote him in full:

"A little stinging is nothing; but there is no doubt that, with anything over a dozen stings or so at a time, the most hardened and experienced bee-man may easily stand, for a minute or two at least, in danger of losing his life.

"So it happened to me once. I had gone to look at a neighbor's stocks. The bees were as quiet as lambs until I came to the seventh hive; and then, with hardly a note of warning, they set upon me like a pack of flying bull-dogs. It is long enough ago now, but I can still give a pretty accurate account of the symptoms of acute formic acid poisoning.[5] It began with a curious pricking and burning over the entire inner surface of the mouth and throat. This rapidly spread, until my whole body seemed on fire, and the target, as it were, for millions of red-hot darts. Then first my tongue and lips, and every other part of head and neck, in quick succession, began to swell.

Bee venom does not contain formic acide Author

My eyes felt as though they were being driven out of my head. My breathing machinery seized up, and all but stopped. A giddy congestion of brain followed. Finally, sight and hearing failed, and then almost unconsciousness.

"I can just remember crawling away, and thrusting head and shoulders deep into a thick lilac bush, where the bees ceased to molest me. But it was a good hour or more before I could hold the smoker straight again, and get on with the next stock."

IDIOSYNCRASY

Idiosyncrasy, in medical language, means a peculiar, greatly increased reaction exhibited by individuals toward certain mental and physical (or better, physiological) agencies. Mental idiosyncrasy often manifests itself as a reflective response to certain stimuli transmitted more by psychic than by corporeal or material means. The channel of contact is our senses, often are extremely hard to explain. I can understand people fainting from the only visual or acoustic, not necessitating a material contact. Such occurrences sight of blood-we can justly ascribe it to a subconscious, rather justifiable fear-but what if someone swoons every time at the sight of a beet root? Many ailurophobes (cat fearers) become nauseous and faint if they enter a room where a little kitten is hidden. People of this type will detect the presence of a cat in a room without seeing or hearing it. Their only other sense is that of smell... but cats have no odor perceptible to the normal human being. Is it a supersensitivity of their olfactory senses of magnetic influence? The late S. Weir Mitchell related the case of his uncle, an ailurophobe, who was expected to visit his father (Mitchell's). Before his arrival they had hidden a small kitten, with a saucer of cream, in a closet. The uncle was taken into this room on the pretense of being shown some interesting books which he had been particularly anxious to see. He sat down, in great anticipation, to inspect the books; suddenly grew pale, started to shiver, and said, "There is a cat in this room." They tried to convince him that he was in error, but he became so nauseated that he had to leave the room, when he quickly recovered.

Mitchell was so much interested in ailurophobia that he sent circulars all over the world in the hope of obtaining some useful information which would help him to solve this puzzling question. He received 159 answers.

A physician reported a case to Mitchell, that of a secretary of a scientific society, who, while reading a report during a meeting, suddenly stopped and said, "I cannot go on-there must be a cat in the room." After a search, the cat was found under the topmost seat of the amphitheatre. (The number of these cat fearers is "legion": Napoleon, Oliver Goldsmith, Buffon, Noah Webster, Meyerbeer, Alphonse Daudet, Hilaire Belloc, and many others.) Rolleston, as proof that this idiosyncrasy has a physiological basis, mentioned two patients with antipathy for cats, who also exhibited a great skin sensitivity to cat extract. After they had been desensitized with minute doses of a special extract from cats, their antipathy disappeared.

Then there are people who feel a sense of horror and faint even from the odor of roses or apples. Many other similes could be mentioned. These are accentuated reflex actions of the spinal centers.

From the viewpoint of a neurologist, I mention here a certain fear of bees, amounting almost to an obsession, called *apiphobia*. (Roch favors another term, for linguistic reasons: *melissophobia*.) A reasonable or unreasonable fear or dread, a morbid dislike of any animal or insect which might injure you, is only natural. The number of those who fear bees is but insignificant compared with the many millions of stanch melissophiles. If we carefully consider the anaphylactoid phenomena, it is very hard, almost impossible, to distinguish between idiosyncrasy and anaphylaxy. No dividing line can be drawn between the two manifestations. There is not a single case which could not be explained by either of the two. In the event that we might provoke a debate, no matter which side our opponent chooses to defend, we should not have the least trouble, taking the opposite view, in overthrowing his arguments with convincing, well-supported, and reasonable counter arguments.

It is rather difficult in some instances to explain a visual or acoustic phenomenon as anaphylaxy, which is the only occasion when we are compelled to use the word idiosyncrasy. When it comes to material contact, which also includes the olfactory senses, we cannot differentiate between the two. Idiosyncrasies can be divided into three classes:

1) Idiopathic
2) Acquired;
3) Hereditary.

Certain passages in this section about idiosyncrasy may have appeared to be outside of our subject, but still they will be serviceable in explaining some peculiar symptoms which manifest themselves as effects of bee stings as well as in the therapy with bee venom.

I quote some cases which are rather typical of idiosyncrasy: L. J. B. Braun, of South Africa, reported as follows:

DECREASED AND INCREASED SENSITIVITY

A woman of 32 lived in a district where there were many bees. She was stung several times and each experience was more frightful and terrifying than the previous one. She was firmly convinced that the next experience would be fatal. She consulted Braun a week after her latest experience and was still entirely exhausted and terrified. She had been stung seven times in the preceding nine years and each time by a single bee. A minute after the sting a hot flush spread all over her body, her face became suffused; she experienced a choking sensation, and great irritation to cough. Her neck and face began to swell. In the abdomen, intense bearing-down sensation, like labor pains, developed. The tips of her fingers and toes were of a deep blue color, and there were urticarial wheals, and general swelling all over the body, starting from the site of the injury. Her mental anxiety was great; she felt that she would choke at any minute. There was violent trembling, and the patient soon fell into a coma and remained in that state usually for three or four days. This state wore off only gradually. Braun was later successful in desensitizing the patient with gradually increasing doses of bee venom solution, which he prepared and standardized.

Zangolini, in the *Gazette Médicale de Paris*, reported an interesting case:

A young man of 36, of very athletic build, was stung by about three or four bees on the dorsal surface of the right hand. In an instant, his eyesight became obscured; he lost all his powers; the whole body was bathed in profuse perspiration; his face was extremely blue; and he complained of intense headache, oppression and feeling of great anxiety. He was carried to his bed; had a very high temperature; his body was covered with blisters. An hour later, all symptoms disappeared. (Apparently a case of idosyncrasy or anaphylaxy.)

F. W. Fitzsimons received the following letter from a lady who was stung by a bee. It is a typical example of extreme idiosyncrasy.

"I live in a place where bees are plentiful. I have been stung several times and each time the sting affects me worse. Recently a bee stung me on the thumb through my glove and five minutes afterwards my whole body, from head to feet, was covered with a rash and I was swollen all over and felt dreadfully ill. The soles of my feet pained me very much, and I could neither walk nor sit up. I felt faint and everything turned black in front of my eyes and I had terrible pain in the abdomen and was shaking so much that I could not hold a glass, much like a bad attack of ague. This lasted about three hours, the swelling gradually getting worse. After that the pains got better and I became able to see clearly, but then breathing became difficult and I felt as if I was going to choke and that my throat and chest were closing. During breathing, there was a funny noise in my chest. This lasted for about three hours. I always have a very bad cold after these attacks. It is now four days since being stung, and I do not feel myself yet."

Gilbert Brown, of Australia, also reported a typical case of extreme sensitivity to bee stings:

A male patient had been stung by bees four times in the previous 12 years. Immediately after only one bee sting, he experienced nausea, faintness, cold extremities, collapse and complete unconsciousness. His color was whitish-gray; his body, cold and moist; pulse and heartbeat, feeble; respiration, shallow. There was always very little local reaction, a small wheal, at the time of injury, and also later. Patient usually responded to stimulants and recovered in several days.

P. Carton's observation is worth mentioning on account of its broad symptomatology.

A young woman was stung by one bee on the external margin of the palm of the hand. She had lancinating pains, throbbing, and intense burning in the whole arm. A sensation of anguish and faintness obtained. Constriction of the throat developed. Five minutes later, there ensued extensive urticaria; mouth and nasal mucosa became swollen and painful; severe cough developed. Face became distinctly blue; the eyes, congested. Vomiting, burning of the esophagus and stomach, painful breasts, suffocating, constriction of the chest, and difficult respiration were reported. Pulse could not be counted. Patient recovered two hours later, after stimulants had been administered.

Perrin and Cuènot suggested that persons with idiosyncrasy or extreme hypersensitivity to bee venom should be desensitized with a dilute solution of bee venom, injected in gradually increasing doses.

While we are discussing the subject of idiosyncrasy, I wish to mention a rather curious observation which has immunological as well as neurological interest. G. H. Stover, of Denver, Colorado, in the Johns Hopkins Hospital.

Bulletin, reported:

"A woman, thirty-five years old, single, consulted me for a rather unusual swelling on her right cheek, following a bee-sting injury received several days before. Her face was considerably swollen and she felt some unpleasant constitutional symptoms. Five days later, she had fully recovered, when she made the very interesting statement that she never before had been able to eat honey, even the smell of it nauseated her, but after she was stung, developed a craving for it and ate it with complete satisfaction." Stover finished his report: "Will some of the immunization experimenters throw a light on this occurrence?"

ALLERGY

Allergy, a term suggested by von Pirquet, means altered energy, or the altered reactivities of the organism to certain proteins after it has passed through a previous introduction of the same substance. It may be an important phase of a certain kind of immunity, but the general understanding is an increased sensitivity of the human organism to certain proteins (allergen) against which it was previously sensitized. I wish to touch the subject only lightly.

There is really no difference between allergy and anaphylaxy. If I put allergy under a special heading, it is only for the purpose of enumerating in this group conditions caused by airborne antigenic molecules produced by:

1) Substances adherent to the bee (proteins);
2) Its venom
3) Pollens attached to the sting or other parts.

Ellis and Ahrens, of Minneapolis, in a very interesting article, mentioned two cases which clearly demonstrated these allergic effects:

An adult, male, age 34, in May, 1930, while working with bees, was stung on left temporal region. An hour later he complained of constriction of the throat, erythema around the neck, itching and burning. Later he had chills, perspiration, difficult breathing (gasping for air). The difficulty in breathing returned every night for a long time.

A male, age 33, beekeeper, worked in a cellar containing many dead bees. He developed a cough, with profuse watery secretion from the nose, lasting several weeks. A year later, he noticed distinct symptoms of hay fever, accompanied by bronchitis, every time he worked around the bees. Had several asthmatic attacks during the time he was in contact with them, even in proximity with any bee material, such as hives or frames. He was compelled to give up his occupation.

Ellis and Ahrens were unable to find any references in medical literature to human hypersensitiveness to airborne allergen of bee origin.

Two other cases came under their observation, with an opportunity for careful diagnosis, study, and successful desensitization. Both were very sensitive to this type of allergen. Attacks of asthma were initiated when near bees or any object which had been in contact with them. They also cited a case of asthma induced during a car ride by a robe which had been used, a short time before, to cover a hive of bees for transportation.

Douglas F. Gibb, of Manitoba, reported the following:

A girl of seven was playing in the garden. A bee became entangled in her hair and stung her. The mother, over the telephone, consulted a doctor, who advised her to apply a solution of bicarbonate soda. She telephoned a second time, 15 minutes later, asking the doctor to call at once. On arrival, he found that large lumps had formed all over the body of the patient who exhibited furthermore every symptom of well-established hay fever. She complained of tickling and burning of lumps had formed all over the body of the patient who exhibited furthermore every symptoms of hay fever. She complained of tickling and burning of the nasal mucosa, she sneezed continually, following which there was a scanty flow catarrhal condition spread rapidly over her pharynx. Soon the condition became of secretion from the nose and eyes. Very itchy urticarial wheals appeared. The complicated with a typical asthmatic cough.

Gibb gave her 1:1000 epinephrine solution hypodermically, sprayed the throat and notes with saline solution, and applied calamine lotion on the skin. After the injection, the hay fever symptoms were less severe. Later on, patient had another coughing spell. He sprayed her again with ephedrine solution, which brought relief. Gibb suggested that the bee might have injected some pollen which developed the hay fever.

Benson and Semenov, of Portland, Oregon, reported an interesting case:

A beekeeper had consulted them three years previously, with typical complaints of hay fever, which he attributed to bee stings. The attacks commenced in April or May, even as late as June, and lasted until October, or, in other words, until the end of the bee season.

Patient had started beekeeping 18 years before. In the first year, he suffered numerous stings—as many as 75 a day-without any unusual consequences. The second year, he noticed increasing distress after each sting. By the end of the third year, his reactions became worse and he determined to discontinue his occupation. Each sting was followed by severe irritation of the mucous membranes of the eyes and nose, violent sneezing, and obstruction of the nasal passages. The acute attacks cleared up in a day or two, followed next day by a greenish nasal discharge. Some attacks simulated asthma, once he even thought that he had pneumonia.

The patient was desensitized by subcutaneous inoculations of special sting and body proteins of the bee. The results were entirely satisfactory. Soon afterward, he was stung, on one occasion, by 25 bees without any ill effect. (Such allergy of the respiratory tract and skin is not uncommon. Author.)

CHAPTER REFERENCES

ARTHUS, M. De L'Anaphylaxie a l'immunité, 1921.

AUBRY. Quoted by G. Legal, Thèse de Paris, 1922.

BAUDISCH, H. Bienenstich, Prag. Med. Wchnschr., 31, 1906.

BENSON, R., and SEMENOV, H. Allergy in its relation to Bee Stings, J. of Allergy, I, 1930.

BERG, R. Ein Fall von Idiosyncrasie gegen Wespengift, Berl. klin. Wchnschr., 1204, 1920.

BRAUN, L. J. B. Notes on Desensitization of a Patient hypersensitive to Bee Stings, South African M. Rec., Capetown, 23, 1925.

BROWN, G. Med. J. Australia, Sydney, Dec. 1931 (quoted by Cleland).

CALMETTE, A. Les venins, les animaux venimeux et la serotherapie antivenimeuse,

CARTON, P. Menace de mort par une piqûre d'abeille, Vie et Santé, 3, Août, 1927.

CLELAND, J. B. Insects in their relationship to Injury and Disease in man in Australia, Med. J. Australia, Sydney, Dec. 1931.

COOKE, R. A. Cutaneous Reactions in Human Hypersensitiveness, Proc. N. York Path. Soc., XXI, 1921.

DENYS, J., ET VAN DE VELDE, H. Sur la production d'une antileucocidine chez les lapins vaccines contre le Staphylocoque Pyogène, Cellule, Lierre et Louvain, 1895.

DENYS, J. A propos d'une Critique dirigée contre le pouvoir bactericide des humeurs, Cellule, Lierre et Louvain, 1924.

DOLD, H. Immunisierungsversuche gegen das Bienengift, Ztschr. f. Immunitätsforsch. u. exper. Therap. Jena, 26, 1917.

EDWARDES, T. The Lore of the Honey Bee, Lond., 1925.

ELLIS, R. V., AND AHRENS, H. G. Hypersensitiveness to airborne bee allergen, J. Allergy, 3, 1930.

FITZSIMONS, F. W. Snake Venoms, their therapeutic uses and possibilities, South African M. Rec., Capetown, 3, 26, 1921.

FLURY, F. Über die chemische Natur des Bienengiftes, Arch. f. exper. Path. u. Pharm. Leipz., 85, 1920.

FLURY, F., U. ZANGER, H. Lehrbuch der Toxicologie, 1928.

GAY, F. P. Tissue Resistance and Immunity, J. Am. M. Ass. Chicago, Oct. 1931.

GIBB, D. F. Anaphylaxis from Pollen, introduced by a Bee Sting, Canada M. Ass., Oct. 1928.

GOETZ, A. Generalisierte Urticaria, Deutsch. Med. Wchnschr. Berl. u. Leipz., 55, 1929.

GREGG, A. L. Anaphylaxis from Bee Stings, Lancet, Lond., March 1932.

JOBLING, PETERSON, EGGSTEIN. Mechanism of anaphylactic shock, J. Exper. M. N. Y., Oct. 1915.

KRITSCHEWSKY, J. L. A Contribution to the theory of anaphylactic shock, J. Infect. Dis., Chicago, 1918.

LEGAL, G. Contribution a l'étude des Condition de gravité des piqûres d'Hymenoptères, Thèse de Paris, 1922.

MACKAY, H. Severe toxemia following Bee Stings, Canada M. Ass. J., Nov. 1924.

MEIGS, G. S. The relation between allergic intracutaneous reaction and symptoms of Anaphylaxy, J. Inf. Dis. Chicago, 15, 3, 1904.

MITCHELL, S. WEIR. Cat-Fear, Ladies' Home Jour., March 1906.

MUCK, O. Eine übersehene Bienengiftstudie, Wien. Tierärztlich. Monatschr., 1, 1922.

NEISSER, M., U. WECHSBERG, F. Über Staphylotoxin, Ztschr. f. Hyg. Infectionskrankh., 36, 1901.

DECREASED AND INCREASED SENSITIVITY

PERRIN ET CUÈNOT, A propos de 13 observations nouvelles d'hypersensibilitié au venin d'abeilles, Rev. Méd. de l'Est, 60, 1932. Contribution a l'étude du pouvoir anatoxique et de la phylaxie, J. de Physiol. et Path. gen. Par., I, Sept. 1931; II, Dec. 1931; III, Mars, 1932. La metathèse, modalité nouvelle de la protection contre le toxique, ses application pratique, Bull. gen. de Thérap. (etc.) Soc. de thérap.... Par., 4, Avril 1931.

RICHET, C. Anaphylaxie. Par., 1913.

ROLLESTON, SIR H. Idiosyncrasies, Lond. 1927.

RYLE, J. A. Anaphylaxis from Bee Stings, Lancet, Lond., March 1932.

SOLLMAN, T., AND PILCHER, J. D. Endermic Reactions, J. Pharmacol. and Exper. Therap., Baltimore, 9, 1917.

STOVER, G. H. Antitoxic Relation between Bee Poison and Honey, Johns Hopkins Hosp. Bull., Nov. 1898.

THOMSON, F. About Bee Venom, Lancet, Lond., Aug. 19, 1933.

VAUGHAN, V. C. Protein Split Products in Relation to Immunity and Disease, 1913.

VAUGHAN, W. T. Allergy and Applied Immunology, 1931.

VON HOHENHEIM, THEOPHRASTUS (PARACELSUS). Schriften, Leipz., 1921.

WATERHOUSE, A. T. Bee Stings and Anaphylaxis, Lancet, Lond., II, 946, 1914.

WEIL, R. The Nature of anaphylaxis and relationship between anaphylaxis and immunity, J. Med. Research, Boston, XXVII, 4, 1913.

WELLS, G. H. The Chemical Aspects of Immunity, 1929.

ZANGOLINI. Symptômes d'empoisonnement par piqûres d'abeilles, Gaz. Méd. de Par., 1857.

ZINSSER, H. The more recent developments in the study of anaphylactic phenomena, Arch. Int. Med., Chicago, 16, 1915.

Chapter VIII The Treatment of Bee Stings

Langer thought it a very curious fact that, in spite of all beekeeping literature, the bee sting is treated like a step-child and the medical fraternity seems to be just as much afraid of the subject as it is of the stings and their consequences, and in general, physicians know less about the subject than many laymen.

The management, respectively the treatment of bee sting injuries, is carried out in two directions: attention to 1, Local effects; and 2, General effects.

TREATMENT OF LOCAL EFFECTS

The treatment of local effects has two purposes; namely,

A. To treat the effects of the local inflammation; and

B. To destroy or neutralize the venom.

Treatment of Local Inflammation. To treat the inflammation and check its progress antiphlogistic measures are employed. Disinfecting the wound is unnecessary as bee venom is an antiseptic in itself. The application of cold, vinegar, alum acetate, Eau de Cologne or alcohol is useful. Hot fomentations will help greatly to alleviate the pain. Old popular remedies are: wet earth, crushed raw potatoes, poppy seeds, honey, figs, onions, garlic, cauterizing the wound with a burning cigarette, cigar, or heated wire, or rubbing it with a wet cigar. Cold has no permanent destructive effect on the sting. If you spray the wound with ethyl chloride, it will freeze and deaden the pain as long as the effect of this agent lasts, but as soon as this wears off the full strength of the venom is felt.

J. F. D. Donnelly, in an article which appeared in Nature, in 1898, stated that he considered cocaine a specific for bee stings, and not only as a temporary relief. He was convinced that it has power to destroy entirely the poison of the sting. He experimented by using a one-sixth grain tablet of cocaine on a lady who had been stung very badly. The stings, as a rule, had a very severe effect on her, not only causing her local pain and swelling but making her sick for several days. Donnelly dissolved the tablet in a few drops of water and applied it to the sting. It immediately relieved the pain and the second application, several hours later, effected complete relief. Donnelly had similar experience with another case. After that, he kept a bottle of a very strong solution of cocaine on hand, which always proved efficacious. It should be applied immediately, but sometimes Donnelly applied it as late as seven hours after the sting had been inflicted and even then it brought considerable relief.

Neutralizing the Venom.-To prevent the absorption of the venom, are of very little value. The channel which the *Lancet* bores is so minute that sometimes physical means are employed (suction). Most drugs recommended after the removal of the sting even the small opening closes and drugs hardly reach the injected venom to counteract its effect. Pliny admitted that he had no remedies for bee stings, and even today we should concede that we are only little better off. We have no more chance of preventing the absorption of venom after a sting injury than we have of frustrating the soporific effect of morphine by external means, after it has been hypodermically administered.

Alkalies, especially ammonia and lime water, or hot magnesium sulphate compresses, are considered useful and are supposed to counteract the acid poison. Halogen compounds (chlorine, bromine) would undoubtedly destroy the venom, if contact could be accomplished. The use of an oxidizing agent, like potassium permanganate, has a scientific basis. Legal recommended 2 percent hypochlorite of lime, which should be used in freshly made solution, as nascent chlorine gas has diffusible power and is likely to be effective even at a distance from the point of sting inoculation. Calmette advised the use of 1 percent chromic acid, the same as for snake bites. Acid phenique in alcohol is very popular in France. Mentholated or camphorated vaseline is very good for the pruritis. Spirit of turpentine and acetic acid are sometimes employed. Plain laundry blueing, rubbed over the sting injury, is supposed to be helpful.

The most logical procedure seems to be the injection with a hypodermic syringe of a neutralizing substance into the wheal, but this is likely to prove more painful. Then too, the local symptoms develop so quickly that if a physician is not available immediately these applications would be useless. As a rule, people expect the effects of the stings to wear off anyhow, and do not take recourse to inconvenient or costly measures. There is an old saying, "Take out the sting, don't rub, and forget it." (Rubbing spreads the venom and causes more rapid and intense effects.) Cicero, almost two thousand years ago, remarked, "To mind a bee sting is a truly feminine trait."

We must not forget that the bee, after she has inflicted a sting, in the majority of cases is "anchored." As previously described, the sting apparatus is easily detachable and, although the bee has departed, the *Lancet*, poison bag, glands, even part of the chitin covering, will be left in the wound. The apparatus automatically, without the bee, drills itself deeper and the poison bag, in an identical manner, pumps its contents into the wound, so the sooner the sting is removed, the better. It is best to scrape it off with a knife or with the sharp finger nail, but never with two fingers, as we are likely to apply pressure on the sac and inject the remaining contents into the wound.

I also mention another fact which has medical interest; namely, that instances have been reported where buried stings were found in broken combs and persons eating such honey suffered bad injuries in their mouths. As the sting is always accompanied by the poison bag, an extracted sting capable of inflicting a wound weeks later. Though the venom is volatile, its strength is well preserved in honey.

TREATMENT OF GENERAL EFFECTS

The treatment of the general effects depends on clinical manifestations. Prompt attention is essential, especially with very sensitive subjects where a previous injury or several former injuries have already caused repeated alarming symptoms. In such instances, it is not advisable to lose valuable time and wait for the appearance of the symptoms but it is better to intervene immediately to prevent the expected, and in all probability, serious general effects.

A successful preventive measure has been tried in cases with previous desperate symptoms, which were possibly due to idiosyncrasy or to an anaphylactoid state. Dr. Braun, of Capetown, desensitized patients with peptone or intravenous administrations of calcium. He also injected at intervals a diluted solution of bee venom of standardized toxicity, gradually increasing its dose. In the event that a strong reaction resulted, he used adrenalin to counteract it. Braun prepared a toxin by grinding the whole sting apparatus in saline solution, then filtered and diluted it to a definite standard of toxicity. The standardization was done by rubbing one drop of this solution on the scarified (blood must not be drawn) area of the sensitive patient. The effects were carefully observed, recording a definite reaction in a definite time. The experiment was successful. After desensitization, he exposed the patients to bee stings and while formerly they had reacted violently, it took as much as ten minutes to see the first signs of a reaction, and even this was extremely mild.

W. R. Jones, of Seattle, who was also successful in desensitizing patients with gradually increasing doses of bee venom, suggested that the initial dose should be weaker than normal venom. Perrin and Cuènot likewise succeeded in desensitizing patients who were oversensitive to the effects of the venom, by injecting a weak solution, gradually increasing its

138

strength. This precaution, they thought, might be very valuable in certain cases.[6]

It is interesting to note that immunity to bee venom does not protect one from the effects of wasp venom. F. Thompson exposed himself to wasp stings and found he soon acquired immunity to them. He stated that there was a family resemblance between the two venoms but that they must differ in some respect.

To prevent absorption, in the event of expected grave symptoms, we must use the same first aid measures that are applied in snake bites. A small cut, under novocaine anesthesia and suction, by apparatus, or by mouth, can be applied. Of course, the venom has no toxic effect on the tongue or on the membranes of the mouth if there are no sores or cuts present, salivary and digestive ferments destroy it. If the injury is on the limb, a tourniquet might be applied above the location of the sting, but it must be released every ten or fifteen minutes for about a minute at a time. (Reports were published that suction by mouth produced untoward effects. Author.)

In connection with our effort to arrest the absorption of the venom, it is interesting to note the important physiological experiment made by Czyhlarz and Donath of Nothnagel's Clinic in Vienna. They strangulated the leg of a guinea pig high above the knee, so tightly that there was no possibility that blood or lymph could flow in a centripetal direction. They then injected a more than lethal dose of strychnine below the constriction, which ordinarily would have killed the animal in a couple of minutes. The ligature was kept on for several hours and after it was removed, the animal remained well. F. K. Kleine's experiment was very similar. He noticed even on very tight constriction of the limb, traces of strychnine in the kidneys and blood. Possibly, an osmosis took place, in spite of the tight constriction. It seems that, just as in bacterial infections, certain haptophore cells (Ehrlich) bound the toxin, and the organism had time to immunize itself through the gradual influence of the smaller amount of poison. In brief, when the full constriction was removed and the entire toxic effect of the larger amount of poison invaded the organism, the system had already been immunized through osmotic absorption.

---

[6] Benson and Semenov used sting and special body proteins of the bee in their procedure with considerable success. Ellis and Ahrens, also, successfully immunized patients hypersensitive to air-borne bee-allergens

THE TREATMENT OF BEE STINGS

Meltzer and Langmann made similar experiments with snake venom, and found that in constricting an extremity of an animal, even after the removal of the constriction the procedure markedly retarded the fatal action of the venom. The same method transformed an effective minimum dose of strychnine into an ineffective subminimum dose.

If we are too late to administer preventive measures, our duty is to treat the general symptoms according to their importance and urgency. Alcoholization is a most valuable first aid; whiskey and brandy are usually at hand. Strong hot coffee or tea often helps. Spirit of nitrous ether or aromatic spirits of ammonia, one or two teaspoonfuls in water, are effective; one will find useful any cardiac stimulant (spartein, camphorated oil) except caffein, which greatly increases blood pressure and may cause hemorrhage. In case urgent detoxication of a very sensitive organism is imperative, the following routine is recommended:

1) Tourniquet or a suction apparatus if the sting injury is on an extremity.

2) Internal alcoholization.

3) Intravenous administration of physiological saline solution.

4) Antivenomous or some polyvalent serum. This will considerably inhibit the neurotoxic effects and lessen the degree of hemolysis.

5) 20 c.c. of blood of a healthy, well-immunized apiarist, injected into the muscles of the injured.

F. J. Mainggolan, of Batavia, East India, reported five cases of various stings which were greatly relieved by subcutaneous injection of 2 c.c. of omnadin and suggested its use in any insect poisoning. T. Freedman, of South Africa, praised, too, the effect of omnadin. Freedman used omnadin for two years in all acute infections. The absence of anaphylactic shock and other unpleasant symptoms makes omnadin very desirable as it is supposed to reduce temperature and the patient feels stimulated. (Omnadin is a sarcine vaccine composed of various animal fats and bile lipoids as well as a relative protein substance derived from metabolic products of nonpathogenic schizomycetes. It also contains the basal elements of all those antigens which play an immunizing rôle in infectious diseases.)

Many authors consider epinephrin as a specific for severe constitutional disturbances caused by bee stings, especially when the symptoms correspond to those of typical anaphylactic phenomena. Adrenalin and pilocarpin injected hypodermically will accomplish a similar purpose. Pituitrin is often useful. A. E. Mahood, *Lancet*, July 21, 1934, praises the use of milk of magnesia as greatly relieving both the local and the general symptoms.

I may just as well make brief mention that many remedies have been suggested, to be applied on the skin and ward off bee stings. The principle is about the same as when using citronella, made from Ceylon grass, yielding a pungent volatile oil, to which mosquitoes have quite an aversion. Wintergreen is considered effective for this purpose and is supposed to prevent the bees from stinging.

Fabre suggested the following prescription:

R Aetheris acetici	5.0
Olei Eucalypti	10.0
Eau de Cologne	40.0
Tinct. Pyrethri	50.0

M. et. Sig. One part to 5 parts of water. Rub in before exposure

CHAPTER REFERENCES

BRAUN, L. J. B. Notes of desensitization of a patient hypersensitive to bee stings, South African M. Rec. Capetown, 23, 1925.

CZYHLARZ AND DONATH. Ein Beitrag zur Lehre von Entgiftung, Centralb. f. innere Med., 13, 1900.

DONNELLY, J. F. D. Wasps and Bee Stings, Nature, 435, 1898.

FREEDMAN, T. Non-specific vaccine Therapy with Omnadin, South African M. Rec. Capetown, 6, 1932.

JONES, W. R. Bee Sting Treatment, Northwest Med. Seattle, 25, 1926.

KLEINE, F. K. Über Entgiftung in Tierkörper, Ztschr. f. Hyg. Infektionskrankh. Leipz., 36, Geneesk. Tijdschr. v. Nederl. Indie., 824, 1932.

MAINGGOLAN, F. J. Use of Omnadin in bites of wasps, bees and other insects, Geneesk. Tijdschr. v. Nederl. Indie., 824, 1932.1901.

MELTZER, S. J., AND LANGMANN, G. Is living animal tissue capable of neutralizing the effects of Strychnine and Venom? Med. News, Nov. 1900.

PERRIN et CuÈnot. Le traitment de l'hypersensibilité au venin d'abeilles, Bull. gen. de ther. (etc.) Par., 183, 1932.

THOMPSON, F. About Bee Venom, Lancet Lond., 2, Aug. 19, 1933.

PART II:
ARTHRITIC AND RHEUMATOID CONDITIONS
APITHERAPY

PART II: INTRODUCTION

It is far from the writer's intention to present an elaborate study of arthritic and rheumatoid conditions, but if we undertake to treat these ailments with injectable bee venom there are certain phases relative to their terminology, etiology, symptomatology, and pathology which have to be jointly discussed, besides the method of the procedure, the critical interpretation of the value of the venom and the justification of its use.

In the previous chapters, I used my best efforts to give a fairly concise study of the venom, for the purpose of familiarizing ourselves with the chemical nature and the physiological effects of the substance. The history of the venom and its traditional use since time immemorial has had a universal medical interest. To comprehend fully its chemistry and physiological action, necessarily demanded a brief discussion of animal venoms in general, and the place of bee venom among them. A dissertation on the fundamental principles of immunity, etc., was indispensable. The physiological effects of bee venom, I thought, could best be understood by acquainting ourselves with the effects of bee sting injuries.

The short description of the treatment of these accidental injuries was probably welcomed by colleagues in the rural districts, not only as a coadjuvant to bee venom therapy but because they are bound to be called upon to treat such emergencies, with all their innumerable complications. Our city confrères, on the other hand, if they have any intention of undertaking the administration of these same treatments, and venture to impersonate the bee, will have a chance to treat, occasionally, injuries they themselves inflict. Before discussing the therapy with injectable bee venom, it is essential to treat, first, the subject of arthritic and rheumatic ailments in general.

And now to make a clean breast of it, I must confess the subject has always touched me deeply. The inexpressible agony, the hopeless martyrdom of the maimed and doomed victims, has always aroused in me a great compassion. I have seen too many wretched examples of this "hell on earth." A medical man never feels more keenly-and certainly not for such an almost endless period-the inadequacy of his power than when confronted with these accursed and hapless creatures. The sensation is comparable only to that of a bird with clipped wings, which is eager to fly. We have to go back to the old classics if we want to obtain a well-drawn narrative, depicting both the tortures of the victims as well as our "crippled" powers. But let Odysseus speak, after his descent to Hades:

143

INTRODUCTION

"Moreover I beheld Tantalus in grievous torment, standing in a mere and the water came nigh unto his chin. And he stood straining as one athirst, but he might not attain to the water to drink of it. For often as that old man stooped down in his eagerness to drink, so often the water was swallowed up and it vanished away, and the black earth still showed at his feet, for some god parched it evermore. And tall trees flowering shed their fruit overhead, pears and pomegranates and apple trees with bright fruit, and sweet figs and olives in their bloom, whereat when that old man reached out his hands to clutch them, the wind would toss them to the shadowy clouds," "... and... then for the first time, it is said, the cheeks of the Furies were wet with tears."

"Yea and I beheld Sisyphus in strong torment, grasping a monstrous stone with both his hands. He was pressing thereat with hands and feet, and trying to roll the stone upward toward the brow of the hill. But oft as he was about to hurl it over the top, the weight would drive him back, so once again to the plain rolled the stone, the shameless thing. And he once more kept heaving and straining, and the sweat the while was pouring down his limbs, and the dust rose upwards from his head."

And while we are with Homer, let us hear how Lady Circe "spake unto him" describing Scylla and Charybdis to Odysseus: "... and all about is a great heap of bones of men, corrupt in death, and round the bones the skin is wasting.... Thereby no ship of men ever escapes that comes thither, but the planks of ships and the bodies of men confusedly are tossed by the waves of the sea and the storms of ruinous fire." And to it, we may add the legend of Hercules and his "Twelve Labors," ...the strangling of the Nemean lion ... the killing of the Lernean hydra... the capture of the man-eating mares of Diomedes... the cleaning of the Stable of Augeas... procuring the golden apples of Hesperides... or even the story of the "Knot of Gordius."...

But I behold, with mental vision, the sign: "No Trespassing."... So let us go up... or down... I apologize for losing my way... to earth and resume our subject. The difference in atmosphere will be hardly noticeable.

Chapter IX Arthritic And Rheumatoid Conditions:
Their Relationship To Bee Venom
SURVEY OF SITUATION

Unquestionably, there is no other subject in medical science which has been as widely discussed and more written about, in both the domestic and foreign literature, than this mass-group of ailments. This stands to reason, as without doubt they constitute not only the largest but also the most difficult chapter of medicine. They touch more fields of diverse organic diseases other malady. Their etiology is obscure, imperfectly understood, than any and, on account of this fact, the treatments are deplorably inadequate; likewise their nomenclature is in a perfectly chaotic state, subjected to continual controversies. Correct terminology is impossible without an exact knowledge of etiology. Last but not least, there is the uncertainty of the pathological conditions. And while we are doing our utmost in an honest effort to clear all these obscurities-at the same time searching for proper methods of treatment-the scourge is progressing like an avalanche, carrying along the unfortunate and hopeless victims.

Lewellys F. Barker said: "Despite the real progress which has been made, it must be confessed that the arthropathies are still veiled in deplorable obscurity. The dimness, while due chiefly to our inability to look at the processes from an etiological viewpoint, is in some extent dependent upon an intervening dust cloud of terminology. In no part of medicine, perhaps, have names been used less satisfactorily than in arthropathies." Nichols and Richardson also admit that considerable pathological and clinical confusion prevails about the whole subject.

There are no two countries which have even nearly similar terminology. If it would not occupy so much space, I would group the American, English, French, German, Austrian, etc., terms in parallel positions to view and compare their relative divergencies. There are classifications, subclassifications, cross-classifications, subdivisions, etc.: exogen, endogen, chronic, acute, subacute, primary, secondary arthritism and rheumatism; then osteoarthritis, periarthritis, perichondritis, synovitis, chondroarthritis, polyarthritis, arthritis deformans, alterativa, sicca, exudativa, productiva, etc., atrophic (proliferative), atonic, metabolic, traumatic, infective, suppurative, etc.; tubercular, syphilitic, gonorrheal, pneumococcal, scarlatinal, dysenteric, hemophilic, serum arthritis, climacteric, menopausal, arthropathia ovaripriva, arthritis of pregnancy, tabidorum, etc.; endocrine arthralgias: thyroid, adrenal, hypophysis; gout (arthritis urica), Heberden nodes, myalgia, myositis, neuralgia, sciatica, neuritis, spondylitis, von Bechterew's disease (spondylarthritis ankylopoetica), iritis rheumatica, etc., etc.

Then we are confronted with the difficulties of the synonyms. Arthritis deformans, rheumatoid arthritis and osteoarthritis are synonymic; so are atrophic, rheumatoid and proliferative arthritis; hypertrophic, degenerative and osteoarthritis are synonymic with some authors and distinctly separate diseases with others.

A correct diagnosis, of course, is a *conditio sine qua non. Qui bene diagnoscit, bene sanabit!* The treatment obviously cannot be started without a correct diagnosis.

Let us now carefully and critically review the whole complex situation. Figuratively, we had better remove to a safer distance from this region of confusion, in an effort to occupy a little "higher" place, so as to gain a better perspective and a more "liberal" outlook.

The enormous number of arthritic and rheumatic patients confidently await relief and cure from the efficiency of our treatments. Intelligent treatment is entirely dependent on a discerning diagnosis. So far, so good! But our real hardships just commence. For example, we have to name a certain disease of these groups. The terminology depends absolutely on a proper diagnosis. The diagnosis again is contingent on the subjective and objective clinical findings, past history, etc., supported by physiological, pathological, chemical, bacteriological, and other researches. When the correct diagnosis has been made, we are able to name the malady. One part of the naming is the easiest: we know that it is arthritis, rheumatism, neuritis, etc., but the difficulty is in—let us call it—the cognomen which designates its origin, type, or possibly degree, etc.

The main confusion in the nomenclature is that the majority of the terms, so far applied, classify the diseases from different viewpoints. Some terms are suggestive of clinical findings (e.g., progressive); pathological conditions (inflammatory, exudative, proliferative, sicca, etc.); topographical, respectively anatomical, considerations (lumbago, occipital neuralgia, sciatica, spondylitis, etc.); causal (traumatic, endocrine, post-operative, serum arthritis, etc.); some refer to the time, its duration (acute, subacute, chronic, etc.); some designate dynamic conditions (ankylotic, deformans, contractive, etc.); others, the chemical (urica) or bacteriological aspects (suppurative, infective, pneumococcal); some refer to their

146

distribution (polyarthritis), age (malum coxae senilis, neonatorum), to sex (climacteric, ovaripriva), then hereditary, and many other designations.

Finally with this I really should have started-the term "arthritis" is itself a misnomer. In the great majority of cases, there is no inflammation. "Rheumatism" is also a very poor term. "Rheuma" (derived from the Greek "rheo"-flow, flux) means some mystic humor in the joints or muscles... and there is no more "humor" in the disease than we doctors are "humorists" while treating it. The sardonic remark of a certain "joker" (?), that the first and only worthwhile progress physicians have made in the last two thousand years in combating "common cold," was that they gave it the name "coryza"; so I think it is really high time to commence to make some progress also in the "treatment" of rheumatoid conditions, by straightening out their nomenclature. H. K. Craig thought that, of all the words in the verbal armamentarium of a physician, none is more deserving of condemnation than rheumatism.

Now for a fairly accurate description of the next complex procedure which is necessary to make a correct diagnosis!

First, a "conventional" search for "occult" focal infection is essential. We have to ask the dentist for a thorough examination of the teeth and also for a dental radiograph. X-rays of the joints and, at least, of the intestinal tract are necessary. The rhinologist and laryngologist must conduct a thorough examination of the accessory sinuses and tonsils. If he attends also to the ears we are saved the trouble of sending the patient to an otologist. The female adnexa very often hide some infective foci and a gynecologist's advice is prerequisite. The urologist has to make a thorough examination of the prostate gland and the seminal vesicles, and so forth.

After another specialist has put the patient through metabolism tests, a fractional test meal, etc., to find out if any faults of metabolism are present, or whether there are some dietetic errors, the patient is sent to an endocrinologist to determine whether the condition is attributable to some endocrine imbalance. The advice of the neurologist is also indispensable as arthritis is often caused by nervous or mental strain or by some other neurotrophic disorders. In over 50 percent of the cases we find hereditary disposition. When all these preliminaries are finally completed, other inquisitorial procedures must be adopted. We must ask the assistance of the bacteriologist to search carefully for bacteria in the blood, synovial fluid, lymph nodes, etc., to find out whether any streptococcus hemolyticus or viridans, etc., are present. Some specialists find, in the intestinal tract, pathogenic streptococci in over 90 percent of arthritic cases. (I am convinced that in healthy individuals or in other non-rheumatoid ailments, the

147

percentage is just as high.) Cruickshank plainly controverts the possibility of such infections through the intestinal tract.

After the bacterial tests are concluded, the serologist is supposed to prepare the proper vaccine. Full blood count, Wassermann test, sedimentation rate, complement fixation for gonorrhea, renal function and sugar tolerance tests must be made and the relative presence of uric acid, blood nitrogen, blood calcium, blood sugar, determined. The chemical relationship of the increase or decrease of plasma proteins, fibrinogens, globulins, and albumins must be definitely ascertained. We know that in various constitutional diseases the fibrinogens and globulins are increased and the albumins decreased to a fair extent.

By this time, possibly the correct diagnosis has been completed. Several specialists have to attend to various disorders: to drainage of the infective foci, to gynecological and urological conditions, renal functions, the blood, the heart, etc. Likewise, if there is an imbalanced endocrine state, it must be corrected. Traumatic disorders, deformities, contractions, have to be rectified by the orthopedic surgeon. Immunological, dietetic, medicinal treatments must be started. Of course, we cannot do it all. The patient often needs colonic irrigations, hydrologic, physiotherapeutic measures like diathermy, various radiant lights, etc. For mechanical readjustment, to allay pain, reeducate lost functions of the muscles and passive movements, we have to employ osteopaths or even masseurs. A foot specialist is often needed. Flat feet and fallen arches are a frequent cause of arthritis. The druggist and orthopedic shoemaker must also have their apportionate share. Sometimes we need even an artist or a mechanic to design proper splints. We had better mention another very important assistant who may be indispensable; namely, the banker to finance the whole "trip." Only the poor undertaker is cheated because these conditions "only" cripple and very seldom kill. There is even a traditional belief that rheumatism prolongs life-a proof of the kindness of providence and of the saying that every cloud has a silver lining! Less than one percent of all death cases are arthritics or rheumatics. They all stay with us for a long time and... Is it any wonder that most arthritics refuse medical assistance? And we are subjected to such cynical backbiting: "Doctor, you don't know what causes arthritis, you don't know how to cure it-all you know is that I have it!" [7]

B. L. Wyatt stated that while about 400 physicians specialize in this branch, there are 800 qualified technicians of physiotherapy, 18,500 chiropractors, 7,600 osteopaths, and innumerable masseurs. Millions take faith cures. Lately there has been a regular pilgrimage to a village doctor in Canada who-as they tell me-treats sometimes 800 to 1,000 patients daily, just by manipulation.

Many patients finally give up all treatments entirely, assume a fatalistic attitude they simply resign themselves, invalided, crippled physically and mentally, to endure the tortures and agonies of their afflictions-firmly convinced that their ailments are intractable and incurable. A great part of the medical profession is of the same opinion. And remember, it is not only a medical but a great humanitarian, economic, and social problem. In England alone, in one year, among 3,500,000 members of the various labor organizations, 370,000 were incapacitated by arthritic and rheumatoid diseases, one sixth of all disabilities. Over two million pounds were paid in compensation for this group of disabled workers during the same period; besides, about three million work-weeks were lost and figuring on the average four pounds a week, it meant another loss of twelve million pounds. This was the loss incurred by the laboring class only.

Let us now analyze the causes of this critical situation. No doubt the subject is enormous and so extremely complex that it seems beyond the faculties of any physician, however competent and experienced he may be. He cannot see the forest for the trees. Teamwork, of course, is necessary and unavoidable. But, in spite of all progress, intense study, honest effort and continuous scientific research, the fundamental uncertainties do not seem to become lucid.

---

[7] Or the statement of someone who defined medicine as "the art or science of amusing the sick man with frivolous speculation about his malady and of tampering ingenuously till nature either kill or cures them"

CARDINAL ERRORS

The three main errors are the following:
a)   diagnostic;
b)   loss of time;
c)   therapeutic.

The treatment of arthritis and rheumatism places a great demand on the physician but, let us be fair, much greater on the patient. The art of healing is a three-cornered battle: the participants are the patient, the doctor and the malady. If the patient and physician are in accord and harmoniously fight the disease as a common enemy, the prospects of victory are fair and bright; but how often, too true, we have to tussle "single-handed" with the patient and malady, joined like two confederates, and not infrequently the patient is the more troublesome of the two. Of course, in such cases failure, defeat, even real calamity is inevitable. *Inde iræ et lacrima!* (Hence this rage and weeping.)-Juvenal, I, 168. Close collaboration between the patient and doctor is imperative.

Diagnostic Errors

Discussing the fallacies of diagnosis, the first and main mistake is that we look at these conditions as diseases. Arthritis and rheumatism are not morbid entities, not diseases in the strict sense, just local manifestations of systemic disorders. Our chief attention must be directed and concentrated on the causative factors-most of the time the effects will take care of themselves.

When the old "furnace," even the whole "boiler room," is full of suffocating smoke, the grates covered with clinkers, and there is no heat because of poor combustion, all the "stoking and poking" or adding and changing of "fuel" will not correct the situation. If you are inexperienced, you will blame it on the old "furnace" or on some of its parts-it is simply sick, maybe even dying—and you might, if Cicero is correct (*consuetudo quasi altera natura*-habit is second nature), fill up the "furnace" with aspirin and salicylates, or, if your habits are confirmed, even wrap it in ice bags.

After you are convinced that all these "scientific" exertions are useless, you are forced to send for a common-sense "repairman." He will soon explain to you-without any hesitation-that the "flue pipe is clogged with soot from using bad coal and not giving enough draft," will clean it out for and the "sick furnace" will blaze up in a couple of minutes-all is well and there is plenty of heat; and while you stand there, confused and humiliated after paying his small fee (which he is almost ashamed to accept), he will even make a diagnosis for you after the cure (his method differs even in this particular), and will tell you that although the "furnace" is old, it is of excellent "make" and if you give it good "hard coal" and plenty of air (he does not know as much about oxygen as we do) you will have no trouble with it and it will last 50 years longer.

After this little parable (may it be useful!), let us resume our discussion of arthritic and rheumatoid conditions. The organism in most of these cases is not more pathologically sick than the other "furnace." In the most painful myalgia and sciatica, we will not find the minutest structural changes in the tissues. Auerbach, Bing, Schmidt excised, under local anesthesia, such affected muscles and nerves; the result of their examination was negative. Abderhalden, who was greatly interested in the subject, personally examined sections of uncured, severely inflamed sciatic nerves, where the patients had died from some other cause, and could not find even the slightest pathological changes in the nerve tissue itself. Of course, an atrophy of muscles and nerves, as a consequence of a protracted chronic involvement is another matter, but any long-lasting inactivity will produce similar results.

Undoubtedly the main symptoms of rheumatoid ailments are pains of various intensity, but if all our attention and attempts are directed toward the alleviation of pain, the whole procedure will be wrong. If the treatments are not based on etiological principles, but on concurrences, they will be only conjectural-in plain English, "guesswork."

The disappearance of the symptom (pain) does not by any means indicate a cessation of the disorder. Often enough, for certain reasons-possibly due to some "error" in treatment-the symptoms may disappear and the condition is worse than it ever was. "Recurrence," accordingly, is only the reappearance of pain, the symptom, but not by far a change in the condition which was present even when there were no apparent manifestations. Clinical interpretations are not always physiological and, still less, pathological elucidations.

Pains are undependable anyhow-often even misleading. Pain localized in the upper interior end of the tibia may signify a disorder in the hip or in the arch of the foot. Pains on the pectoral or dorsal regions, even on the arms or legs, are not infrequently mere reflex manifestations of some thoracic or abdominal disturbances-in a word, they are symptomatic and not idiopathic pains, and are obviously due to adjacent nerve roots in some cerebra-spinal areas.

Our efforts to concentrate on the removal of pain which is only a symptom and not the cause of the trouble will lead us to commit, also, other errors. In rheumatic fever, some will administer salicylates or other antipyretics, whereas a pyretic treatment is requisite. The fever, in these cases, is a physiological-or call it therapeutical-but not a pathological process. No wonder that, working against Nature, these treatments will leave behind an army of permanent cardiac victims. West, for six years Medical Registrar of St. Bartholomew's Hospital, London, where the patients suffering from rheumatic fever were treated with frequent doses of sodium salicylate, found that in 1,137 cases, which is a large enough number for statistical classification, over 70 percent developed heart disease in some form or other.

When we neglect to supply proper oxidation and elimination of waste through lack of exercise and misuse of food-which may, also, be our own fault (as it often is)—and when, as a consequence of unfortunate complications, some additional contributory exogenous causes aggravate the already existing unsound conditions and we burn up with fever-and when Nature tries to assist us by rectifying the whole desperate situation with violent exercise (exercise is the same chemical act as fever)-then we criminally use our "fire extinguishers." Do the same thing to your chef: put out his fire while he is cooking your dinner. If you watch his expression and read his thoughts, you have before you, in effigy, our friend Nature. Your chef, like Nature, has put to use a physiological, serviceable and not a pathological, destructive fire, so why not leave both of them alone? You don't wish to starve or remain ill?

How sensible is the procedure of our other friend, the bee! Through "sanguificating" treatment, she will adjust the disorder, just as though she were an emissary of Nature. It is not surprising that Terc, Keiter, and others often repeated the statement that they considered bee venom a specific for both rheumatic fever and the consecutive endocarditis, myocarditis, pericarditis, etc., because fever and pain generally disappear within a few days-it seems as though there were no further need of them-and the patients usually recover without cardiac effects.

But we have to return to the place where we started, namely, the first error, and, at the same time, conclude with the statement that arthritism and rheumatism are only pathological conceptions and not diseases.

Loss of Time

The second error is the loss of time. Quick diagnosis and early treatment are very essential. *Bis dat, qui cito dat*! (He gives twice who gives promptly!) In case of a "regular" fire, we must extinguish it at the start here is our chance-and not wait until there is a general widespread conflagration, because even if we succeed in extinguishing it after tremendous effort, we have to expect considerable "ruin." Time is everything in these ailments-we have to treat them in the beginning and not at the end. Over 80% of arthritics improve greatly or recover perfectly if they are properly treated within the first six months. The percentage of favorable results is considerably decreased by delay, and after the condition has existed for several years, the treatments will be incomparatively more difficult. We have to confess that after a duration of four or five years the patients will derive hardly any benefit from the ordinary treatments, and can, still less, hope for a cure.

Therapeutic Errors

The third important error is that we pay too much attention to the removal of positive factors whereas replacement of the missing, negative, essential requirements is often more beneficial. We must not only remove but also add. Building up the body resistance, especially by well directed and sufficient diet, improving the blood and general circulation, plenty of sun, good air and oxygen, will help more than all vaccine therapy.

In suggesting the "replacement of missing, negative, essential requirements," I am referring to a cardinal "faux pas" which is true not only in the management of rheumatoid conditions but also in the entire field of clinical medicine; that is, we are not paying enough attention to the maintenance of the body temperature, which should be confined to a certain limited range, called normal temperature. A deviation from this thermic standard, however slight, is detrimental.

Both physical and chemical forces of the organism function best betwixt and between certain thermic boundary lines. The vasomotor mechanism, circulation, oxidation, cellular activity, nutrition, metabolism, elimination all require what we call normal body temperature. We all pay too much attention to high, and too little to low temperature. We forget that the "dreaded" fever is often only a consequence of or a benevolent substitute for a neglected low temperature. Many maladies could have been prevented if we had not overlooked the low "bank balance" of the body. Low temperature is really the "forgotten man" in medicine. Many of our culpably disregarded and unattended poor subjects are just able to "navigate," whilst their proper quarters ought to be in a hot house or even in an incubator and

153

among these victims, carrying their cross with unconcern, we find plenty of auspicious candidates for rheumatoid ailments-potential rheumatics. There is no better and wider field for preventive medicine!

PRODUCING CAUSES

Reflecting on the etiology of arthritis and rheumatism, we find here the same chaotic state which is characteristic of their pathology, terminology, and therapy; to these we may add also, the prognostic uncertainty. All workers in the field have their own theory, opinion, and, of course, method of treatment. Some blame the entity entirely on bacterial invasion, hidden foci; others again on metabolic disorders, heredity, occupational stress, mental strain, senile changes, postural defects, disturbed endocrine balance, etc.

I am firmly convinced that the main producing cause of these ailments is merely *a local relative state of suboxidation, produced mainly by impaired circulation*. A pathological suppression of a normal flow of blood and lymph will produce an inadequate oxygen supply, be it an idiopathic condition or the result or complication of other unfavorable endogenous or exogenous influences. Insufficient circulation and the consequent relative anoxemia are a great handicap, destructive to all living tissues.

Pemberton said: "The arthritic shows, on the whole, distinctly less blood in the field, closure or narrowing of many capillaries, irregularity and slowing down of blood flow and often a difference in the amount of blood in the venous as compared with the arterial limb of a capillary.... An arthritic maintains at the periphery a temperature lower than that of a normal individual as measured by a thermocouple. The peripheral surface temperature of the arthritic changes less rapidly under the varying environmental conditions, such as cold and heat. This implies a lesser capacity for adaptation to the environment on the part of the capillary beds in the arthritic. This incapacity is doubtless accompanied by added physiologic dysfunction-a deduction which would partly explain the exacerbations experienced by arthritic persons as a result of changes in the weather."

We know that the temperature varies on different parts of the body, which fact must be logically attributed to the content of the blood or to the extent of circulation. In unilateral arthritis, there is not only an occasional difference in the temperature of the affected side, compared with the corresponding normal joint, but even at times a fluctuation is noticeable. The oscillometric test will show a parallel variation. Of course oscillometry will not detect capillary dysfunctions; it will indicate only those of the larger vessels.

The age-old cure, the successful treatment of arthritic and rheumatic ailments with exercise, massage, and heat, is easy to comprehend as they tend to increase circulation. Proper circulation is a most vital factor in every part of the organism. The function of the nerves may cease, as in the case of paralysis, and the system is still able to perform some of its duties, but suspended circulation means a speedy destruction of the tissues mainly due to a lack of oxygen; they simply "suffocate."

The blood, which is really a connective tissue in liquid form, attends not only to the metabolic requirements of the tissues but, also, to their important respiratory function. Heat is produced by combustion, and this requires oxygen. The human organism is nothing else but a superior, complex, internal-combustion engine.

We transform energy into heat and heat into energy-that is motion but we never create new energy. The food is transformed into potential energy-heat and motion.

Liebig was confident in his doctrine that oxidation takes place in the tissues, not in the lungs. The lungs only draw in the oxygen but the blood carries it to the tissues. *Asphyxia takes place in the tissues, not in the lungs.* Gage appropriately called the lungs the carburetor of the organism, providing only the proper air-mixture.

Barcroft, in writing about the function of the blood, said that oxygen is transferred through the capillary vessels to the tissues, unloading the oxygen by diffusion of the gas from the blood to the cells, through the capillary walls. This flux of oxygen will provide the need of the organism. Temperature is an important factor. The blood is different when it reaches the various parts of the organism than when it leaves them, distributing oxygen and carrying away waste, like carbonic and other acids. The diffusion of oxygen, its discharge into the tissues, is a process similar to its influx, its transition through the epithelium of the lungs into the blood stream. Hemoglobin, the carrier of oxygen, for which it has great affinity, is very sensitive even to slight changes, like temperature, acidity or alkalinity. Carbonic acid has great influence on the dissociation of oxygen, but is not a specific; lactic acid has the same effect.

The cells require a certain amount of oxygen. They will take what they need and leave the rest. Increased activity of the organs entails a call for oxygen. If this is not supplied, there will be a disturbed gas equilibrium and asphyxia of the tissues.

The adequacy of the oxygen supply depends absolutely upon the rate of blood flow, which again depends on the pressure of the vessels. The response to the call for oxygen is at a maximum after the action of the organ has passed off, and the call will continue for some time after the actual work has been performed.

Loevenhart thought the mechanism of oxidation the most fascinating theme in the entire domain of chemistry. Lavoisier was already convinced that there is constant oxidation within the body, from which it derives the necessary heat. Oxidation in the body requires a much lower temperature ($37°$ C.) than the same process outside of the body, because of an oxidizing enzyme (oxidase).

From a hemodynamic point of view, the circulatory speed is a very essential factor. The most important "transportation" function of the blood circulation, next to nutrition, is to convey oxygen to the tissues and remove CO_2. Speed is just as important in efficient transportation as the "cargo." If the amount is insufficient, it must be supplemented by speed to maintain the proper balance. In anemic conditions or when the demand of the tissues for oxygen is great, as during or after exercise, the circulatory speed is high. The speed can be determined not only by physical (hemodrometry), but also by chemical means. The quantitative correlation between oxyhemoglobin and CO_2 is a safe estimate of the circulatory speed. The more and the less CO_2, the slower the speed, and vice versa. The difference between the two is an accurate speedometer of the blood circulation. In anemic conditions, as mentioned above, there is little difference between the oxyhemoglobin of the arteries and the CO_2 of the veins, indicating high circulatory speed.

The heart, of course, as a pump, the propeller of circulation, is an all important factor in circulatory speed. Next is the peripherical resistance. Here again, the capillary meshes, on account of their almost imperceptible size and considerable distance from the heart, play an essential part. Naturally the lumina of the vessels, their elasticity, the quantity and quality of blood, together with the demand for oxygen, will all influence the motion of the circulation. It may be normal, fast, slow, or an alternating type. The latter condition is usually attributable to vasoneuritic influences.

In arthritic and rheumatic conditions, the circulatory speed is ordinarily low, which is also one of the important causative factors. In infective arthritis, the speed is increased, because of fever, which is already a defensive response. In arthritis deformans, gout, on the other hand, the circulation is again very slow.

The purpose of the centuries-old treatments of arthritis and rheumatism with mechanical and thermic measures is, as already stated, to accelerate the circulatory motion, relieving the peripherical resistance-which is, at the same time, an automatic labor-saving expedient for the overtaxed heart.

Krogh, of Copenhagen, laid great stress on capillary circulation, both as to the caliber of the vessels and the regulating mechanism. A proper diffusion rate for oxygen and the right oxygen pressure are important factors oxygen consumption. A state of contraction or relaxation of the capillaries very material. The dilatation of the arterioles will raise the pressure in the corresponding capillaries. They contract by their own elasticity. In resting muscles, the capillaries are in a state of contraction and, to a certain degree, closed to the passage of blood. Gentle massage, tetanic stimulation and contraction of the muscles will open these capillaries. Oxygen pressure in resting muscles is very low, but in working muscles approaches very exercise in open air. Active muscles during exercise mean increased "critical" closely that of the blood. This explains the vital importance of wholesome blood circulation and a more rapid and sufficient oxygen distribution. *Not so much the lungs as the tissues of the organism benefit by the enhanced oxygen supply.*

Clinical hyperemia and anemia are due mainly to the changes in the caliber of the capillaries. Good color and good circulation mean open capillaries; pale tissues and poor circulation, closed capillaries. (It will not be very long before most diseases will be explained as a lack or an over-supply of oxygen, a function attended to by the capillary circulation. A. T. Livingstone suggested years ago that neurasthenia, headache, neuralgia, neuritis, hysteria, chorea, asthma, spasm, convulsion, paresis, and insanity should be treated by correcting abnormal states of the capillary circulation.)

According to Goldschmidt and Light, external and internal influences have marked effect upon the blood flow through the peripheral parts of the body and on the consequent variability of the gaseous content of the venous blood, oxygen saturation and carbon dioxide content. If the arm is exposed to high temperature, hyperemia, vascular dilatation will result and the increased oxygen content will average the oxygen saturation, 88%. According to Wells, hyperemic tissues contain more oxygen and less CO_2 than normal blood.

Let us ascertain now the correctness and accuracy of these statements with convincing arguments and a sound process of reasoning, make proper deductions, draw logical conclusions and apply them to our subject.

The circulation of the joints is, in general, very limited. Tendons have poor blood circulation and cartilages, none at all. A scanty blood supply reaches the joints and their immediate neighborhood through the medium of fine capillary vessels. The oxidation and metabolism are restricted, even normally. In myalgia cases, if we carefully investigate, we find that the most sensitive spot is at the arthral insertion of the tendons to the bones.

The synovial fluid, an indispensable substance in all joints, is also absolutely dependent on good circulation. It requires only a minor functional disturbance in an important part of the organism to produce incalculable, harmful consequences. Sometimes a trivial mechanical dysfunction may cause incomparably great local damage.

We can divide the causes producing these detrimental changes into two classes: a, exogenous; and b, endogenous.

Exogenous Causes

Any little interference with the capillary circulation will produce important pathological disturbances in the motive mechanism of the body. If the circulation is impaired, the joints and their coverings, the muscles, tendons, nerves, are deprived of their nutrition and the necessary oxygen supply. Bacteria, also, grow best in a medium low in oxygen.

Sometimes it might be a mechanical, and frequently, a thermal influence: exposure, chills, cold, draft, damp atmosphere, etc.; other times, occupational, industrial, social, and domestic unfavorable conditions. Farmers, drivers, launderers, workers in damp rooms and cellars, often acquire arthritis and rheumatism.

Undoubtedly the great majority of chronic rheumatic and arthritic conditions is due to exposure to cold. Sleeping in cold, damp beds, lying on the ground, etc., frequently produce rheumatic fever. This fact might also explain some phases of "fever." The human body not only possesses a certain amount of heat, but according to the law of physics, it also radiates heat. If the body is chilled, this radiation is checked and the body temperature will automatically rise.

Rheumatic ailments are prevalent in moderate climates. In very cold or tropical regions, they are rather uncommon as the atmospheric variations are not so extreme. There is no explanation necessary for their absence in tropical provinces. In cold countries, again, the inhabitants are well protected by furs and warm clothing. They seldom change the type of wearing apparel;

the body is always kept warm. Their food contains plenty of fat, which is also helpful in the production of necessary warmth.

The conditions which assist or obstruct the process of oxidation are manifold. An efficient or deficient blood circulation is, of course, a primary and vital consideration. There are numerous circumstances which influence circulatory efficiency or deficiency, sometimes known, but frequently concealed or not wholly understood. Atmospheric conditions—not only temperature, but barometric pressure, humidity, even the velocity of the air current, are essential factors. *Excessive humidity will not only influence the respiratory function of the skin but also the influx of oxygen through the membranes of the lungs and even the dissociation of oxyhemoglobin in the tissues*, all resulting in suboxidation. Extreme humidity or draft will greatly retard the proper supply, distribution and absorption of oxygen, and undoubtedly the elimination of carbon dioxide; therefore, rheumatics and arthritis feel even the approach of humid spells, become listless, tired, lose their appetite; their pain increases as the result of oxygen deficiency on account of both the regional and the systemic influences. Chilling of the body is besides injurious, not only on account of the contraction of the capillary circulation, but because the organism is deprived of the necessary heat which is indispensable for proper oxidation.

The etiology of "common cold" can be logically explained by the same theory. Chilling of any part of the body will deprive the tissues of a certain temperature necessary for proper oxidation. The bacterial phase is just incidental, a mere complication.

Perfect oxidation is, so far, the only cure for tuberculosis. The remarkable results achieved in treating surgical tuberculosis by exposure to sunlight are partly due to increased circulation, partly to the energy and ability of the sun to generate hemoglobin, the carrier of oxygen (the same process which creates chlorophyl in plants). The healing power of artificial fever, like the introduction of malarial infection for the treatment of paresis, etc., is based on the same principle. Physiotherapeutic measures are hand-made or machine-made fever.

The uniform functioning of the skin has a general physiological importance. Much arthritis and rheumatism is caused by a lack of excretory and oxidizing facilities in the skin. If the respiratory power of the skin and the secretory efficiency of the sweat glands and ducts are impaired, it might result in temporary or permanent dysfunction, producing indirectly harmful effects on the whole organism, especially on the motive mechanism. Sometimes we even notice that arthritis develops in joints over which the skin has been destroyed by a previous traumatic injury, forming scar tissue, which is unfit to attend to the duties of normal skin.

Faulty obliterative structural conditions, like scoliosis, flat feet, traumatic injuries, etc., often produce or complicate circulatory impairment and cause, indirectly, rheumatoid and arthritic ailments. It is an old saying: "We grow old because we stoop, rather than we stoop because we grow old."

Hard water we could also include as a frequent exogenous cause. The prevalence of arthritis greatly varies even in nearby localities on account of drinking-water. This is clearly due to a lack of iodine content in the soil, which, also, is the cause of the deficiency of iodine in the agricultural food products, both vegetable and animal. Grain grown in these so-called "goiter belts" is entirely destitute of iodine. Lambs, pigs and calves are all born goiterous and show signs of thyroid insufficiency; the sheep shed their wool, pigs and calves are deficient in bristles and hair, and suffer from malnutrition and maldevelopment (Llewellyn).

Goiter and acute or cardiac rheumatism are coexistent in these districts, and it is not surprising that the administration of iodine is beneficial to goiterous and rheumatic conditions, as both are produced by the same deficiency. A lack of nitrogen, calcium, and phosphorus in the soil and water will produce similar adverse influences in the fauna and flora of such regions, the absence of these oxidative catalysts indirectly favoring rheumatoid conditions.

Endogenous Causes

Poor quality and quantity of blood, infective foci, stagnation caused by lack of exercise, imbalanced endocrines, pregnancy, menopause, nephritis, and many other conditions are all endogenous contributory causes. For instance, among 58 women who had been treated with deep X-ray therapy, resulting in artificial sterility, Aschner found 34 arthritics. Gout during menopause was known to Hippocrates. Poor circulation is a natural consequence of old age, or maybe just vice versa. The aged, especially, suffer from arthritis. In youth the constructive processes predominate; in old age the destructive ones are more active. Mild arthritics are stiff in the morning, but during the day, when they use their motive apparatus, their circulation is improved and they often become entirely free from pain. Convalescent states, pneumonia, influenza, dysentery, accidental injuries are often harbingers of polyarthritis. No need to explain any further this development except to say that it is not due only to absorption of toxins but is mainly the consequence of impoverished circulation and consecutive anoxemia.

ARTHRITIC AND RHEUMATIOD CONDITIONS

Millions of people become infected with gonorrhea and only in a comparatively small percentage is there a complication of arthritis. If it occurs, it must be due to defective distribution of blood and a lack of local defensive mechanism. The same applies to grippe and other infectious diseases, even to infective foci.

The blood pressure of arthritics is usually low or at best, normal. High blood pressure is exceptional. Women, on account of the lower hemoglobin content of their blood, are considerably more frequent sufferers from chronic arthritis than men. According to some authors, like Llewellyn, women are five times, and, according to Bannatyne, six times more susceptible to chronic arthritis. There is no other constitutional disease where sex has a more pronounced influence. Bannatyne found in 95% of his rheumatoid arthritis cases more or less advanced anemia and a certain amount of leukocytosis, already a defensive effort of the organism. Anemia is, of course, not the consequence of arthritis but the reverse. Metabolic disorders, which according to some authors are the primary causes of arthritis, in the majority of cases are also due to the curtailment of the general circulation. Other pathological states are likewise unjustly accused.

Hypothyroidism, as already stated, will produce suboxidation. Graves' disease is often complicated by chronic arthritis. Thyroxin is a powerful oxidizer. Llewellyn thought that thyroid inadequacy and rheumatoid arthritis are closely linked, on account of an endocrine-autonomic imbalance which influences the sympathetic-hormone mechanism, in which process the adrenals and pituitary undoubtedly participate. Acidosis, which we so often find in chronic arthritic, but more frequently in acute inflammatory rheumatoid conditions, is, also, due to oxidative deficiency. Hyperthyroidism— which Kocher called thyrotoxicosis-and fever might both be merely defensive measures of the organism.

Varicosity frequently precedes arthritic and rheumatoid conditions and they are often closely associated. No need to explain that in such disorders stagnation of the circulation, directly, and impaired oxidation, indirectly, are the causative factors.

A frequent and important source of impaired circulation is the vasomotor constriction of the fine capillary vessels produced by the sympathetic nervous system. *This is a more common cause of arthritis and rheumatism (and possibly of hypertension) than we suppose.* Raynaud's and Charcot's arthropathies, and syringomyelia are considered of neurogenic origin. Whether it is a primary or secondary condition, an arterial spasm or

161

abnormal vasodilator response is another issue. A great deal of arthritism accompanies nervous states.

Psoriasis, the prevalent skin disorder, so far regarded refractory to treatments, is also caused by contraction of the capillary circulation. The nerve endings and capillary vessels of the epidermis are defective; therefore it is not surprising that psoriasis often accompanies arthritis. The etiology of psoriasis is considered rather doubtful. Some authors favor a parasitic theory; others say it is a neurogenic condition, as its appearance is generally symmetrical and often can be traced to some nervous disorder. Again, others give a hereditary-dietetic explanation.

Bourdillon, in 1888, was the first to notice the connection between psoriasis and the arthritic conditions. Psoriasis arthropathica (arthritis psoriatica) is a frequent combination. Psoriasis and arthritis are usually worst in the spring and fall. Peschel described repeated recurrences of psoriasis and arthritis at exactly the same time. Falk, also, noticed in 14 out of 29 cases of arthritis psoriatica the identical phenomenon. Exacerbation of the respective symptoms and also recurrences often occur simultaneously. On the other hand, according to Asberger, some observers at Dr. Bier's clinic noticed that when psoriasis improves arthritis becomes worse, and vice versa. We have to suspect that the concurrent changes in both conditions must be due to the central nervous system. Even topographically, in many instances, there is a parallelism in the outbreak of both diseases.

It is a rather peculiar fact that, while arthritis predominates in women, the complication of arthritis and psoriasis occurs more frequently in males. Adrian reported 87 cases of combined arthritis and psoriasis, 68 of which were men and 19, women. The percentages were 78 and 22 respectively. Falk, in 29 cases, found 22 men and 7 women; that is, 76% men and 24% women. The congruity of percentages is worthy of note.

Bucky and Müller, during their X-ray research work, found that there is a special connection between the skin and the autonomic nervous system. As proof, when they injected a nonspecific protein, like aolan, into the skin, a local leukocytosis and a corresponding dilatation of the splanchnic vessels resulted. If certain branches of the sympathetic nerves were severed and they injected aolan into the skin which was originally controlled by these cut branches, there was no leukocytosis, while it did develop on other skin surfaces.

Neuwirth and Weiss achieved remarkable results in treating climacteric arthritides by packing the abdominal regions and the thighs in hot Pistany mud. These authors suggested that the intense and protracted hyperemia and hyperthermia penetrate the deeper tissues and the parenteral absorption of protein bodies promotes endocrine activity. Likewise, the energetic stimulation of the skin powerfully influences the endocrine glands and the vegetative nervous system.

An angiospastic condition of the hypertonic capillaries will result in stasis and in poor nutrition of the joints and muscles, producing consequent untoward metabolic changes. Next to the asthenic, chlorotic, and lymphatic individuals, the nervous excitable types are most disposed to be sufferers from rheumatoid ailments. They are distinctly spasmophile subjects. In such states, we may often observe fluctuations, manifestations of changes-for better or worse-and, although on superficial observation the cause may seem to be obscure, it can be easily explained by the alternation of the neuropathic conditions. If we are optimistically disposed, we may frequently "blame" our treatments for the conspicuous, sudden improvement. Numerous authors rationally attribute the cause of arthritis deformans to the influence of the central nervous system, induced by anxiety, prolonged nervous strain, or sudden shock.

Capillary circulation is a favorite topic of many research workers. It is rather surprising how much the reflex influence on capillary circulation is still disputed in medical literature. All one has to do to test this reflex action is to place one hand in cold or hot water and observe the contraction or dilatation and the decrease or increase in the velocity of the capillary circulation of the other hand. The ophthalmologist fully comprehends the significance of this reflex correlation.

Rowntree and Adson, of the Mayo Clinic, performed bilateral lumbar sympathetic ganglionectomy and ramisectomy for the relief of polyarthritis. Their first patient was a woman of 34 years, a stenographer. In 1917, she was injured in a railroad accident and confined to bed for a considerable length of time. When admitted to the hospital she had been suffering from generalized arthritis for six years and was entirely incapacitated for work. She gave a typical picture of chronic polyarthritis: cold, clammy hands, and all extremities cold and cyanotic, which signified a constriction of the arterioles, capillaries, and venules of the skin. Her hemoglobin was 65%.

The operation at first consisted of the removal of the second, third, and fourth lumbar sympathetic ganglia and of the division of the corresponding rami to the hypogastric plexus. This made quite a striking change in the patient's condition. After the operation her feet were dry, normally pink and had a pleasant sensation of warmth. The pains disappeared entirely and also the sizable tophi on the great toes. Was soon able to walk two miles without effort.

Of course, the operation had no effect on the upper extremities. The hands were quite a contrast, cold and clammy, distressingly painful. Temperature of the hands was 9° C. lower than that of the feet. Patient asked for a cervical sympathetic ganglionectomy to obtain relief.

In another article, Rowntree and Adson gave a summary of the second operation performed on the same patient. She returned to the hospital in October, 1928, and stated that she had experienced a complete cure from the hopeless arthritis deformans of the lower extremities, which had persisted for six years prior to the operation. She described the sensation from waist down as "cozy" during the two and a half years following the operation. Patient lived in the northern part of Canada, did plenty of walking during the cold winters, without even the suggestion of a return of the arthritis in the lower extremities, which had a pleasant warmth, without pain in the joints.

The upper extremities were diametrically opposite, in bad condition. Could type only with one finger. The shoulders, elbows and hands gradually became worse, with intense pain. Her hands were cold, clammy, bathed in perspiration. A typical configuration of arthritis deformans; no grip in either hand. The operation was performed November 3, 1928, in which the cervical and first and second thoracic sympathetic ganglia were removed. Immediately the hands became perfectly dry, warmer and of normal pink color. Could make a fist and grip a hand. The elevation of temperature in both hands was striking. Patient was dismissed January 7, 1929. Returned in March, with arms much improved, better muscular tone, hands warm and dry, fingers more shapely. Adson performed 16 similar operations, 14 lumbar and 2 cervico-thoracic sympathetic resections, resulting in distinctly beneficial neuro-circulatory changes.

These reports are unusually instructive as they prove that arthritis deformans is due to the vasoconstriction of the sympathetic nerve endings, producing ischemia and, indirectly, suboxidation.

PATHOLOGICAL CHANGES

We have discussed so far the main causes of arthritis and other rheumatoid conditions, suggesting that *they are due to suboxidation*, produced by impaired circulation, respectively a defective distribution of blood and lymph.

Now what are the effects and consequences of defective circulation and insufficient oxidation which, at the same time, are the indirect causes of arthritis and rheumatism?

They are:
a- Disturbed local metabolism; and
b- Bacterial growth.

Disturbed Local Metabolism

The disturbed local chemistry of the muscles and joints is a great factor in hindering their normal function and altering their structure. The increased CO_2 concentration, the precipitation of calcium and magnesium elements, lacto-phosphate of lime, etc., the subsequent ossification of the joints, are the effects of the underlying pathological causes. The blood flow beyond the area of the local lowered circulation may be normal again.

While normal or high temperature saves the tissues from the harmful lime salt deposits and other metabolic waste, low temperature is conducive to the formation of such deposits, the accumulation of acids, even calcareous concretions, producing arthritis, rheumatism, fibrosities, neuritis, gout, etc. In animal experimentation, through ligation of the arteries as a consequence of disturbed and lowered blood and lymph supply a calcareous or bony overgrowth will result-in brief, hypertrophic or osteo-arthritis.

The colloidal chemistry of muscles and joints explains the pathology of rheumatism and arthritis. Muscles especially play a more important part in producing these conditions than we realize. As a proof, some authors claim that in 90% of so-called sciatic neuritis cases the pathological state is not in the nerves, but in the muscles. We know the greatest lack of oxygen and, likewise, of hemoglobin is near bones and joints, while the major part of the body metabolism—over 50% of all physico-chemical processes of the organism-takes place in the muscles, which include the heart, gastro-intestinal and respiratory musculature.

The molecular, chemo-thermodynamic mechanism of oxidation creates our energy. Lactic acid, this product of tissue metamorphosis, which is formed in an anaerobic way from carbohydrates (glycogen), is easily

165

oxidized and is the greatest creator of muscle energy. Muscular contractions are produced through osmotic processes. The anoxybiotic "glycogen-born" lactic acid (the quotation marks are my own), in explosive contact with oxygen, creates and supplies not only the thermic heat of the body but also the kinetic energy. Is it chemistry or perhaps physics, like friction? As interesting and as important as this metabolic study may be, it is much beyond our subject.

Lactic acid, which has an intensely acid reaction, is easily neutralized by salts, and is their natural solvent. The greatest portion is oxidized, transformed into CO_2 and water which are eliminated through the lungs and skin. If lactic acid, which we may consider as potential energy, is not oxidized, in a word, not consumed, it will form deposits. The muscles become rigid, shortened, and contracted—especially the flexors, which are stronger— causing considerable dysfunction and pain. These same pathological processes will also influence the joints.

Defective circulation, lack of oxygen, will materially retard the consumption of lactic acid. Fatigue is nothing else than an accumulation of this substance. During epileptic convulsions, a large amount of lactic acid is produced in the muscles; consequently, the victim feels great tiredness and exhaustion after the attacks. We know that in muscle-weak individuals the muscles and joints become tired very easily on account of faulty elimination of this substance, as the result of defective circulation (insufficient oxidation). While the muscles of a normal, robust individual, whose circulation is active -possibly through training-and who, therefore, has plenty of oxygen at his disposal, will not become sore after walking a long distance, an asthenic person, with atonic muscles, covering the same route, will complain of "pains and aches." The asthenic person has another handicap, too, because in the majority of cases he is less protected by a fat covering, and is deprived of the necessary heat, which greatly assists oxidation.

From a pathological standpoint, there is no better explanation for rheumatism and arthritis than the accumulation (suboxidation) of lactic acid-the identical condition present in rigor mortis. A muscle contraction is really a brief, short-lived, transient rigor mortis, during which the amassed lactic acid is used up by oxidation, generating heat and energy. A relaxed muscle is one from which the lactic acid has been eliminated.

The systemic salts (sodium, potassium, calcium, etc.) play an important rôle in these metabolic processes as neutralizers of lactic acid. If the salt equilibrium of the organism is disturbed, the condition may have considerable harmful consequences. According to some authors (Peritz) the

166

salt deficiency will produce, even through reflex action of the sympathetic nerve system, a contraction of the capillary vessels.

It is rather interesting that, years ago, the followers of the chemical school, who attempted to explain rheumatoid conditions by claiming that they are caused by metabolic changes, favored lactic acid as materies morbi. Prout, Todd, Williams, Fuller, Headland, Spencer Wells, Richardson, Foster, all favored the lactic acid theory. Recently Wilde, Peritz, and others have supported this belief.

Richardson, in 1856, reported that he injected the substance into the peritoneal cavity of experimental animals, producing swelling and pain in all joints. Balthazar Foster, in 1874, described his clinical experiments. He gave lactic acid internally, with the result that patients complained of acute pains in the joints and limbs. When he discontinued administering the substance, the pains stopped. He repeated this procedure several times; and when he gave lactic acid the pains invariably reappeared, the joints became swollen, red, hot and painful, with raised temperature of 101° F. Foster firmly believed that rheumatoid conditions are produced by lactic acid.

Wilde thought that lactic acid has been very much neglected lately. It is all uric acid today. He called attention to the fact that uric acid is an abnormal product, while lactic acid is always present in the system. Exercise raises the temperature by reason of excessive lactic acid. Uric acid contains lactic acid. While lactic acid is more painful in the system than uric acid, it is a vital necessity, but if the circulation is unaffected, it is doing no harm. Wilde, as a proof, mentioned one of his experiences, that of a lady, whose skin had been inactive since infancy. Otherwise, she was robust and took a great amount of exercise. The joints were free, but if she were confined to bed for a week, for some reason lithic deposits appeared in all large joints as evidence of their existence, but as soon as she resumed her exercise, they disappeared and she had no gout, swelling, or pain.

Cajori, Crouter, and Pemberton found that the blood, urine, and sweat of those suffering from rheumatoid ailments and normal persons did not show any difference with regard to their lactic acid content. Of course, the sweating experiment, induced in an electric baking apparatus, is not an infallible proof against the theory. Lactic acid is an unstable substance, combines, and dissociates very readily. It is possible that the effect of heat hastened its oxidation, which might explain its absence in the sweat.

Circulatory disturbances will also produce lowered sugar tolerance, with the natural consequence of diminished sugar utilization. The organism can utilize glucose to a certain degree, that is, until it reaches its sugar tolerance. In animals, according to Woodyatt, we can inject intravenously chemically pure glucose, and its material part will be utilized until it reaches the saturation limit. In dogs and rabbits, 0.8 gram of glucose per kilogram of body weight can be injected for seven hours without producing glycosuria. Defective sugar utilization will result in a delay or stoppage of sugar removal. This principle is applicable not only to the general system but also to localized areas. In local ischemic portions of the body, the glucose will not be utilized, that is oxidized, and retention will be the logical consequence. Glucose, remaining for a longer period in any tissue, will unquestionably have harmful effects. The constriction of fine capillary vessels, whether produced by internal or external influences, will result in general or local suboxidation, underconsumption and a decreased removal of sugar. We know that more than three-fourths of arthritics suffer from low sugar tolerance. While in diabetics there is increased elimination of sugar, in arthritics it is just the opposite. This is the reason that we rarely find severe diabetic conditions complicated by arthritis.

Joint fluids also are closely dependent on the blood. If proper glycolysis is missing, it is due to lack of leukocytes. Suppurative joint fluids have low sugar content, high acidity and abundant leukocytes. Cajori, Crouter, and Pemberton said: "Joint fluids contain (1) nutritive, (2) harmful substances. Little is known of its function; probably it has a lubricating rôle. Cartilage contains a considerable amount of glycogen. After glucose ingestion, the rise in blood sugar is promptly followed by a rise of sugar concentration in joint fluids."

Pemberton remarked in another article: "Joint fluids are in very close communion with the blood stream. Sugar ingested by mouth may reach the joint fluids almost immediately and in such concentration as even to exceed that of the glucose of the blood. Glucose is necessary for the nutrition of the avascular central portion of articular cartilage. It is clear that glucose and presumably other products of normal digestion may reach the from the intestinal tract to detrimental substances." joint fluids in excess amount...also the way is open to the joint cavity from the intestinal tract and detrimental substances.

Changes in the synovial fluid will disarrange all joints. Its chemical composition, its viscosity, due to its mucin content, its sugar concentration, carbon dioxide, uric acid, nitrogen, etc., are all influenced by the blood circulation. Purin metabolism, the trans formation of purins, depends on the action of enzymes, which are supplied by the blood. When the system, for instance, is slow to remove uric acid by oxidation, there will be retention and deposits. The same applies to nitrogen, which will be retained by delayed and defective excretion. In gout we find monosodium urate in the joints. Gout is a typical disorder produced by suboxidation. It is a chemical arthralgia. Though it is considered that it is caused by defective purin metabolism or by some food idiosyncrasies, often accompanied by eczema, migraine, etc., the underlying indirect cause is suboxidation. Gouty subjects have subnormal temperature and, as a rule, very inactive skin.

In England, gout is very prevalent, mainly on account of badly heated houses. Part of the body may be warm from the fireplace, while the feet are cold. Wilde was convinced that the widespread belief that gout was caused by port wine is a delusion. On the contrary, the inhabitants of England suffer from subnormal temperature, which is more a producer of than excessive drinking. Alcohol raises the temperature and increases gout metabolism. Prohibition would only increase gout, and Wilde was convinced that more arthritis is caused by too much food than by the consumption of alcoholic drinks.

Any abnormality of the synovial fluid, either as to quantity or quality, abnormal deposits of glucose or mineral elements, will greatly contribute to the dysfunction, stiffness, and pain in the joints. A decrease in quantity will result in lack of lubrication; an increase, in hydrarthrosis, which is, also, a hindrance to their proper functioning; the muscular, tendinous, pericapsular and nervine tissues will all be influenced. The pathological changes, as a rule, correspond to the degree and chronicity of the disease. Necrosis of the cartilages is not infrequent.

The success of some practitioners in injecting a large amount of normal saline solution into the proximity of the seat of the disorder, affording sometimes a surprising relief, may be explained as the flushing of the toxic substances and metabolic wastes.

Finally, I mention another fact, which might have some contributory effect in aggravating rheumatoid conditions, namely, the faulty removal of dead cells from the organism. These cast-off cells must be eliminated. Active circulation of blood and lymph is certainly helpful in the proper discharge of this function.

Bacterial Growth

Inadequate circulation and lowered defensive power will favor bacterial growth, especially in the joints, on account of their anatomical structure.

But bacterial growth is not the producing cause of arthritis, only a secondary, intervening, or at best, an interdependent consequence of insufficient oxidation and scanty blood supply.

The omnipresent bacteria, these remarkable colonizers, can be compared to downright opportunists: when and wherever they "spy" a suitable, expedient spot, they will encamp.

The streptococci of chronic arthritics, compared with other streptococci, always have a low virulence; increased circulation and a consequent elevation of the body resistance may easily destroy them. In acute arthritis of the young, they are of a more fulminant type. Chills, high fever, and acute pain accompany them. In the old, they are just the resultant local manifestations of systemic disorders. The symptoms are those of long-standing, true toxemia: low fever, clammy hands, inactive skin, poor complexion, lack of appetite, etc. Intestinal absorption may contribute to the production of such somatic states, but some authors doubt it.

Infective foci undoubtedly produce arthritic and rheumatoid ailments. These secondary infective arthritic conditions are plain and simple metastatic processes; the transference of infective (not septic) substances-by the blood vessels or lymph channels-from the septic foci to the joints could result just as well in an endocardial, meningeal, pleural or peritoneal invasion if the circulatory and oxidizing facilities of these organs were as inadequate as those of the joints. Under such conditions, the organism is in an anaphylactic state, sensitized by the gradual absorption of protein substances from the "smoldering" focal infection. Chvostek even suggested the possibility that arthritis is not caused by bacteria but by the toxins produced by them. The removal of an infected focus is often followed by recovery. Another consideration is whether such toxemia is not caused by lack of proper circulation. In the majority of cases, this is true. In certain parts of Russia, arthritis is very uncommon and pyorrhea universal. It is proof that local foci do not always have harmful effects when the circulation and oxidation are not impaired. *Sapienti sat!*

Nasal, pharyngeal, dental focal infections, those originating in the respiratory or abdominal organs or anywhere else, may and will produce absorption of toxic substances and secondary rheumatoid states, but, on the other hand, we must take into consideration another eventuality—that, while the organism is preoccupied in a defensive effort to combat these invasions, through mobilization of its blood supply as a pyretic measure or by producing antibodies, there is a possibility of a corresponding neglect to other superseded organic parts. Under such circumstances the joints are deprived of their prerogatives, the necessary blood and lymph supply to which they are fully entitled, more so because their blood supply is generally limited-on account of their anatomical construction, as already stated. I might just as well mention here a rather peculiar phase, namely, that bacterial toxins which contribute to the production of rheumatoid conditions show special affinity to sensory nerves and only rarely touch the motor nerves, as diphtheria and tetanus do.

The bacteriological theory of rheumatoid conditions has many followers and a wide application. Often, valuable time is lost by administering vaccines, debilitating the patients, wasting their energy and resistance, which they so badly need. We are still far away from success in curing arthritic and rheumatoid ailments, either by active immunization with isolated bacteria or by passive immunization with sera. Disturbed defensive mechanism is more detrimental than the focal infection. Co-existence is no evidence. A streptococcal etiology, even of acute inflammatory rheumatism, has yet to be proven. The "lock and key" analogy is very enticing, but as a rule we find that the key does not fit and the "research" for a master-key is just a futile attempt.

Cause of Pain

Before concluding this particular section which treats the pathological changes in arthritic and rheumatic conditions, I wish to touch upon another rather pertinent question-what causes the pain in these ailments?

Physical pain as an abnormal sensory impression is discomforting and distressing... we can add just as many adjectives as its quality, intensity and duration will warrant... and the number is infinite! It might be tenderness, numbness, smarting, or annoying soreness; a burning, throbbing, lancinating sensation; even a tormenting, excruciating, crucifying pain-finally, agony and hell, terrific, dreadful and indescribable.

Now what is pain? It is a "telepathic" (in the strictest sense of the word, tele, Gr.=far off; pathos, Gr. = suffer) alarm, announcing a disturbed molecular equilibrium. The perception of pain is a subjective impression caused by objective mechanical or chemical stimuli, conveyed by the recipient sensory nerves to the sense-perceptive center of the brain.

Unquestionably, it is a protective mechanism of great biological utility. Pain is our best friend (this allusion is not made from a material standpoint, with the meaning that it brings us patients); it signifies and informs us that there is some anomaly either on the periphery or in the interiority of the system. It is really an S O S call of the organism, which alarm will not stop until relief is obtained.

The most illustrative physiological definition would be that pain is "pressure." There are very few... if any... painful impressions which we could not explain with this one word "pressure." Whether it is an injury, inflammation, congestion, new growth, collection of metabolic waste, or any one the of innumerable other conditions, the pain is induced by pressure on terminal filaments or on the sensory nerve proper. (To discuss hyperesthesia, paresthesia, hysteria, sensations simulating pain, etc., is much beyond our plan.) If medical men would always keep this in mind... in all their professional work... and, instead of inhibiting the perceptive center, would pay all attention to treating, not the effects, but the causes-which would consist of removing the pressure, it would mean the betterment and great advance of medicine.

Pain, in our case, relates to joints, bones, muscles, tendons, cartilages, synovial membranes, even to the subcutaneous tissues, and the skin itself. A lack of oxidation, the accumulation of CO_2 and other metabolic wastes, or a local anemia, constriction of the capillary vessels, arterial and venous blockade, interfering with the propulsion of blood and causing passive congestion a back pressure without inflammation, or an active inflammatory condition, will all produce pressure on the nerve endings, and cause pain. May I add here, with regard to articular pain, that the ache, though it seems to be located in the joints, is only in their proximity.

The defensive (curative) power of the organism will make a strong effort to remedy any such abnormal pathological conditions and will try to overcome them by enforced circulation.

Pain-conducting is not, however, the sole function of the nerves; the irritation will possibly even provoke simultaneously, through a protective reflex action, a capillary dilatation and an increased supply of needed blood. Active and passive movements, force or any tension (like weight-bearing), will only increase the pressure on the peri and intra-articular sensory nerves. There is almost a temptation to divide arthritic conditions into two groups: I, arthritis, where the energy reserve is sufficient to make an attempt to overcome pathological conditions, and may even succeed; and 2, arthrosis, where there is not sufficient power in the organism and, therefore, it is unable to combat the disease. It is possible that the more active inflammatory character of arthritis and rheumatism of the young, in contrast with the torpid course and progress of similar conditions in older subjects-without inflammation, with no raised, but even lowered temperature-can be explained by the presence, decrease or absence of the defensive mechanism in the system.

Predisposing Influences

Undoubtedly, there are predisposing influences in certain organisms which are conducive to the acquirement of these diseases. Individual constitution is often even more important than etiology. The following is a summary of the main groups:

1) Hereditary tendency; which especially favors their development.
2) Female sex; much more susceptible than the male.
3) Poor metabolism, defective elimination, acid diathesis, endocrine imbalance, etc.
4) Chlorotic, anemic, asthenic individuals, with poor nutrition, weak muscles, thin fat covering, etc.
5) Stout people, with poor circulation, who are easily bruised and fatigued, and have poor musculature.
6) Nervous, irritable types (angiospastic).

CURATIVE EFFECTS OF BEE VENOM

And now for the bee venom therapy! My highly respected and esteemed reader, I fully comprehend your thoughts. You expect me to say that all the enumerated difficulties which a well-educated and intelligent physician cannot overcome without the assistance of a whole army of specialists, our poor, insignificant little friend, the bee, will do all by herself! Far from it, sorry to disappoint you, but I can tell you right now that she will do surprisingly more for you than you expect.

What is to be taken away, you must do yourself. Search for and remove all exogenous and endogenous contributory causes and she will do the rest. Rather odd, isn't it?

I have too much regard and consideration for you to anticipate that will just take my word and will use this little-known, unaccepted, and almost unheard-of remedial agent without obtaining a proper explanation. It would be rather an effrontery or insult on my part, which is the least of my intentions. I am firmly convinced that you would never expose your patients to such risk and danger.

Before I give an explanation of what contributes to the production of these unique curative effects of bee venom, for your satisfaction I just mention the fact that the remedy has been used by hundreds of physicians all over Europe, in well-known clinics and hospitals of highest repute, in thousands of cases, and *not a single instance has been reported where it has done any harm or produced injurious effects*. The administration of this remedial agent must commence with a minimum amount and the divided doses must be increased gradually, both with respect to the number of injections and the concentration of the solution. We shall discuss all this in Chapter XI.

The curative value of bee venom is due mainly to its hemorrhagic and neurotoxic properties-especially to the former.

The *hemorrhagic effect* of bee venom is not only a powerful action on blood itself, stimulating the circulation, but also on the blood vessels. This is the best explanation and interpretation of its efficiency. *Bee venom accelerates and intensifies the circulation, and dilates the capillary vessels. It has a distinct endotheliolytic action, to such an extent that it opens the capillary walls, enabling the blood cells to transmigrate into the tissues.* This will result in an increased metabolism and, on account of the greater supply of oxygen, in an adequate oxidation, additional heat supply, improved elimination of accumulated waste, and destruction of bacterial growth-in other words, required to correct the existing harmful pathological conditions and to restore the disturbed normal physiological state.

Necropsies of animals, after severe bee venom intoxications, show abundant blood effusions in all cavities of the organisms and hemorrhages of the mucous and serous surfaces, hepatic and peritoneal bleeding. Very often a leakage of blood can be found outside of the capillaries which form hemorrhagic areas in the tissues. The strong effect of the venom on menstruation, which we will describe later, is due to this property.

The physiological effects of bee venom can be best compared with those of histamine, which produces a noticeable dilatation and relaxation of the arterioles and capillaries, increased circulatory speed of the blood stream, lowering the arterial and increasing the venous pressure. After a hypodermic injection of histamine, even to the naked eye the dilated capillaries on the face and finger nails are plainly visible. In the whole body, it produces a sensation which is comparable to the "hot" climacteric flushes. Ruhmann thought that urticaria of the skin is due to the effect of histamine.

Pogany proved that histamine, administered intravenously in experimental animals:

1) Dilated the arterioles and capillaries, and increased the capillary pressure, which influenced the venous pressure.
2) Caused contraction of the veins.
3) By contracting the veins of the lungs, produced stagnation in the right heart.

Pogany found, also, that the syndrome was similar to that of Basedow's disease, and both conditions exhibited great sensitivity to adrenalin.

Deutsch, likewise, found that histamine has a distinct vasodilator effect on the small vessels, at the same time provoking a reflex central irritation. He thought that, so far, histamine excels all known remedies in the treatment of arthritis and rheumatism. Injected into the painful muscles, it has remarkable alleviating power, which is not due to any direct anesthetic effect, but can be attributed only to vasodilator action. In exposure to cold, especially in inactive states, there will be a lack of histamine in the cells of the organism, which, when replaced, will relieve spasm and pain. The usual empiric, symptomatic treatments of arthritis and rheumatism with physiotherapeutical measures (massage, spas, local irritants), mechanical, thermic, electric, and actinic treatments, have only one purpose-to increase circulatory speed, produce hyperemia and histamine. The circulatory speed of the rheumatic and arthritic is, as a rule, diminished and histamine produces a derivative action.

Harmer and Harris used 1:1000 histamine-acid-phosphate in nor mal saline solution, in their injections for clinical experiments. The most striking effect was the dilatation of the minute blood vessels of the skin, associated with an increased rate of blood flow. Reddening of the skin, and the raising of its temperature were the manifested phenomena; the increase of the limb volume was ascribed to the same cause. Subcutaneous veins assumed an increased tone. Blood pressure, both systolic and diastolic, fell slightly. Transudation of fluid from blood vessels into tissue space definitely increased, attributed to the intensified permeability of the vessel walls. Pulse rate was augmented by about twenty beats a minute. The respiration rate was usually not affected. Injected intravenously, the effects were complete in about three to four minutes. These effects occurred even in doses 500 times smaller than those used in animal experiments.

If we carefully observe the physiological effects of histamine, we cannot fail to notice their great similarity, almost identity, to those produced by bee venom, which would explain the action, utility, and efficacy of the venom in the management and treatment of arthritic and rheumatoid conditions.

The *neurotoxic effects* are like those of many other venoms of the same type. Arndt-Schulz's great homeopathic theories were that 1, diseased organs are more sensitive to drugs than healthy ones; and that, 2, small doses of poison are stimulants while large doses paralyze. Both points are not only plausible but very true and are especially applicable to our subject.

We often find that toxic substances, if given in carefully graduated doses, produce a sedative effect upon the nerve centers and act as a physical and mental tonic. Many poisonous drugs have beneficial effects. The same can be said of bee venom. The hemorrhagin, an important component of bee venom, will dilate the capillaries and make them permeable to blood. The neurotoxic action is similar, since by paralysis it releases the capillary constriction of the nerve endings of the sympathetic nervous system. It produces an intrarachidian anesthesia, paralyzing the peripheral terminals of the sensory nerves. In addition, it has a powerful tonic effect.

Whether there is a specific action as in the case of foreign protein therapy, as some authors believe, is irrelevant-the main consideration is efficiency. Pemberton remarked that the nervous system is importantly concerned in arthritis. Sharp anxiety and emotional strain often produce surprising, temporary benefits. We cannot exclude the conjecture that the psychic influence, which is supposed to accompany the nonspecific protein injections, may also constitute a part of the reactive mechanism when the injections with bee venom are given.

(C. Flandin, of France, and his associates recently achieved remarkable results in the treatment of arthritics with Chinese acupuncture. This age-old procedure was employed in China and Japan for thousands of years and consisted of driving gold or silver needles into the tissues with a mallet or by twisting. If the involvements were more extensive, they used many needles, leaving them in place for hours, even days. This method was revived many times during past centuries; Dr. Louis Berlioz, father of the musical composer, was one of those who used it with great success, not only in arthritic and rheumatoid conditions, but for many nervous afflictions, like hiccups, asthma, hemiplegia, contractures, etc.

The French author's success was so striking that they were convinced it could not be attributed solely to local counterirritation but to some reflex action of the sympathetic nervous system. They applied only superficial punctures of rather short duration, stressing the importance of precise topography, which is yet undefined.)

The parenteral application of foreign substances has a specific omni cellular effect, possibly on the endocrines or on other glands, bone marrow, spleen, etc., and, also, on the pyrogenic center, promoting oxidation. Their ability to arouse universal protoplasm activity accounts for the invigorating and tonic effects which they produce and, also, for their indirect influence on certain local pathological disturbances which, perchance, may exist.

Keiter, for many years collaborator of Terc, who administered bee venom in thousands of cases, frequently stated that when anemic people were treated with it he often noticed remarkable improvement in their condition. It apparently had the same effect as intravenous injections of iron and arsenic. Keiter, also, noticed that if the treatments were given to women, even between menstrual periods, they showed temporary menorrhea. In pregnancy, this sometimes led to abortion. It is possible, as already mentioned, that some fatal cases of bee stings reported in older persons, after only one sting, were due to cerebral hemorrhage.

Whether there is any special selective affinity of bee venom to the sugar content of the blood and joints is yet to be proved. So far, to my knowledge, nobody has considered the question but I strongly suspect that bee venom may have some physico-chemical effect on the glucose of the organism, possibly even as a catalyzer. I wish I could experimentally support this statement but to my regret I cannot, and, therefore, I have to leave this, another fertile field, for the physicist and biochemist.

R. T. Woodyatt said: "In the body, a special glucolytic enzyme (alkali carrier or intensifier) destroys the glucose selectively. All sugar must become glucose before it is destroyed. Alkali administration may also increase glucose utilization. It might be conceived that the cells contain molecules of a glycolytic catalyst or enzyme. As fast as glucose molecules enter the cell, they come into collision with the catalyst molecules, perhaps combining with them, and as a result of the encounter the glucose molecules would be dissociated into unsaturated fragments or ions. From the moment of union or dissociation they would cease to behave as glucose molecules." (A fermentative splitting is required before sugar can be oxidized, which Woodyatt appropriately called "dissociation.")

According to Cohnheim's theory the muscles form a glycolytic enzyme for which the pancreas supplies an essential activator. Allen suggested that the pancreas supplies an amboceptor, which is necessary for a proper colloidal sugar combination. Landsteiner thought that chemical changes alone may be sufficient to account for specificity, but another question is still open, whether physical properties play any part in determining specificity, like electric charges, ionization of an amphoteric electrolyte. Professor Rosenbach, of Berlin, suggested that the biologist should not be satisfied to describe just the stabile symptoms. A functional diagnosis is important. Kinetic factors, dynamic conditions, the consideration of harmonious synergy are essential. May we apply this to the effect of bee venom? As Hopkins stated, dynamics of living matter must always remain beyond the reach of chemical studies since at the moment when chemical methods are applied the materials ceased to be alive.

Does the effect represent the transmitted, concentrated, dynamic energy of the sun? Meyerhof thought the difficult question of what purposes the chemical exchange of energy serves cannot yet be completely answered. The study of some measured exchanges of energy has led to the fundamental problem of cell energetics, namely, the storage of the sun's energy in green plants. The greatest part of radiant energy can be changed into chemical work under proper conditions. Possibly, some time, we shall succeed in explaining the utilization of oxidation energy in the chemical metabolism of cells.

The new cosmogonic theory of nuclear physics is building an intellectual "bridge," linking the material and nonmaterial... and "something" with no dimensions may assume a three-dimensional existence... and electro-magnetism can be converted into matter in the form of pairs of electrons and positrons.... Why could not the action, also, be reversed and matter be converted into radiation? According to Einstein, the modern interpreter of the major mysteries of physics, substance and energy are the same and theoretically one can be converted into the other.

No doubt, we have made tremendous progress and advancement in the knowledge of the physical and chemical nature of matter, but we are yet in utter darkness with respect to some occult power and its laws, which harmoniously control, regulate and coördinate the vital functions. All phenomena cannot be explained by physics and chemistry. There are some other basic, yet-to-be-discovered, extra, or better call them, supreme vital forces to be considered. We are more than physico-chemical automata. The study and interpretation of vital forces still remain "open"-so far defying all known analytical methods.

Recent biological studies link plants and animals more closely. Porphyrin, the base of red blood-cells, is also the base of chlorophyl, the green coloring matter of plants. Chlorophyl is derived from the energy of the sun. The combined with iron, while the porphyrin of green plants contains magnesium. only difference in these two substances is that porphyrin of the blood is combined with iron, wile the porphyrin of green plants contains magnesium.

C. B. Coulter, of Columbia University, extracted cytochrome, a pink pigment found in all living creatures which use oxygen. This fact establishes a powerful relationship between the chlorophyl-green plants and red-blooded animal life.

We know the marvelous effect of bee venom on honey. Honey will keep for centuries without fermenting and fouling, due not only to its high sugar concentration, but also to the action of the venom which it contains only in a very minute quantity. Possibly, beekeepers who are saturated with bee venom have no lowered sugar tolerance, no delayed sugar elimination, but sufficient potential capacity to utilize sugar. This may be one of the reasons why they do not suffer from rheumatic ailments.

Bees feed only on the purest pollen of flowers. They convert or distil from this substance, in their mysterious alchemic laboratory, the venom. And what is pollen? The endocrines of the plants and trees.

Terc, more practical and rational than scientific, used bee venom for over 40 years, successfully treating thousands of cases, but never approached the subject for a theoretical explanation. He was interested only in therapy and clinical results, reminding me of an excellent cook who uses the fire for his art but is not interested in its chemistry.

CHAPTER REFERENCES

ADRIAN, E. D. The nervous mechanism of pain, Univ. Coll. Hosp. M., 1929.

ADRIAN, E. Über Arthropathia psoriatica, Mitt. a. d. Grenzgeb. d. Med. u. Chir., Jena, 1924.

ALLEN, F. M. Studies Concerning Glycosuria and Diabetes, Boston, 1913.

ASBERGER, A. Über den Zusammenhang des Psoriasis mit Gelenkerkrankungen, 1927.

ASCHNER, B. Klinik und Behandlung Menstruationstörungen, Stuttg. u. Leipz., 1931.

BANNATYNE, G. A. Rheumatic arthritis, its pathology, morbid anatomy and treatment, London, 1904.

BARCROFT, J. The respiratory function of the blood, Cambridge, 1914.

BARKER, L. F. Differentiation of the diseases included under chronic arthritis, Am. J. M. Sc., Phila., Jan. 1914.

BEHAN, R. J. Pain, 1922.

BERGMANN, N. Über Psoriasis und Gelenkerkrankungen, Diss., Berl., 1913.

BERLIOZ, L. Mémoire sur les maladies chroniques, les evacuations sanguines et l'acupuncture, Rev. d. Alcaloides, Oct. 1928.

BOURDILLON, H. Psoriasis et Arthropathie, Thése, 328, Par., 1888.

BUCKY, G., UND MÜLLER, E. F. Strahlende Energie, Haut und autonomes Nervensystem, München. Med. Wchnschr., 22, 1925.

CAJORI, CROUTER AND PEMBERTON. The alleged rôle of lactic acid in arthritis and rheumatoid conditions, Arch. Int. Med., Chicago, 34, 1924.
The physiology of synovial fluid, Arch. Int. Med., Chicago, 37, 1926.

CARRIER, E. B. Studies on the physiology of capillaries, Am. J. Physiol., Baltim., 61, 1922.

CECIL, R. L., AND ARCHER, B. H. Classification and treatment of chronic arthritis, J. Am. M. Ass., 87, 1926.

COATES, V., AND DELICATI, L. Rheumatoid Arthritis and Its Treatment, London, 1931.

COHNHEIM, J. Gesammelte Abhandlungen, Berlin, 1885.

CRAIG, H. K. Rheumatism, N. York M. J. (etc.), Sept. 1917.

CRUICKSHANK, J. The bacterial flora of the intestines in Health and Chronic Disease, Brit. M. J., Lond., Sept. 29, 1928.

DEEKS, W. E. Suggestions on the nature and treatment of rheumatism, N. York M. J. (etc.), March, 1906.

DEUTSCH, D. Histamin zur Therapie rheumatischer Erkrankungen, Med. Klin. Berl. u. Wien, 41, Oct. 1931.

FALK, N. Psoriasis arthropathica, Arch. f. Dermat. u. Syph. Wien u. Leipz., 129, 1921.

FISCHER, A. Blutbefunde bei rheumatischen Erkrankungen, Rheumaprobleme, 1929.

FLANDIN, FERREYROLLES ET DE LEPINAY. Traitment des algies par l'acupuncture chinoise, Bull. et mem. Soc. Med. d. Hop. de Par., May 1933.

FORSBROOK, W. H. C. A dissertation on Osteo-arthritis, London, 1893.

FOSTER, B. The synthesis of acute rheumatismus, Clin. Med., Lond., 1874.

FREEDLANDER, S. O., AND LENHART, C. H. Clinical observations on the capillary circulation, Arch. Int. Med., Chicago, 29, 1922.

FREUND, E. Lehrbuch für Gelenkserkrankungen, Wien, 1929.

GAGE, W. V. The relation of capillary caliber to normal and pathological sensation and function, Med. Rec., N. Y., Sept. 1917.

GLOVER, J. A. A report on Chronic Arthritis, Ministry of Health Rep., 52, Lond., 1928.

GOLDSCHMIDT, S., AND LIGHT, A. B. A method obtaining from veins blood similar to arterial blood in gaseous content, J. Biol. Chem., N. Y., 64, 1925.

HARMER, J. M., AND HARRIS, K. E. Observations on the vascular reaction in man in response to histamine, Heart, Lond., XIII, 1926.

HOPKINS, SIR F. G. The problems of specificity in biochemical catalysis, Oxford, 1931.

KEITER, A. Rheumatismus und Bienenstichbehandlung, 1914.

KROGH, A. The supply of oxygen to the tissues and the regulation of the capillary circulation, J. Physiol., 52, 1918.

KROGH AND VIMTRUP. The Capillaries, Special Cytology, I, 1932.

LEWIS, TH. Studies of Capillary Pulsation, Univ. Coll. Hosp. Mag., IX, 2, 1924. The blood vessels of the human skin and their response, London, 1927.

LIVINGSTONE, A. T. The capillary and venous circulation in relation to disease, N. York M. J. (etc.), Nov. 29, 1919.

LLEWELLYN, L. J. Aspects of Rheumatism and Gout, London, 1927.

LOEVENHART, A. S. Certain aspects of biological oxidation, Arch. Int. Med., Chicago, 152, 1915.

LOMBARD, W. P. The blood pressure in arterioles, capillaries and small veins, Am. J. Physiol., 29, 1912.

MEYERHOF, O. Chemical dynamics of life phenomena, 1924.

MÜLLER, E. F. Strahlende Energie, Haut und autonomes Nervensystem, München. Med. Wchnschr., 22, 1925.

NATT, A. G., AND BOYD, L. J. The Pathology and Pharmacology of Apis Mellifica, J. Am. Inst. Homeop., 16, 1923.

NEUWIRTH, E., UND WEISS, E. Zur Behandlung chronischer Arthritiden der Frauen mit Schlamm, Arch. med. Hydrol., 3, Nov. 1933.

NICHOLS, E. H., AND RICHARDSON, F. L. Arthritis deformans, J. Med. Research, Bost., 16, 1909.

NOBL, G. Zur Kenntniss der Psoriasis Arthropathie, Arch. f. Dermat. u. Syph. Wien u. Leipz., 123, 1916.

PAP, L. Endocrine arthralgia, Orvosi hetil., Budapest, Oct. 1931.

PAUL, G. Das Wesen der Hautimpfung und ihre Bedeutung für die Bekämfung des chron. Rheumatismus, Wien, Med. Wchnschr., 14, 1927.

PAVY, F. W. On Carbohydrate metabolism, etc., Lond., 1906.

PEMBERTON, R. The significance and use of diet in treatment of chronic arthritis. N. York State J. M., 26, 1926.
Arthritis and Rheumatoid Conditions, their Nature and Treatment, 1930.

PERITZ, G. Der Muskelrheumatismus, Ergebn. der Ges. Med., 3, 1922.

PESCHEL, E. Psoriasis und Gelenksrheumatismus, Diss. Berl., 1897.

POGANY, J. Die Wirkung des Histamins auf die Blutgefässe des Menschen, Zeitschr. f. ges. Exper. Med., Berl., 75, 1931.

RICHARDSON, B. W. The cause of coagulation of the blood, Astley Cooper Prize Ess., 1856.

ROSENBACH, O. Energetik und Medizin, 1904.

ROWNTREE, L. J., AND ADSON, A. W. Bilateral lumbar sympathetic ganglionectomy and ramisectomy for polyarthritis of the lower extremities, J. Am. M. Ass., 88, 1927.
Polyarthritis, further studies of the effects of sympathetic ganglionectomy and ramisectomy, J. Am. M. Ass., July 1929.

ROWNTREE, ADSON, AND HENCH, P. S. Preliminary results of resection of sympathetic ganglia and trunks in 17 cases of chronic "infectious" arthritis. Amn. Int. Med., Nov. 1930.

RUHMANN, W. Die örtliche Histamin Einwirkung bei Muskel rheuma, München. Med. Wchnschr., Dec. 1931.

SCHMIDT, A. Der Muskelrheumatismus (Myalgie), 1918.

THRAENHART, Bienenstichbehandlung gegen Rheumatismus, Schweiz. Bien. Zeit., 1921.

UMBER, F. Zur Nosologie der Gelenkserkrankungen, 1929.

WALTER, H. E. The Human Skeleton, 1918.

WELLS, G. H. Chemical Pathology, 1925.

WEST, S. The form and frequency of cardiac complications in rheumatic fever, Practitioner, London, 1888.

WILDE, P. The Physiology of Gout, Rheumatism and Arthritis, London, 1921.
The pyretic treatment of rheumatism and allied disorders, London, 1928.

WOODYATT, R. F. Diabetes (Wells' Chem. Path.).

WOODYATT AND SANSUM, J. Biolog. Chem., N. Y., 30, 1917.

WYATT, B. L. Chronic arthritis, fibrosities, Diagnosis and treatment, 1933.

ZIMMER, A. Die Behandlung der rheumat. Krankheiten, Leipz., 1930.

.

Chapter X Apitherapy

GENERAL PRELIMINARY COMMENTS ON THEATMENT AND ITS TECHNIC

Bee venom for therapeutic purposes is administered by the injection of the substance into the intradermal tissues, faithfully imitating the action of the natural bee sting. I would also suggest the general acceptance of the term "apisination" for the procedure of inoculation with bee venom.

The technic is very simple. The water-clear solution is supplied in half c.c. and one c.c. ampoules and administered with a one c.c. correctly graduated Luer syringe. The usual dosage is 0.1 c.c. This amount, when injected into the intradermal strata, forms a "wheal." *It is a general rule never to use more than 0.1 c.c. in one wheal.* If we increase the dosage, it must be regulated in two ways:

1) By the gradual increase in the number of wheals, 1-2-3 or 2- 4-6, etc.; or

2) By gradually increasing the concentration of the solution.

By increasing the number of wheals, we obtain a larger surface action, a very important factor. When referring to a certain dosage, we have to mention only the number of wheals and the degree of concentration. If we say one wheal, it means O.I c.c. of venom of a certain concentration; ten wheals, one c.c. The most appropriate distance between the individual wheals is between one-half to one inch, depending on the number of wheals and the expected reaction. If we are near a reactive state and the wheals have a tendency to spread over a larger area, we must accordingly select a surface sufficiently large to prevent as much as possible their confluence.

For the site of the injections, we must select the extensor surfaces of the body, *carefully avoiding flexor surfaces* on account of the thin quality of skin and proximity or presence of arteries, veins, and lymph vessels. This is one of the prime considerations during the administration of treatments. An arterial or intravenous injection may produce a too rapid absorption; no local, but violent general effects; even the danger of an embolus. Some authors prefer the skin near the involvement of the respective joints (periarticular), e.g., wrist, elbow, knee, spine, etc. (loco dolenti). As a rule, the dorsal surfaces of the arms and legs, shoulder blades, or sacral region are used. As we sometimes have to expect a certain temporary disfigurement of the skin, hardening, pigmentation, and later desquamation of epidermis, when treating women, we must consider the fact that, on account of "décolleté," this may be objectionable.

As mentioned before, a one c.c. graduated Luer syringe is used, aspirating as much of the venom as we require for the number of wheals we intend to form. The most practical needle for the purpose is a specially constructed one of very fine gage (No. 27) with a very short bevel. Above the distal end of the point of the needle, at 1.75 millimeters distance, there is a small protruding knob which will prevent any deeper penetration of the skin and will accomplish our purpose of reaching the germinative strata of the intradermal tissue. In case we do not have a special needle, any fine gage, short bevel needle will serve the same purpose.

Scratch the ampoule with a file, which must be sterilized with the syringe and needle, above its shoulder, tap the head, and it will break off at the mark of the file. The syringe can be filled with or without the needle. After we have aspirated the required amount from the ampoule, the balance of the solution should not be used unless there is another patient available to whom it could be immediately administered, of course, with another needle. The strict warning not to use the remainder of the solution should be heeded, as *the substance quickly deteriorates if exposed to air*. The writer is using every effort to persuade the manufacturers to dispense the substance in rubber-sealed vials, which would enable us, by piercing the diaphragm, to withdraw any desired quantity and use the balance some other time, which would mean considerable saving. If we can have a bottle with a rubber diaphragm, the solution will have to be aspirated first with the help of an ordinary needle, to be substituted later by the special one, before the injection. All other rules, especially those of asepsis in hypodermic administrations, must be scrupulously carried out. Before use, hold the syringe vertically, needle point upward, and press on the plunger until all air is expelled. A few drops of the solution escaping through the needle will generally indicate that the air bubbles have been expelled.

The sterilization of the syringe and needle must be done only by boiling. Autoclaving a certain number of needles may also be practical. *No alcohol and, of course, no tincture of iodine must ever be used* either for disinfecting the syringe, needle, or the skin, as alcohol destroys bee venom very rapidly. This a very essential point. For disinfecting or cleansing the skin surface, our choice should be benzine, ether, chloroform, or acetone. Before administering the injection, it is always advisable to let the patient lie down, as in any regular hypodermic injection, to avoid possible needle-shock.

It is important that the skin should be stretched to give the needle a necessary resistance; otherwise the elastic skin will give way and the needle will not reach the intradermal layer. The stretching of skin depends on the choice of location. If we apply it on the upper or lower extremities or over joints, we grasp the patient's arm or leg below the site selected for the injection and, by a pull, stretch the skin downward between the thumb and the rest of the fingers of the left hand. If we administer the injection on other parts of the body, the best procedure is to stretch the skin horizontally between the thumb and index finger. The needle must be inserted into the outstretched skin with a sudden thrust-the knob of the special needle will prevent deeper penetration. After the needle has been inserted, a very slight withdrawal is sometimes necessary, depending entirely on the thickness of the skin. The syringe should be held between the thumb and middle finger of the right hand and applied vertically, reserving the use of the index finger to exert the necessary pressure on the top of the piston to express the required amount of the solution, which, as I have already mentioned, must be always 0.1 c.c. for each individual wheal.

An intradermal injection demands much more pressure than a hypodermic, more even than local infiltrations for skin anesthesia, on account of the greater resistance which is encountered; the subepidermal tissues are rather tough and resistant. The syringe must be absolutely airtight; likewise the needle firmly attached, or else it will result in a leak, possibly both ways—through the needle attachment and along the piston. If the needle has no Luer connection, "back-fire" can be anticipated. The procedure is a crucial test for a good Luer outfit.

Continuous sterilization will in time produce a leakage in the best Luer syringe. I suggest boiling the syringe and piston together, which will eliminate considerable erosion caused by boiling water, and it will remain airtight much longer. Experiments have proved that sterilization is just as effective whether boiling is done with the syringe and piston separated or inserted.

If we follow these rules, using a very sharp needle (which should be honed before use), and pierce the skin with a quick thrust, the manipulation will be absolutely painless, and the subsequent injection of the venom be only slightly felt. Of course, a lot depends on the individual sensitivity of the patient, but it does not hurt so much as a normal hypodermic injection when a solution is used which has no sharp, inflammatory effect. The injected quantity is so minute and the time required is so short that the sensation is almost negligible. Higher concentration produces a sharper sensation; but by that time the patient has become so used to it that it is hardly felt.

The next important consideration, outside of the number of wheals and the higher concentration of the solution, is the time interval between the administrations. The interval of time depends entirely on the adopted plan and on the reaction obtained from the last apisination. The reactions manifest themselves immediately and by gradual development attain a fairly complete state. Usually within ten or fifteen minutes after the injection, we have a fairly accurate picture. Then we can decide upon our future program.

The final purpose of the treatments in chronic cases is complete immunization of the patient to bee venom and, of course, the sooner we reach the point the quicker we are able to afford relief or cure. *We must start with a minimum number of wheals and also the weakest concentration of the solution* to test the tolerance of the patient and only then gradually advance. Immunization involves a certain time. In mild cases we may sometimes succeed with an energetic treatment, but in old chronic cases we have to expect delay and must not try to beat time by too forceful measures. Our motto should be: "Make haste slowly."

Referring to the interval, if we administer a certain number of wheals in the morning and there is no reaction, we may treat the same patient again in the afternoon with subsequently increased number of wheals, or a proportionately higher concentration and near-minimum number of wheals. For instance, if our last dosage was I-10 (ten wheals of I. concentration), we may give for our next dose II-2 (two wheals of II. concentration). This will often considerably shorten the whole course of treatment, and, as said before, the quicker we reach a reactive state, the earlier improvement will manifest itself, especially in more acute cases. In old chronic cases, we have to follow our predetermined plan.

Contributor Note:

See the annotations for Roman Numeral conversions on page viii.

Wheal: a suddenly formed elevation of the skin surface : Welt especially a flat burning or itching eminence on the skin. [58,59]

We must always bear in mind that our aim is immunization of the patient to bee venom, which is apparently-analogous to immunization to rheumatism and arthritis. The best guide in our progress is the reaction when and how it manifests itself.

The reactions are:

A, Local skin reactions;
B, General systemic reactions;
C, Focal reactions (in the affected joints or seat of pain).

These reactions we might consider as immunity reactions though they are really not. Rheumatics and arthritics have a certain degree of apparent immunity to bee venom, as has already been stated, dependent absolutely on the state and duration of morbidity. Light cases react soon, require less treatment; in old chronic cases, the reactions will be delayed and they will require longer treatment. When we arrive at the reactive state, we reach the limit of their presumptive immunity. This is just what we are after. It means that we are making progress and approaching results; the organism is already capable of reacting locally.

To clarify matters, we had better discuss the reactions:

Local Skin Reactions. The skin is an important, visible organ in all immunity reactions. In bee-venom treatments, the skin reactions are very serviceable. The systemic reactions have a rather secondary importance, because if we slowly, gradually, and carefully progress in the administration of treatments, they are almost entirely lacking, depending mainly on the visible, responsive, and illustrative skin reactions. We can distinguish three relative phases in their development, identical to those produced by bee stings.

If we view the behavior of reactions, we notice:

1) Progressive state, from the time of the injection to its complete development.

2) Stationary state, when there is no more essential change in the reaction.

3) Retrogressive state, gradual disappearance of reactive symptoms.

The speed of development, duration of the reaction, and its vanishing are very characteristic and instructive. They have to be carefully and closely observed and recorded. The skin reactions in our treatments are, as a rule, dependable—they are influenced only by our solution and the systemic conditions; the topographical influences are negligible, which is quite unlike the usual bee stings. We do not inject intravenously or on the eyelids, lips, ears, tongue, etc.

APITHERAPY

The reactions are, for us, a combination of speedometer, dynamometer, measuring rod, road sign-and will even act as traffic lights. In contraindications, we shall distinctly see the "red light," but if we carefully observe the important "regulations" of the treatment, during its whole course the green light will never change, and we may go ahead.

In rheumatics, at the beginning we will hardly notice any reactions, and if they develop they will appear slowly and disappear quickly. Later, through increased dosage, the local reactions change; they gradually increase in intensity, develop more quickly, remain longer in a stationary state, and recede only slowly.

A normal reaction can be described as follows: On the place of injection a wheal forms, a small elevation of the skin with a whitish center, similar to an infiltration in local anesthesia. It will soon be surrounded by an inflammatory ring and a gradually developing, circular edema. It is a leukocytic concentration, a phagocytic defensive effort of the organism. The edema is a collection of plasma fluids-a physiological "blockade"; a battle is being waged between the invading substances and the lytic enzymes. Sometimes the surrounding skin shows a goose-flesh appearance, which quickly disappears and is followed occasionally by a moderate urticaria. The edges of the wheals, which are supposed to include the surrounding inflammatory area, in the beginning are round; later, when spreading, they are apt to become serrated (saw-edged). This would suggest that the inflammatory process encounters a certain resistance in the skin and its progress is uneven. Still later, especially when approaching the state of reaction (which we call a prereactive state), these wheals have a tendency to become confluent and form one large plaque. The spreading tendency is already noticeable in the previous injections and we have to distance the individual wheals accordingly. Usually about one inch distance is sufficient. The formation of the wheals into one common plaque is a very encouraging sign, as it usually indicates improvement-even, in light cases, a final cure. I cannot lay enough stress on the importance of a slow, gradual, progressive and comfortable immunization-especially in more chronic cases which always consumes a certain time, corresponding to the nature of the disease. The progress must be made with arithmetical accuracy. If we unduly force the treatments, intense itching and urticaria may develop around the wheals with the possibility of other systemic disturbances. Of course, individual sensitivity, idiosyncrasy, or, on the other hand, excessive, though only assumed tolerance, will considerably modify the development of the symptoms. The appearance of the reactions, local, general, or focal, should be no cause for slowing down, still less for interrupting or discontinuing the treatments; just the contrary-we have to persevere in our chief aim to reach a higher, complete, this time real, immunization. The local inflammatory phenomena will gradually disappear; some elevation, hardening and pigmentation may remain. These occasionally last for several weeks. The systemic and focal reactions will also gradually subside.

The control and thorough observation of the local reactions is important. The character, size of the individual wheals, the time of their appearance, rapidity of their growth, their confluence and subsidence-in a word, all clinical and pathological changes-have to be minutely observed and carefully recorded. We will notice that cases of similar morbidity or chronicity will produce wheals of corresponding behavior. These records will be of considerable assistance to us in making plans and shaping the course for future proceedings, in addition to their value as diagnostic and prognostic aids.

May I give here a simple and appropriate illustration? Arthritis and rheumatism in the feet and knees are quite frequent. In certain instances it is doubtful whether these involvements are attributable to injuries or are rheumatoid conditions, possibly both. The first injections will clear up this question. If they are due to postural defects, the reactions will be those of a normal person, that is, of fair intensity. If it is a true arthritic condition, it will show only a slight or no reaction at all, on account of a certain degree of pathological immunity; and even more, not only the character of the morbidity, but, also, its extent. Naturally the later we reach the reactive state, the more resistant and obstinate is the case. If the reaction is very violent, infinitely stronger than a normal one, it will be a warning, suggesting idiosyncrasy or one of the previously mentioned trio: tuberculosis, lues or gonorrhea-often not suspected. These may provoke not only violent local but also alarming general reactions. I cannot emphasize enough the importance of commencing the treatments with only one or two wheals of the weakest concentration, on account of the possibility of provoking unexpectedly severe reactions.

General Reactions. The manifestations of the general symptoms, compared to the local ones, have only secondary importance. In mild cases, the limit of pathological immunity is easily reached with hardly any noticeable systemic disturbances. In chronic, old cases longer and less intense treatments are required.

189

The general reactions usually appear at the height of the local ones and, as a rule, accompany the confluence phenomena. A distinct parallelism between the intensities of the two reactions is very striking. The appearance of the focal reactions is also almost simultaneous.

The ordinary general symptoms are dizziness, headache, nausea, perspiration, slightly raised temperature and, rarely, diarrhea. There is sometimes somnolence, occasional restlessness and disturbed sleep. The patient often notices a bitter taste in the mouth on account of the absorption of venom.

Polyuria always follows the administration; the quantity of urine shows a marked increase, as the venom is a strong diuretic. At the beginning of the treatments the urine is dark yellow. In advanced pathological states, it is brownish red with brick dust sediment, and has a strong "urinous," ammoniacal odor. This condition gradually clears up during the progress of the treatments and is accompanied by a corresponding improvement in the general feeling.

Urticaria is rarely noticed and only in sensitive patients. The venom has decided influence on the menstrual flow, the menses usually appearing earlier. In the event of dysmenorrhea, this condition will greatly improve. If the menses manifest themselves, it is no reason to postpone or interrupt the treatments. In pregnancy, the utmost precaution is advised.

The general symptoms gradually pass off and seldom give any cause for anxiety.

Focal Reactions. As already mentioned, we often notice, especially in arthritic conditions, an exacerbation of pain and swelling in the affected joints, sometimes even a slight rise of temperature. This ordinarily coincides with the height of the local and general reactions, but passes away in several days and is followed, as a rule, by improved motility of the joints.

COURSE OF IMMUNIZATION

It is imperative to keep, beside the usual clinical records, careful and exact memoranda of the dosage, the intervals between the injections, and the demeanor of the reactions. Mathematical accuracy will be required; these notes will clearly indicate our progress, will present a true picture of the pathological changes, likewise be our guide in the future regimen. Let us now consider the phases we have to pass through during the course of treatments:

APITHERAPY

First Stage. At the start, when dealing with a real rheumatic we find an apparent, relative state of immunity-pathological immunity. We may safely exclude natural immunity, which is rare, or acquired immunity, that of beekeepers, who hardly ever suffer from rheumatism.

We gradually "step up" in our systematic, progressive immunization. The wheals, if we deal with a true rheumatic, will scarcely show any reaction at the beginning. If they show slight reactions, their appearance will be tardy and they will disappear quickly. Later, the wheals will show a stronger and gradually increasing reactive tendency. We are then in the prereactive state. Finally, depending greatly on the pathological conditions, we at last reach the first reaction. If the case is a light one, we already notice considerable improvement. The general feeling of the patient is better, pain decreased, joints are more mobile, sleep and appetite improved, and psychic depression decidedly diminished. In general, the outlook is encouraging.

Sometimes, we may encounter just the opposite, a considerable exacerbation of pain and swelling, which is produced by the focal reaction. This, as mentioned, is far from being a discouraging sign as it wears off in several days and results in marked improvement in the affected joints.

In neuralgia, myalgia, myositis and neuritis, we may even reach by this time-that is, by the end of the first stage-a recovery. The last named group is the first, among all rheumatoid involvements, to respond and yield to the medication, as the pathological immunity is not high and requires shorter and less intensive treatments.

Let us assume now that we are dealing with a mild case. The patient, at the end of the first stage, may be perfectly free from all morbid symptoms-to use a common phrase, "cured." Our aim has been achieved but the treatment is not yet completed. We should bear in mind the fact that the principal object immunization. Even if we reach such a state, we must not forget that all immunity wears off; we have to continue our treatments, to secure one of higher degree, making allowance for the expected loss, which would be equivalent to a recurrence of the disease. This will involve only a limited amount of effort and time. If we treat a more chronic type, the first reactions will yet be delayed and a longer treatment required to obtain them. After the reactions finally manifest themselves, often accompanied by general and focal reactions, we have reached the end of the first stage.

Second Stage. In the second stage, we have to pass again through another state of immunity, but this time it is an acquired (artificial) one. The initial stage we call the first postreactive state. We have to step up gradually in our immunizing procedure toward the second reactive goal. During the major part of this stage, we find again slow reactivity or no response at all. Sometime later we notice, once more, a livelier reactive tendency of the wheals—exact repetition of what we experienced toward the end of the first stage the reactions become more intense, the individual wheals show a tendency to get confluent; we have then reached the second prereactive state and approach the second reaction.

By this time, even fairly chronic cases will show considerable improvement or can be considered cured. The same rule which was suggested for light cases, at the end of the first stage, is applicable here; namely, we must augment the immunity with a short additional treatment to insure against the loss, that is, to prevent a recurrence. Therefore it is practicable to pass through a part of the second postreactive state, which is in the third stage. General and focal reactions are more frequent at the end of the second than at the end of the first stage.

Third Stage. Only where the malady has existed for several years, do we have to go through the entire third stage; as a rule a short part of it will be sufficient even in most chronic cases. The respective phases are similar to those of the first and second stages. Finally we reach the third prereactive state and soon afterwards the third reaction. It will be only rarely necessary to pass the third immunity reaction or through the third postreactive state. Not only is it probable that the most exceptional chronic types will be cured, but we have provided plenty of security against a recurrence of the ailment.

In every instance, several months or a year later, depending on pathological conditions, it is advisable to give a short "after cure," a repetition at least of some of the stages. Of course, we are confronted with a considerably smaller degree of pathological immunity and can progress more rapidly, both as to the number of wheals and the concentration of the solution. The stages will be considerably shorter. It is impossible to establish standard or routine treatments; the modus operandi must be individual and not schematic. Terc often mentioned the fact that patients under treatment knew very well what the reactions would mean to them and exhibited remarkable courage and endurance, tolerating the torture and agony of being exposed daily to 150 to 200 stings, anxiously anticipating the desired response and eventually the end of their suffering. They realized that when they became sensitized to bee stings they were more like normal persons. When they reached the reactive states, local, general and focal, they always looked forward to great improvement or a deliverance from their afflictions.

The chart on the next page illustrates the various transitional stages in the course of treatments.

SUMMARY

1) Initial injections will produce-even without reaction-improvement of the general condition; pain is lessened; appetite and sleep are considerably improved.

2) Postreactive states generally show most marked improvement.

3) The less advanced the case, the quicker the reaction and recovery.

4) The more chronic the case, the more tardy the reaction and recovery.

APITHERAPY

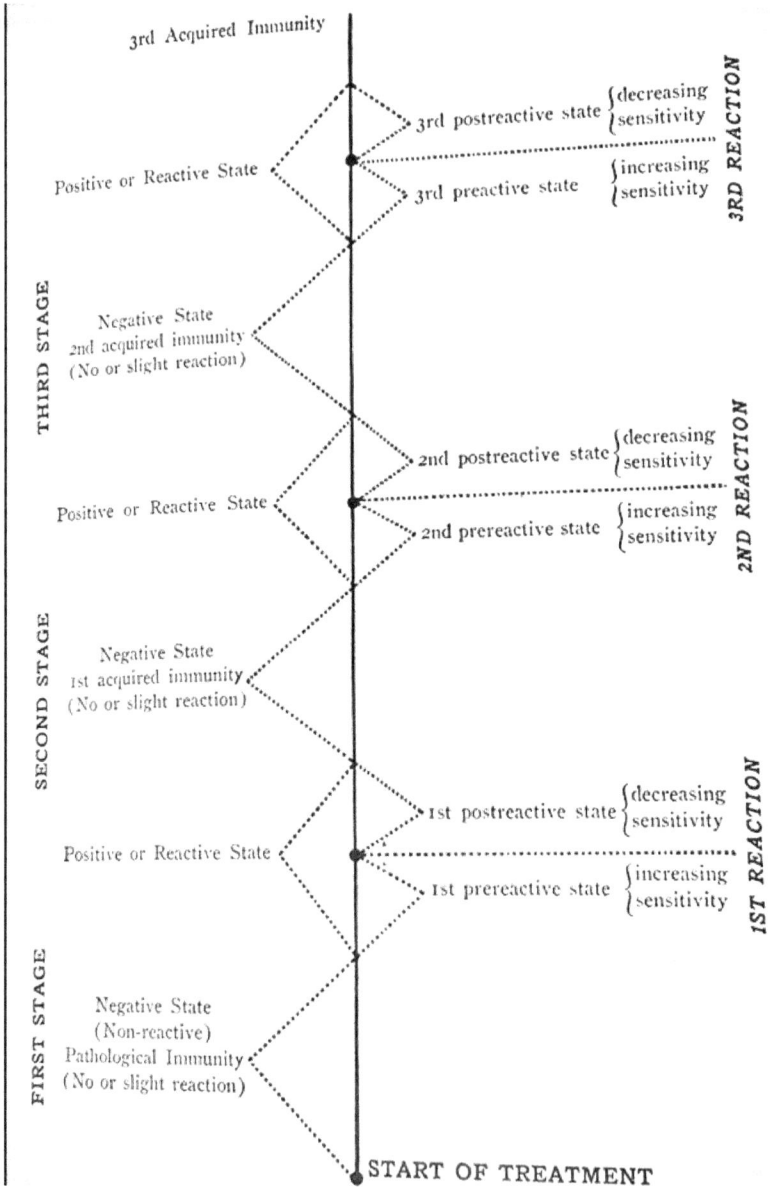

Figure 1 Graphical Chart Illustrating the Various Reactions and Different Stages

194

After each recovery another shorter course (after cure) is advisable to prevent recurrences. The time and duration of these courses depend entirely on the former character and chronicity of the case.

EXPECTED RESULTS

FIRST STAGE

During or by the end of the first stage rheumatic, neuritic, and acute arthritic cases will show a great improvement or recovery.

SECOND STAGE

During or by the end of the second stage the average milder chronic cases will show great improvement or recovery. We may expect not only local, but general and focal reactions.

THIRD STAGE

During or by the end of the third stage even advanced chronic cases will show considerable improvement or final recovery. General and focal reactions are more frequent.

Chapter XI Treatments with Injectable Bee Venom

In giving an outline of treatments, the three main considerations are the number of wheals, the concentration of the solution, and the intervals between the injections. All these are dependent on many modifying circumstances. Experience is the best teacher. Mistakes and errors are bound to occur at first but by close observation the necessary experimental knowledge will soon be acquired. A proper perspective and a systematic, judicious conduct of the treatments will be most helpful.

It advisable to eliminate all other medication as much as possible. Alcohol during the treatments, even in small quantities, is strictly forbidden, because it destroys the effects of the venom. This is the reason that alcoholics are just as resistant to the stings as the bees are anxious to sting them. (In severe bee-venom intoxication, on the other hand, alcoholization is the best remedy.) Calmette, in antivenin administration, prohibits the use of alcohol.

In case of extreme nervous reactions, disturbed sleep, etc., some bromide or other sedative is indicated. If the local reaction is very annoying, and there are considerable soreness, itching, and swelling, some local astringent, salicyl alcohol or a mentholated ointment, is suggested.

Physical therapeutics, diathermy, ultraviolet rays, hydrological measures, massage, exercise to restore the lost functions of the joints, to break down adhesions, to reeducate the wasted muscles, elevate the skin reaction, allay pain, etc., are not only not contra-indicated but they may be considered as necessary supplementary measures.

No special diet is required during the treatments, but if a certain diet has been previously prescribed it may be continued, or, in fact, any diet adapted to each individual case.

If any other treatment should be indicated, for instance, the removal of infected foci, it will be only too helpful.

TREATMENTS WITH INJECTABLE BEE VENOM

To gain a clearer understanding of the treatments I divide this chapter into four parts:

INJECTABLE BEE VENOM, describing the different preparations in use.

CONTRA-INDICATIONS.

INDICATIONS, describing also the treatment of individual groups.

CASE REPORTS, giving the various methods of different authors and their results.

INJECTABLE BEE VENOM

Before we proceed to discuss the therapy of the various rheumatic and arthritic groups with injectable bee venom, let us first describe the preparation itself, its dosage, and the manner of administration. There are, so far, two preparations in general use: *Apicosan* and *Immenin*.

Apicosan is made in Bielefeld, Germany, by Dr. August Wolff (Chemische Fabrik Vinces). It is marketed in I c.c. ampoules, five or ten in a box. The solution is a water-clear fluid and it comes in three concentrations:

I. Mild, containing one unit per ampoule.
II. Medium, containing three units per ampoule.
III. Strong, containing nine units per ampoule.

In every box of No. I concentration, there is a test ampoule, containing less than one unit, in brown colored glass (the other ampoules are colorless). Its use is always essential before starting the treatment, to determine if the patient exhibits any special hypersensitiveness to the venom. The test consists of the formation of one intradermal wheal using o. I c.c. of the test ampoule. I emphasize the importance of this precautionary measure.

Immenin is produced by the State Serotherapeutic Institute, of Vienna. It is put up in 0.5 c.c. and I c.c. ampoules, made in five strengths. The unit volumes (they call it Series) are the following:

Series N (neuritic). This is employed for neuritic, neuralgic, and ophthalmic conditions. It is the weakest solution and is also suitable for a tolerance test as a preliminary to treatments.

Series A. Mild,

Series B. Medium,

Series C. Strong,

Series E. Extra, which is the strongest concentration, a multiple of Series C. There is also a Series F., obtainable on special order, still stronger than Series E.

I, II, III of the Apicosan correspond approximately to A, B, C, of Immenin and can be interchanged accordingly.

With the Swiss preparation, "*Apisin*," which, according to directions, is given subcutaneously or intramuscularly, I have had so far no experience, nor have I read any reports of results obtained by others.

A new preparation, called *British Bee Venom*, which was only recently put on the market, is described in chapter 2 (towards the end).

In giving a dosage in the course of treatments, the strength of the solution will be denoted by the Roman numerals I, II, III; the Arabic number will signify the number of wheals. This schematic abbreviation saves time and space in designating the dosage. For example:

I- 4 means four wheals of concentration

II- 7 means seven wheals of concentration

II. III-12 means twelve wheals of concentration III.

Contributor Note:

See the annotations for Roman Numeral conversions on page viii.

Wheal: a suddenly formed elevation of the skin surface : Welt especially a flat burning or itching eminence on the skin. [58,59]

CONTRA-INDICATIONS

Contra indications have to be carefully considered. It is important, not only to treat cases correctly, but also to select them cautiously.

Kidney involvements, albuminuria and hydrops demand vigilance and discretion. Cases with cardiovascular complications, as a rule, are not very desirable, and if such pathological conditions are advanced, the treatments are absolutely contra-indicated. To this group belong: myocarditis, angina pectoris, arteriosclerosis, aneurism of the aorta and, in fact, any chronic cardiovascular condition. Rheumatic inflammation of the heart, endocarditis, pericarditis-acute or chronic-are not only not contra-indicated but are most suitable cases for treatments. Of course, watch out for the trio, the "bête noire" of bee venom therapy: tuberculosis, lues, and gonorrhea. Diabetes is generally a contra-indication, but diabetics only rarely require intense treatments, as arthritis among them is exceptional.

All arthritism caused by endocrine imbalance, like climacteric arthritis, arthropathia ovaripriva, etc., does not respond readily to bee-venom treatment, as the progress of the producing causes remains unbroken. Rheumatoid etiology of course is a peremptory requirement.

INDICATIONS

The ailments listed below are amenable to apitherapy:

Muscular Rheumatism, Myalgia, Myositis, etc.,
Neuritis, Neuralgia, Migraine, etc.,
Acute Rheumatic Fever and Endocarditis,
Acute and Chronic Arthritis,
Arthritis Deformans,
Chronic Surgical Inflammation of the Soft and Bony Tissues,
Iritis and Iridocyclitis Rheumatica,
Dermatoses.

In the following outline I attempt to give, in addition to the indications, a condensed schedule covering the course of treatments for each individual group. Naturally, it is impossible to devise a predetermined, standard routine. The treatments, as already stated, must be individual, not schematic. The clinical symptoms and the reactions in each category are different, and the treatments must be modified accordingly.

The administration requires discriminating judgment, which can only be acquired through practice, experience, careful control, and close observation. Accurate records should be kept, as they will be very instrumental both in the control of our cases as well as in determining the future program. We must not only consider the character of the ailments, which are certainly very multiform, but also pay attention to constitutional states, sensitivity of the patients and all other contingencies.

Muscular Rheumatism, Myalgia, Myositis, etc.

The ailments in this category yield quickly to bee venom therapy, as the pathological conditions produced by ischemia and anoxemia are easily corrected by the powerful hemorrhagic effect of the venom. Chronicity will require correspondingly longer treatments. Subcutaneous nodes, endothelial and perivascular changes, local metabolic disorders, edema, are all consequences of impoverished circulation. Occasional swelling, redness, and pain induced by increased circulation, are due to the curative effort of the organism to overcome the existing deficiencies.

Rheumatoid conditions are often brought on by exposure to cold or dampness, which causes poor circulation, or they may be of mechanical origin, induced by postural defects. In such cases, sometimes infective foci are present, as the ischemic tissues are an excellent breeding ground for microbes. Muscular wasting often accompanies these disturbances, which is only natural.

The marvelous cures of paralytic cases reported by the various Continental beehive "clinics" could be explained as motor paralysis affections due to some interference with the blood supply of certain parts of the nervous system (Volkmann's paralysis). Good results in such instances are obtained very rapidly and are often amazing.

> *Contributor Note:*
>
> *See the annotations for Roman Numeral conversions on page viii.*

The treatment is commenced with I-2, progressing to I-10, then II-2, gradually increasing the number of wheals and concentration until a final cure is achieved. As a rule, in these types it is unnecessary to step up to III concentration, as the final cure is usually reached during or by the end of the administration of series 2. The patient is ordinarily very soon free from pain and complaints. A short additional treatment is imperative for the sake of preventing recurrences. A very appropriate place to administer the injections is one near the seat of the pain (*loco dolenti*).

I wish to make here some general remarks: The improvement, which manifests itself in every respect immediately after the start of the treatment, so noticeable that it is rather surprising. The pathological conditions, due to lack of oxidation on account of impaired circulation, yield very quickly to the distinct and remote effect of the venom, which accelerates circulation and increases oxidation. The remarkable universal improvement is only logical.

The patients, in the great majority of cases, are much impressed and are enthusiastic about the treatments. They notice a sense of stimulation and feel a certain warmth in the body, especially in parts which were previously rather numb. Patients usually describe a general tingling sensation in the joints and limbs, which were formerly rather lifeless. We may generally expect some cheerful reports from them. They are trustful and hopeful. Of course, being relieved from all the impediments and multiform untoward consequences of poor circulation which gradually crept on them almost unnoticed-and caused them so much apprehension, even genuine scare, they become especially enthusiastic.

Many of my patients, without any prompting or suggestion, have made the identical statement; namely, that their eyesight has improved. Women mention, for instance, with what surprising facility they are able to thread a needle, which act, formerly, they were unable to do without glasses or were compelled to ask some one else to do. It is a source of great satisfaction to notice the conspicuous manifestations of improvement.

Neuritis, Neuralgia, Migraine, etc.

The rapidity with which results are secured in this group almost equals that achieved in muscular rheumatism, which disorders as stated in the preceding subdivision, yield readily to bee-venom treatments.

The site of the injections should be near the place of the malady; for example, in neuritis brachialis or antibrachialis, the extensor surfaces of the upper or lower arm of the affected side should be used. In trigeminal or occipital neuralgia, the nape of the neck or the shoulder blades of the afflicted side should be the choice. In sciatic neuritis, the sacral region or the upper extensor surface of the leg is recommended.

The time of the injections in neuritic and neuralgic cases should be late in the evening, if possible, as the administrations have a distinct sedative effect and the employment of other sedatives can be avoided.

Treatment should be commenced with one wheal of concentration I, gradually increasing the number of wheals. It is possible that we may have to step up to 15 or even to 20. In the event that this is not adequate, we may continue with the concentration II, until satisfactory results are obtained.

Heberden's nodes, endocrine or climacteric polyneuritis, are rather resistant to bee-venom treatments. As I mentioned, the state or progress of the producing causes is uninterrupted.

Acute Rheumatic Fever and Endocarditis

The maladies of this group present a grateful field for bee-venom treatments. Terc and Keiter often mention the fact that bee venom can be rightfully considered a *specific in rheumatic fever and endocarditis.*

The treatments are administered on alternate days, starting with concentration I, increasing the number of wheals by two or three, or even more, stepping up to II, or eventually to III concentration. On the days when no injections are given, Kretschy suggested administering antipyretics, if the temperature is high, but when it approaches normal only the venom should be used. The writer never found it necessary to resort to any other accessory remedies; the venom, as a means of pyretic treatment, will reduce the temperature, and also shorten the convalescent period very considerably.

Acute and Chronic Arthritis

A rheumatic etiology is self-understood. The average rheumatoid arthritis is much more resistant to treatment than muscular rheumatism, neuritis, even rheumatic fever or endocarditis rheumatica. The response is much slower. Complete immunization of the patients is essential-they must be "saturated" with bee venom. Traumatic arthritis, on the other hand, responds very readily.

During the treatment of rheumatoid arthritis, we are frequently confronted with more or less severe general reactions, such as nausea, headache, profuse perspiration, diarrhea, and occasional high temperature, but this is no cause for anxiety. It is most important that the treatments should not be interrupted, but the doses should be gradually increased, as the effects will slowly wear off. Exacerbation of the pain is due to focal reactions, which will also soon subside. Patients usually tolerate well these intensified symptoms because they have already noticed a general improvement in the prereactive state; the motility of the joints is freer, appetite and weight are increasing, and sleep is decidedly better.

Bechterew's disease, spondylitis deformans, is included in this group. The results are very good. The distressing characteristic symptom of this disease, profuse perspiration, will quickly disappear. The pressure exerted by the compression and irritation of the nerve roots soon shows a distinct improvement and, also, there is freer motility of the spine. Patients all state that they feel "looser."

Acute and chronic gout, also, belong under this heading. Reports about the results obtained in this class are very favorable, depending, of course, on the chronicity and character of the case.

The treatments for all the ailments constituting this group should be given daily as their course is rather prolonged. It is suggested to start with I-2, gradually increasing by one or two wheals to I-10, and after three or four administrations of I-10, stepping up to II-2, then to II-10, and from III-2 to

III-10, all depending on the case. During the administration of the II series, symptoms begin to improve, but still a higher immunization is necessary.

Contributor Note:

See the annotations for Roman Numeral conversions on page viii.

Several months after the treatment, a second course is suggested, but this will be considerably shorter as the increase of wheals and concentration can be executed with more rapidity, without provoking disturbing general reactions.

I wish to mention here an important point, referring particularly to arthritis of the knee. If only the knee is affected, and no other joints, with few exceptions it is a traumatic condition, which quickly responds to bee venom treatment. With reference to this traumatic origin, Wilde, of Bath, England, with many years experience in treating rheumatic diseases, has said that the knee, being the largest and most exposed joint, and carrying the weight of the body when bent at all angles, is often involved in chronic rheumatic conditions. We must distinguish between these cases and those where the knee joint alone is affected. Many chronic knee troubles are diagnosed as "arthritis" but true arthritis never commences in the knee, the knee remaining the only affected joint. Wilde noticed in many such destructive changes, when other joints remained unaffected, that it was due to a neglected chronic synovitis primarily caused by an injury. A diagnosis of such "arthritis" should always be regarded with suspicion. Not a few of these cases had a good deal of surgical advice before coming to see him. The history of most of them was that some slight sprain or injury had set up a synovitis. I fully agree with Wilde; my observation has been much the same.

Arthritis Deformans

The reactions produced in treating arthritis deformans differ absolutely from those obtained in all other rheumatic ailments. In arthritis deformans, the first reactions appear much sooner, not only the local but also the general and focal. We find swellings in the joints during the reactions, but without any improvement. The postreactive and succeeding nonreactive stages are also extremely short. The reactive and nonreactive phases alternate frequently, and these changes continually repeat themselves during the rather protracted treatments.

While in other groups we can fairly predict the approximate duration of a nonreactive state, in arthritis deformans this is impossible. Therefore, it is advisable to proceed slowly because we cannot foretell when the reactions will suddenly appear. The treatments are usually long because we must proceed leisurely, and of course, the improvement will be correspondingly delayed. A rapid advance may aggravate conditions.

The treatments should be started with concentration I, increasing the number of wheals by one or two, giving the venom daily. The best plan is to ascend to I-10, then from II-1 to II-10, and from III-1 to III-10, or even higher, depending on the chronicity of the case. A second course may be necessary, when the number of wheals can be increased more rapidly. If the increase is gradual, the general and focal reactions are usually absent, but still we notice marked improvement in the general condition and in the motility of the joints. The majority of the workers in the field favor a deliberate treatment, with a gradual increase of the dosage. If we observe Case I of Perrin and Cuènot the course which they employed seems rather forced and drastic.

Women are often subject to arthritis deformans. If it is caused by climacteric or other endocrine disturbances, the treatments will be less favorable. hypersensitive (It is a peculiar fact that many arthritis deformans cases are to tuberculin.)

Chronic Surgical Inflammation of the Soft and Bony Tissues

The beneficial effects of bee venom on nonspecific inflammations of the soft tissues and bones are remarkable. Osteomyelitis, chronic cellulitis, torpid fistulae, etc., which did not respond to surgical procedures, will yield readily to the effect of the venom, as a consequence of "sanguification," on account of its hemorrhagic action. We can notice the rapid disappearance of the pathological tissues through absorption and increased cellular activity. Sometimes violent local reactions are perceptible on the affected parts and this inflammation is characterized by swelling and reddening, which, however, soon subside.

Nowotny's cases are illustrative, showing the distinct absorptive effect of the venom, which, as he himself stated, exceeded anything he had used before.

The principle in treating this group differs absolutely from that which we employ in the management of rheumatic, arthritic, and neuritic ailments. In the former we have no immunizing purpose in mind, only to derive benefit from the hemorrhagic effects of the venom. All further conduct of the treatments should be determined by the produced hyperemia. It is advisable to wait for the next injections until the inflammatory effects of the previous ones have subsided. This should be the only guide in administering these treatments. The number of wheals and concentration should be increased with more or less rapidity until the inflammatory reactions develop. The injections are best applied around the local infiltration to be treated.

Iritis and Iridocyclitis Rheumatica

Iritis and iridocyclitis are rather painful and distressing complications of rheumatism and arthritis and, according to several authors, respond to bee-venom therapy, even when all other remedies have failed.

The treatment is carried out with the weakest concentration, the wheals increased in the beginning by one, later by two. The site of the injections should be on the upper external part of the arm or on the shoulder blades, in either case on alternating sides. Usually about 12 to 15 injections will be sufficient to achieve a cure.

Dermatoses

This subdivision-in the strict sense-does not belong to our subject, but I do not wish to omit the fact that bee venom is also used for various skin diseases. As mentioned before, Lautal, a lay beekeeper, successfully used it in eczema, lupus, epithelioma, and leprosy.

At the present time, the writer himself has several psoriasis cases under treatment, so far with encouraging signs and best prospects for satisfactory results, attributable to the hemorrhagic effect of the venom on the constricted capillary vessels. He will consider it his privilege to publish these reports as well as others at a later date.

Professor Boinet introduced in *The Marseille Médical* (60-1923) two cases of lupus cured by bee stings:

Female, 50. In 1909, erosion on the ala nasi. Patient was treated by the apiculturist, Lautal, for four months. He applied 1500 stings on and around the cutaneous lesions, which resulted in a gradual and perfect cure. No recurrence in 13 years.

Miss R., a girl of 30. In 1911, marked tuberculotic lesions on the face and alae nasi. On the buttocks, a lupus erythematosus, the size of the palm of a hand. The treatment lasted nine months. 4000 stings were applied. Patient perfectly cured. No recurrences.

Vigne and Bougala introduced, at the meeting of the Sociéte de Médicine, Colonial Hygiene d'Marseille, on December 12, 1923, an enormous elephantiasis with diffuse, deep ulcerations of four years' standing. Patient was 45 years old. Entered the hospital on June 25, 1923, with violent pain and immense edema. Approximately 30 to 40 stings were applied daily. Altogether about 4,450 were recorded. There was a great improvement and although the patient was brought to the hospital on a stretcher, on December 12th he walked up two flights to the meeting without difficulty.

Boinet, with the help of Lautal, also introduced, in 1923, his second case of leprosy cured by stings.

A leading physician of Chartrès presented in July, 1923, to the same Society of Colonial Medicine in Marseille, a case of phagedenic ulcer completely cured after 140 stings, applied in 14 séances, on and around the ulcer. Professor Boinet later reported the matter to the Governor of Indo-China, recommending apipuncture, as he was convinced that bee venom possesses great healing power in leprosy, phagedenic and varicose ulcers, eczema, lupus, etc., all so prevalent in the tropics. He ascribed to the venom therapeutic vasodilator influence, phagocytosis, and an antitoxic effect upon microbes, without being able to establish anything positive at that time outside of the actual results.

CASE REPORTS

I am well aware of the fact that the title of this chapter is "Treatments with Injectable Bee Venom" and, being pledge-bound to a certain degree, I ought to observe tradition and confine myself to the subject. But I realize that this new method is yet in its infancy; there is no domestic product at our disposal; to obtain the foreign preparations is somewhat circumstantial and costly, and there are other contingencies to be considered -as my recent experience proved-when I offered a colleague some of the material to help him out temporarily and he refused because it was made in Germany.

For this and other reasons, I deemed it advisable to include in this chapter the case records and methods of physicians who have used or still use live bees in their treatments. Possibly some members of the profession, especially those in the Southern States, where bees can be obtained during the greater part of the year, may be willing to experiment with them. Of course. in the metropolitan district and in larger cities, we are absolutely dependent on injectable venom.

We have to grant Terc the first place, not only because I list the names of collaborators chronologically, but also because of merit.

TREATMENTS WITH INJECTABLE BEE VENOM

Philipp Terc

Terc acquired, without doubt, a great experimental knowledge in the administration of bee stings. He utilized them in thousands of cases, over a period of more than 40 years, applying as many as 150 to 200 stings in one day to a patient. He had innumerable difficulties but his greatest handicap, especially when it came to treating chronic cases, was that he had to stop in the fall and could resume his treatments only at the beginning of the next summer. With mild rheumatics or arthritics the treatments could be completed in one summer.

Terc was an experienced beekeeper. He was in closer contact with the apistic brotherhood than with the medical fraternity. The beekeepers encouraged and assisted him in every possible way. They had unlimited faith and confidence in his judgment and procedure; always extended to him their sympathies during the days of strife and struggle. Most of his work, anyhow, was executed through the coöperation of the beekeepers; from his colleagues, he received only contempt and ridicule. The apiarists knew that his doctrines were both good and true, as none of them suffered from rheumatic ailments. They were all aware of the magic healing power of their mutually respected little friend, the bee. Quite possibly, Terc never thought that someday the production of injectable bee venom would be accomplished, inaugurating a new era and a much simplified technic.

Terc's main endeavor was to procure immunity. To him, immunity to bee venom meant immunity to all rheumatic ailments. In later years, he founded a school in Graz, where he taught his technic to physicians. He gave a full account of his methods and results. Terc always advised the light cases with salicylates or any other drugs, or by physical means, should be administered only in cases which would not yield to any other as bee sting treatments were tedious and inconvenient; he thought they medical agencies.

Plain muscular rheumatism, myositis, myalgia, monarthritis, polyarthritis, difficulties for him. In these ailments, Terc obtained very quick and satisfactory results. Neuritis and sciatica, especially, yielded quickly, and did not require many stings. He emphasized the fact that we must discriminate between rheumatic inflammations of the nerves and other neuralgias. In the latter type, his results were rather unfavorable. Terc had great pride in the excellent recoveries he obtained in inflammatory rheumatic conditions of the heart; the murmurs soon disappeared and the improvements were astonishing.

Terc could never explain the effect of the venom on rheumatic ailments; he was convinced that there was an intimate relationship between the two but always considered it a difficult problem to solve. He thought children old people were poor subjects for treatments. Heart ailments were a positive contra-indication for him-of course, nonrheumatic heart and very affections.

After Terc achieved success in all kinds of chronic cases which previously had been considered incurable and had been given up by others, he concentrated his energy on the treatment of arthritis deformans. This was the height of his ambition, and he was always very proud that he succeeded. He considered arthritis deformans a very peculiar disease, a complex pathological condition, starting slowly, usually without fever, on the upper or lower extremities and, as a rule, symmetrically. For a time, it is at an apparent standstill—to spread again with renewed force all over the body. First it attacks the smaller joints, later the larger ones, finally the internal organs, kidneys, serous surfaces of the pleura, but never the heart as other rheumatic inflammations. The patients gradually become helpless and crippled, awaiting death or the miserable torture of old age.

Terc published many of his case reports. It would consume considerable time and space to cite even a small part of them, so I have selected some characteristic, instructive, and interesting examples which will throw a proper light on his method and results.

Arthritis Deformans

Miss Josephine Goudot, 28 (patient consented to the publication of her name). In February, 1900, without fever, a very painful swelling started in most of the joints of her fingers. Gradually other joints of the upper and lower extremities were involved; later on, her spine. Her chest was very painful with a distinct exudate; there was considerable dyspnea and she was confined to her bed most of the time. Terc was consulted more than two years later, at the end of March, 1902, after all other treatments had given her no relief. The patient was anemic; all her joints deformed, thickened, and painful. Position of the hands was characteristic. Could not stretch her elbows and had occasional spasmodic contractions of the knees. Urine contained albumin.

Terc commenced the application of the bees at the end of March, 1902. The first reaction appeared only after 300 stings. During continued treatment there was no reaction again until after a nontreatment interval when a second one was obtained. These reactive and nonreactive states alternated up to November, by which time she had received 5,600 stings.

Patient had improved considerably. She had recurrences but always lighter and shorter. Terc persevered-notwithstanding all the difficulties of winter application-for several weeks until there was no recurrence.

Albumin in urine had already disappeared in June and also the exudate in the right chest. By the end of September, patient was free of pain, looked wonderful (in spite of the "horse treatment"), walked for hours. Terc warned her about recurrences. The next winter, she felt very well, even reporting that in Trieste she withstood the hardships of a formidable bora (a winter storm blowing from the Alps over the Adriatic).

In March, 1903, she had light recurrences in her fingers and hands, which passed away after a few sting applications. During the following summer, she received a thousand stings. General condition was excellent, but once in a while she developed a slight swelling, in certain joints of the hand, which disappeared in several days. Immunization had to be kept up for several years.

This arthritis deformans was very interesting from both a practical and theoretical viewpoint. The patient had been bedridden for almost two and one-half years, was treated for four years, and received altogether 15,000 stings, but became perfectly well and all joints diminished in size. Terc thought that this one case ought to advance bee-venom therapy from the place of unbelief and ridicule to a higher and more exalted position.

Mrs. N. F. was also an interesting case. Terc had success fully treated her husband, a physician, for arthritis. She was bedridden, emaciated, fingers and toes in a clawlike position, perfectly deformed. Not a single joint was exempt. Patient was hardly able to move, had no appetite, and was sleepless. There was albumin in the urine.

She started treatment in the month of May. Terc increased the number of stings very rapidly. In the first week, she received 100 stings. Later on he gave her 120 to 150-once even 220-a day in two sittings.

General condition greatly improved, albumin in urine disappeared. Gradually, the pains left her, the thickening of the joints and deformity regressed. Up to August, she had received 7,000 stings. She looked fine, felt excellent, attended to housework, and was able to walk for hours. Patient stood the treatment exceptionally well, was very enthusiastic about bee-sting therapy, and Terc remarked that he never could give her enough stings.

Mrs. M. P. Patient was brought to him from far-away Hungary and carried on a stretcher from the railroad station to the hotel. She was emaciated almost to a skeleton and suffered from arthritis in all her joints;

was feverish, with severe gastric and intestinal catarrh. Terc thought her "a heap of misery," and hated the idea of sending her back on such a long journey, as he expected that the treatment would take a few years considering the usual interruptions.

After several thousand stings, the patient was relieved of all her pains, her joints loosened, and he massaged her atrophied muscles. Three months later, she was able to walk and looked fairly well. Went home but her husband failed to pay the rather large bill. Next spring she again begged Terc to resume the treatments, but he refused.

Muscular Rheumatism and Complications

Muscular rheumatism offers a very great field for bee stings, no matter how old or chronic the cases may be.

J. P., male, 60 years old. In the spring, while perspiring and in thin clothing in an open carriage, he contracted severe muscular rheumatism, which proved to be quite stubborn. Joints were free. Internal medication, electricity and spas gave no results. Patient could not leave his bed. First consulted Terc in August. Was emaciated, feverish, had no appetite, was sleepless on account of pains which kept up day and night. His hands were powerless, certain groups of muscles atrophic, could not write or even hold a spoon in his hand, besides he was tortured by muscular cramps.

On account of his advanced age, Terc started treatments very carefully and to his joy found that after only 160 stings the patient manifested his first reaction. After two weeks' treatment, there was no more fever, his sleep was normal, appetite improved, and pains quite tolerable. Up to November 15, he received about 1,000 stings, and felt perfectly well; paralysis of the muscles was cured by faradic current. Next year, to preserve his immunity, he received about 100 more stings. Lived 25 years longer, always free from rheumatism.

Dr. G. H. Two years previously had had very severe arthritis. In spite of former treatments, a mitral insufficiency remained, the arthritis and muscular rheumatism became chronic. The stiffness and soreness of the muscles of the neck and head made breathing difficult. Chest was stiff as armor, walking quite impeded. Patient was depressed and emaciated. Someone suggested bee sting treatments to him. He was willing to submit to the "experiment" only after he had no other hope for recovery. During the summer, patient received about 1,000 stings. By fall, he was walking around and during the winter took up ice sports and felt fine. For the next two years, he took light after-cures of about 150 stings each summer. Afterwards, perfectly well.

Inflammatory Rheumatism and Arthritis

Mrs. P. Suffered for weeks from acute rheumatism, with affection of the heart. High fever. Could not tolerate drugs. After 600 stings, she had a perfect cure. No recurrence for ten years. She then acquired another attack of acute rheumatism. Drugs did not help her. Returned for bee-sting treatments as a last refuge. A week after the treatments started, fever entirely disappeared, and in three weeks was perfectly cured. Patient was discharged with the promise to return occasionally to refresh her immunity.

Mrs. M. G. had repeated attacks of arthritis and muscular rheumatism, endocarditis and pericarditis, marasmus, dyspnea, and fever. Could not endure drugs. During the whole summer, Terc applied bee stings without interruption. Altogether she received about 2,000. Was perfectly cured, no pain or dyspnea, heart murmurs almost gone.

K. J., student, 17 years old. Since his sixth year, had suffered from a very painful rheumatism. Patient was pale; suffering expressed on his face. In 1908, had a very serious attack, all joints were involved, high fever, endocarditis, and pleurisy of the left side. He was carried on a sheet from one bed to another, writhing with pain and in constant agony. Terc hesitated to start the treatments as he was afraid that they might contribute to an almost unavoidable fatal ending. The parents insisted, for they had nothing to lose. Terc started treatments carefully, twice daily. A week later, fever receded; two weeks later, entirely disappeared. Soon, patient received 40 to 60 stings daily. In four weeks, left his bed. Treatment was continued until 1,800 stings had been applied and immunization was entirely successful. Patient received 200 stings the next two summers, was climbing mountains and riding a bicycle.[8]

Female, 60. Terc had treated her 25 years previously for arthritis. She was well until 1907 when she again developed arthritis and sciatica, and was in bed for seven months. Patient begged him for morphine injections to alleviate the pain, at least until the next spring when the treatments could be started. They were commenced in the spring. Four weeks later, left her bed and in two weeks resumed her vocation. During the summer, she received

---

[8] Such cases should be tested every year for immunity, which eventually has to be renewed.

altogether 1,000 stings. Patient, while formerly almost emaciated to a skeleton and utterly despairing, recovered perfectly by fall, was well nourished, with rosy cheeks.

J. B., 29 years old, railroad locksmith. Suffered repeated attacks of rheumatism. Later arthritis in both knees. Had hospital treatment without success. Terc was first consulted on a New Year's day and found the patient, who lived in a cellar, bed ridden, emaciated, feverish, bathed in cold perspiration. Both knees quite swollen and painful. His family took care of him. He was afraid of losing his job so Terc took pity on him and started the applications, which were difficult, because of the fact that it was a most unfavorable season for bee treatments. Up to January 17th, the patient had 70 stings without any reaction or relief. The winter turned out to be unusually severe and the treatments had to be discontinued. Terc in the meantime tried all other remedies without success. Treatments were resumed again on March 6th. Up to the 26th of April, he received 250 stings. Only after the 90th sting did a reaction appear. By the end of April, he was able to leave his bed. Patient was treated until the end of May, when he resumed his work. During the summer, and until the end of November, received over 1,000 stings. Was free from attacks for five years, when, after a severe exposure, had another attack of rheumatism and endocarditis. In two weeks, he received 100 stings, recovered perfectly and was well afterwards.

This proves that only part of the immunity has to be restored and, also, how quickly a recurrent rheumatic endocarditis responds to a short treatment. Years ago, Terc was called to attend a woman in Spielfeld Castle, who had been suffering from inflammatory rheumatism for eight weeks. Was treated, *lege artis*, up to that time. Patient had heart murmurs, emaciated, could not move in bed. She heard of his cures and begged him to help her. Terc at first was unwilling to comply with her request especially when the mistress of the castle sneeringly asked him: "How can you have the courage to torture a dying patient with bee stings?" Nevertheless, he started. He remained with the patient for half a day-first he put on one, half an hour later two, and an hour later two more bees, which produced no feeling in the patient and no reaction. Next day, he continued the applications, the head gardener, who was also a beekeeper, putting the bees on. In three weeks, the "dying patient" left her bed, perfectly cured, without a heart murmur.

Polyarthritis

Mrs. M. F., 42. Patient was sick for six years. Tried every possible remedy, spas, etc. Emaciated to a skeleton, all joints swollen, thickened, and deformed, could sleep very little. Treatment was started in August. Up to October, she received about 1,700 stings. Went home for the winter, looked very well, and was without pain. Next spring, she had 300 more stings. Looked fine, although the deformities of the joints remained and she walked with some difficulty; she had no recurrence or pain for years. The only thing patient regretted was that she had not started the treatments earlier.

TABLE SHOWING TERC'S RESULTS

Ailment	Number of Cases	Cured	Improved	Unimproved
Rheumatoid heart affections	48	36	7	5
Muscular rheumatism	253	212	41	0
Chronic arthritis	186	151	35	0
Arthritis deformans	17	6	6	5

In 1912, Rudolf Tertsch, Terc's son, published 660 of his father's cases showing these results:

Perfectly cured	544	82%
Improved	99	Very advanced cases, some interrupted
Unimproved	17	treatments, others gave it up

Iritis Rheumatica

Rudolf Tertsch, an ophthalmic surgeon in the University of Vienna, Assistant to Prof. Ernst Fuchs, the ophthalmologist of world-wide reputation, on the persuasion of his chief made attempts years ago to treat iritis rheumatica with bee stings, but not being an apiarist like his father, he gave it up very soon on account of technical difficulties.

Joseph Langer

Langer, Professor of Pediatrics at the University of Prague, is unquestionably the most prolific writer on the subject of bee venom and one of the first to make a thorough chemical analysis of it. He published extensive physiological and biological experiments and also used bees and their venom in his clinical work.

Langer for a long time used live bees, but found them very impractical for children. They were too much afraid of the bees, complained of severe pain, and could not endure the treatments. He prepared a venom-solution, killed bees in chloroform vapor, and with forceps extracted their stings and poison bags. He rubbed the substance in a China mortar with some physiological salt solution and filtered it, washing off what remained on the with some more saline solution and putting the whole filtrate into a boiling water bath to destroy the minor albumin parts. After filtering repeatedly, he used the solution for injections. Children tolerated the injection much better than adults.

Langer noticed that the same solution produced a different reaction in every case. For example:

Case 1. In 15 minutes, erythema, swelling, painful burning of the surrounding skin, doughy elevation.

Case 2. Erythema the size of the palm of a hand, swelling, painful burning, edema. The erysipelous redness disappeared within 48 hours.

Case 3. Erythema after 15 minutes, edematous swelling only 5 hours later. In 24 hours, all symptoms disappeared.

Langer came to the following conclusions:

1) Terc's method of applying bees is very painful-applicable to adults but not to children.
2) Local influence is very effective.
3) Confirmed Terc's assertion that a rheumatic's reactions are different from those of a normal person.
4) The pain was greatly relieved in both rheumatic and arthritic conditions and the joints became more mobile.
5) Did not notice harmful effects in any case.

Langer's experience was that children suffer mainly from acute rheumatism and arthritis. Chronic form is very rare. The involvement of the joints is, in the majority of cases, symmetrical, which is proof that it has a neurotrophic origin. The joints are swollen, doughy, sensitive, with restricted or no motility. The etiology is unknown, possibly it is thermic or bad hygienic conditions, faulty feeding, or toxic influences, often tuberculosis and syphilis.

Alfred Keiter

Keiter of Graz was a collaborator of Terc. He, also, used live bees, and advised holding the bees with the fingers and not with a forceps, to obtain a more effective sting. Keiter came to the same conclusion as Terc: that real rheumatics react much less to bee venom than a normal person does and that the effects of the stings are, also, less painful.

TREATMENTS WITH INJECTABLE BEE VENOM

Keiter noticed that during the treatments, even after the first applications, improvement was very conspicuous. Patients felt looser in the joints and slept better. He also gave strict warning to look out for tuberculosis, lues, and gonorrhea, as these ailments often give very alarming reactions, emphasizing the diagnostic value of such an occurrence.

Keiter frequently noticed an exacerbation of pain in the diseased joints during the course of treatments, on account of the provoked focal reaction. He looked upon it as a welcome sign, as it always proved to be a forward step to improvement and cure. He found that the patients not only were more comfortable but looked better while the treatments were progressing, comparing the improvement with that produced by intravenous injections of iron and arsenic. Patients felt warmer; they were more jolly and hopeful. Keiter thought that bee venom is very beneficial in rheumatic heart ailments and in anemic conditions. Neurasthenics improved very remarkably and regained perfect health. He advised never to stop when the reactions appear but to force the treatments until total immunity is reached.

While Terc applied the stings on various parts of the body, especially on the back and extremities, Keiter preferred to administer them over the respective joints, loco dolenti, depending on a quicker effect in stirring up a focal reaction.

Keiter considered bees' venom as a specific for rheumatic heart ailments. His results were amazing. The pulse became stronger, slower, more regular, blood pressure increased, murmurs disappeared; heart muscle and dyspnea improved, appetite was better, and in general, patients exhibited considerably more endurance. He also often complained of the handicap of being able to use live bees only during the summer months.

TREATMENTS WITH INJECTABLE BEE VENOM

F. H. Maberly

Maberly described some of his experiences with bee venom in the July, 1910, issue of The *Lancet*.

CASE 1. Maberly related that he saw an old patient of his who, three years previously, had had a severe attack of rheumatism, which later developed into chronic arthritis. He tried spas, physiotherapy and drugs without the least sign of improvement. Patient was 55 years old, and had been pensioned. He steadily grew more helpless and finally gave up all treatments. Legs and arms strongly flexed, chin almost drawn to his chest, was not able to open his mouth more than half an inch. Never was free from pain, and from a fine and active man had become a helpless cripple. Maberly tried to cheer him but the patient seemed perfectly hopeless. The same evening, by chance, Maberly met a bee expert, who, after the case had been described to him, said that it was just the kind for bee treatment. The doctor made arrangements with him to visit his office and apply the bees.

The first treatment was given on October 30, 1910. Patient came to the doctor's office only with the greatest difficulty. His height was five feet and three inches. giving 18 stings weekly. In two months, patient stood five feet five, was able to Formerly his stature was five feet and ten. They persevered with the treatments, hold up his head, open his mouth fully, pains in the joints almost all disappeared.

After this success Maberly became an ardent follower of Terc.

CASE 2. Man, 35. Was laid up three times with rheumatic fever, for six or seven months each time. Joints became increasingly stiffer with every attack. In this case, the bee stings worked marvels. Patient told the doctor that his feet had been stiff ever since the first attack, but when the treatments were completed, he could walk anywhere—in fact he "did about twenty miles every Sunday." Maberly found the ankle movements perfect, patient stood easily on his toes, eating and drinking everything he liked and said that whenever he could catch a bee in his garden he "put it on."

Maberly visited a number of cases with the same bee expert, some were old-standing, chronic rheumatics, both elderly and younger subjects; all did well, though in every instance all recognized remedies had been tried without success. Maberly then quoted some of his own cases:

Mrs. A. Married, 30 years old. Attacked with rheumatic fever while on a holiday 20 miles from home. She was brought back in a motor, delirious, and was confined to bed for eight weeks. The first fortnight her temperature was between 104° and 105°. She had profuse acid perspiration, severe pains in the joints, endocarditis, with left regurgitant mitral murmur. Pains in the joints were very troublesome during convalescence.

Maberly tried everything without any sign of improvement. At last he persuaded patient to try the bees. Five applications completely relieved her, and she has been quite well ever since.

Miss B. 25 years old. Had influenza four years previously, which left her with neuritis of the left arm. It was so painful that she could not even sew without discomfort. Carried her arm in a sling for six months. Tried massage, electricity, various ointments, etc., without any result. At last, she consented to try the bees. Four applications of bee stings completely cured her.

Mr. C. 35 years old. Professional violoncellist. In December, 1909, had influenza, which left him with rheumatic pains in the joints. Patient was advised to take the bee treatments, but preferred to go to a spa, where, during his stay, he contracted rheumatic fever and was laid up for several weeks. When he returned, the pain in the joints was so severe that he could not accept any professional engagement. On February 27, 1910, Maberly commenced the course and applied 15 bees. By March 3rd, patient was able to play at a concert away from his home. The treatments consisted altogether of ten applications of bees. Since then the patient has been quite well.

Maberly was convinced that, though the remedy does not effect a permanent cure in every instance, it will always give a considerable relief even in cases which were considered almost hopeless. He suggested starting the treatments on elderly patients with about six stings for the first three applications, and then gradually increasing the number to a couple of dozen. If too many bees were applied at first, he found that patients became quite ill.

Franz Kretschy

Kretschy, of Vienna, after many years of experimentation, succeeded in producing an injectable bee venom suitable for therapeutic use. In his treatments, Kretschy faithfully followed Terc's principle-that the main purpose is total immunization of the patient.

He started with three intradermal injections of 0.1 c.c. each, gradually increasing the number of wheals and the strength of the solution, carefully controlling the formation of the wheals, their redness, swelling; being also heedful of malaise and other general effects. Kretschy noticed that in cases of similar morbidity, the reactions were also alike. He considered urticaria an anaphylactic phenomenon or an indication of idiosyncrasy. If the reactions were unduly severe, he took it for granted that this was attributable to tuberculosis, lues, or gonorrhea, and considered the occurrence an important differential diagnostic aid, to which fact he referred during the International Bee Conference in 1930.

Herbert Pollack

Pollack, of Munich, contemporaneously with Kretschy, succeeded in producing an injectable bee venom, called Apicosan. He treated his first cases in the Munich Medical Polyclinic under Dr. May and later in the Second Medical Clinic under Dr. Von Muller. Since 1927, he has been a collaborator of Kretschy, in Vienna. Pollack at first used intragluteal injections but later, intradermal wheals, as he found the method more efficacious.

In the Vienna Medical Clinic, under Prof. Strasser, during one year, 100 arthritic, rheumatic, neuritic, and neuralgic cases were treated with *Apicosan*. The results were extremely favorable. In 20 cases of iritis rheumatica, a complication of rheumatoid conditions, he had very good results. He started with two wheals (0.1 c.c. each) of concentration II, and after five or six injections had complete cures in cases which would not respond to any other medication. In neuritic conditions, he used the weakest solution. Pollack reported a case of trigeminal neuralgia which defied all other efforts, even surgical operations:

Female. Suffered for four years from a very severe trigeminal neuralgia. During the four years, she tried every possible treatment without result: first, the usual symptomatic medications, later alcohol injections, and finally operative measures. As the severance of the single branches did not bring her any relief, the extirpation of the Gasserian ganglion was performed without relieving the painful condition. Pollack decided to use Apicosan, without much hope. Already, after the first injections, patient did not complain for ten hours and after every application the painless intervals increased. Following the seventh injection, which was given at 3 P.M., patient remained perfectly painless until the next morning. Slept for the first time in four years without narcotics; even large doses of morphine had not given her such relief. Close upon the eighth injection, the facial "tic" disappeared; two weeks later the sensitivity on pressure and percussion considerably diminished; and in three weeks, after twenty-one injections, she was entirely relieved. Patient's general feeling was good; she increased in weight, her sleep was normal, and she had no recurrence.

According to Pollack, every irritant like Apicosan must be administered in gradually increasing doses until patient reaches immunity. In his four years' experience, he found few recurrences. He thought the treatments increased appetite, improved sleep and were without any danger of anaphylaxy or hemolysis.

Prof. Passow

Prof. Passow, of Munich, used Apicosan in intragluteal injections in three to four day intervals, gradually increasing the doses from 0.3 to 1 c.c. He obtained very good results in iridocyclitis rheumatica and gouty iritis. He was rather doubtful about recurrences.

In neuritis optica, which did not yield to any other remedial measures, Passow obtained very quick cures. He found a slight temperature rising during treatments but no albuminuria and no anaphylactic symptoms. He considered bee venom a remedy worthy of experiment, and suggested a wider field for its application.

Professor Lauber also obtained excellent results in iritis and iridocyclitis cases, where all other remedies failed.

R. Loebel (Hofgastein)-A. Simo (Schallebach)

R. Loebel and A. Simo used Apicosan, even in severe cases of primary and secondary chronic polyarthritis, and obtained good results. It was found to be especially effective in myalgia and neuralgia cases. They thought that it was worth further experiments.

Klemens Wasserbrenner

Wasserbrenner of the General Polyclinic of Vienna (Professor H. Strasser) treated 121 patients during a year with Apicosan: sciatica, 45; plexus neuralgia, 16; intercostal neuralgia, 25; chronic arthritis, 25; arthritis deformans, 10. He used it in three ways: subcutaneously, intramuscularly, and intradermally, but he obtained best results with intradermal administrations. Wasserbrenner usually started with 0.2 c.c. (two wheals) of concentration I, and increased it to 0.5 c.c. (five wheals). In every case the wheals looked different. The local reactions disappeared, as a rule, within 24 hours. Patients manifested considerable pruritus. Reinjections were administered only after the symptoms of the previous injection had disappeared. The local and general reactions were minimal compared to the focal reactions. The pain in the diseased joints increased considerably but usually disappeared in three days.

Wasserbrenner obtained best results in sciatica and other rheumatic neuralgias. There were never any bad effects. In chronic arthritis, especially monarthritis, his results were not so good. In climacteric arthritis, patients showed very little improvement. In arthritis deformans, he had very unsatisfactory results.

Wasserbrenner's article was written in 1928, and he concluded with the remark that he had just learned that a stronger concentration of injectable bee venom was being made which was supposed to give much better results in chronic arthritis.

Jacques Kroner

Kroner, of the Friedrich Wilhelm Hospital, Berlin, used Apicosan in rheumatic conditions. He started with three wheals, o.1 c.c. each, of concentration I, increasing the wheals 5-7-10, etc., continuing with the next higher concentration until he reached immunity. He administered it in two or three-day intervals and never found it necessary to give it longer than two months.

Kroner noticed very strong focal reactions, often chills and high fever in the late stages of arthritis. He considered skin reactions very important. The best results were obtained in muscular rheumatism, neuritis, and sciatica. Kroner admitted that the remedy deserves consideration because it gives chronic arthritics improvement in general feeling, freer function of the joints. He suggested reducing the intake of calories, starting with carbohydrates and albumin, and considered fat as the best food for arthritics.

Kroner delivered a lecture before the Third International Congress for Rheumatism (October 1932), commenting in laudatory terms upon apitherapy. During the same meeting Perrin and Cuènot announced their successes with bee-venom treatments. Both these lectures aroused considerable interest.

Siegfried Becker

Becker, of the First Medical University Clinic of Vienna (Prof. Otto Porges), used Immenin and gave a detailed report of his experiences, observations, and results. He noticed that best results were obtained in neuralgia, especially sciatic neuritis. With toxic neuritis, he had had no experience, as these cases are not generally included in ambulatory material. In polyneuritis, the treatments were not so successful, as these conditions usually are of endocrine origin, mainly climacteric. This group, he thought, was rather resistant to bee venom therapy. The selected subjects were, as a rule, brachial, crural, or ischiadic neuralgias, not in a peracute state. He used weak concentrations to avoid stronger reactions; only if the cases were obstinate and resistant did he step up to higher concentration. An exacerbation of the painful symptoms was often noticed, but generally it subsided very soon. In neuralgia, his results were very good, even in cases which were refractory to all other medications.

The treatments of arthritic cases were difficult and more tedious. Becker had very little experience with acute arthritis, considering the ambulatory character of the clinic. Chronic arthritis with acute exacerbation of the symptoms was more in his domain, both the exudative and fibrous types. In chronic infective arthritis, it was hard to judge the results, as spontaneous remission of the process is very frequent, even without treatment. He often noticed that when a new remedy was used and, by chance, the time of treatment just coincided with the remission which was due anyhow, the optimistic patient overestimated its efficiency and hailed it as a wonder cure. In arthritis deformans, although the number of cases treated was small, Becker noticed a decided, even surprising improvement and he advocated a wider field for bee-venom therapy in such conditions. In arthritis deformans, there is no spontaneous remission of the symptoms and if improvement manifests itself during the treatments, the post hoc, ergo propter hoc principle can be applied. He increased the wheals and the concentration only gradually. Every time he attempted a sudden increase, the patient felt worse. Improvements in this category were comparatively late and slow. A tabulation of his results is given below:

Nature of Disorder	Number of Cases	Good Results	Improvement	No Results
Primary chronic polyarthritis	28	16	9	3
Secondary chronic infective arthritis	20	15	3	2
Bechterew disease	5	4	-	1
Arthritis de formans	10	4	2	4
Sciatica	14	12	-	2
Neuralgia	18	10	4	4
Endocrine polyalgia	25	4	6	15

He recommended bee venom as a valuable weapon with which to combat rheumatism and arthritis, especially in view of the great advantage that there is never any danger connected with the procedure. His results in the various groups were about the same as those of other authors.

TREATMENTS WITH INJECTABLE BEE VENOM

Hans Nowotny

Nowotny, of the Orthopedic Hospital, Vienna (Prof. Hans Spitzy), published in 1932 twenty cases of chronic inflammatory conditions which he had treated during the two previous years with injectable bee venom. He found the results distinctly favorable. I quote some cases of interest:

Man, 40. After amputation of the femur, he was in the hospital three times for an abscess of the stump. In July. 1930, he returned for the fourth time with cellulitis, fistulae, and a hard infiltration the size of an orange. In September, Nowotny gave milk injections and other treatments, without success.

On the 20th of November, 1930, he decided to administer Immenin. He injected intradermally over the infiltrated area five wheals of o.1 c.c. each, concentration I. There was a slight local, but no general reaction.

Three days later, the infiltration was smaller and softer. Continued treatment with concentration II, up to 0.8 c.c.

December, 1930, infiltration disappeared. Patient had no difficulty in walking on his prothesis.

Examined April, 1932. Continuously used his artificial leg without pain, and walked much better.

Man, 45. Was admitted to the hospital September, 1918. Amputation-stump of femur, with cellulitis and osteomyelitis. Was discharged as cured, February, 1920. In June, 1920, returned with severe pain in the stump, especially in the scar. Typical sciatic complaints. In July, 1920, excision of the old scar, resection of the sciatic nerve, normal recovery. Left hospital in September, 1920. In December, 1931, returned to hospital with high temperature and cellulitis of the stump. On incision, one quart of putrid pus evacuated (staphylococcus pyogenes aureus). In January, 1932, drains were removed. Considerably improved but infiltration and thickening of the stump did not show any tendency to recede.

January 20th, Nowotny injected bee venom intradermally into the infiltrated surface. Strong inflammation and swelling on the place of injection, spreading over the major part of the stump.

January 25, 1932, fever, swelling, and redness subsided. Infiltration quickly disappeared. February 10th, patient tried his prothesis. February 20th, was discharged from hospital cured. Walked very well.

April, 1932, reëxamined. Had worn prothesis uninterruptedly, without pain or pressure, was even skiing in the Alps.

Woman, 23. Admitted to the hospital, January 27, 1932. For the previous two years had had pain in right ankle, wore plate for a year. No improvement. Ankle swollen, with dilated veins, slight erythema, infiltrated nodes the size of a hazelnut. Diagnosis: arthritis.

January 27, 1932, 0.4 of concentration I intradermally around the infiltration. Slight local and general reactions. Increased number of wheals up to ten (I c.c.). Wheals were applied on the shoulder.

February 11, 1932, infiltration entirely gone. No pain.

Man, 40. Admitted to the hospital in June, 1930, with compound fracture of both lower limbs. While left limb healed in comparatively short time, the right one, after septic infection, even a year and a half later showed no inclination to close. Decided to give bee venom.

November 4, 1931, 3 wheals of concentration II on the right shoulder.

November 5th, reported twitching in the wound. Administered 4 wheals of II. November 6th, 6 wheals of II. Wound already showed tendency to heal. November 7th, 8 wheals of II on the left shoulder.

November 9th, 10 wheals of II, right shoulder.

November 16th, wound considerably smaller. 5 wheals of concentration III.

Increased doses gradually.

By December 16th, wound entirely closed.

Nowotny thought that bee venom increases the healing tendency in chronic inflammations. The first case cited above proved that bee venom possessed a greater resorptive effect than any other remedy he had tried. The fourth case cited above demonstrated the quick healing power in a wound which had been open for more than a year. He recommended it for treating chronic inflammatory conditions.

Wilhelm Fehlow

Fehlow, of the Surgical Clinic of Berlin University (Prof. August Bier), used bee venom in the treatment of arthritis and rheumatism, and published very favorable results. He could not report good results from Immenin but found Apicosan very effective. His treatments averaged from six to ten weeks. He used Apicosan in the following types:

Polyarthritis. Polyarthritis, primary and secondary infective arthritis, stood the treatments well. In 16 cases of infective arthritis, 7 were very much improved, 2 improved, and there were 2 interrupted treatments. In 3 cases of Bechterew disease, he had one very good result.

Myalgia and Neuralgia. In myalgia, neuralgia, and sciatica, he obtained very rapid and satisfactory results even with short treatments and weaker concentrations. Eleven cases were all cured. Had 3 recurrences, where the immunity wore off.

Arthrosis. In 17 cases of arthrosis, he had 7 surprisingly good results, pain considerably lessened or none at all. Several cases were given up on account of their endocrine origin; they were rather refractory to treatments. Fehlow found that bee venom gave best results in myalgia, neuralgia, and sciatica; polyarthritides were greatly improved. He commented that bee venom was a remedy which, in properly selected cases, gave good results, and, second, that there was absolutely no danger in its administration.

Gertrud Koehler

Koehler, of the 1st Intern. Dept. of Urban Hospital, Berlin (Prof. H. Zondek), treated chronic polyarthritis, arthritis deformans and Bechterew's disease with Apicosan. She was unable to report the cases in detail on account of the limited space granted for the article, but summed up her observations by stating that the remedy favorably influenced all the symptoms in those conditions; the swelling and pain of the joints gradually subsided and their improved motility was very noticeable.

Maximilian Grünsfeld

Grünsfeld, of Vienna, in his report did not give the number of his treated cases, but stated that he considered bee venom a very valuable remedy in rheumatic and neuralgic conditions, suggesting a hot full bath during treatments to secure a freer movement of the joints.

Grünsfeld urged that the treatments should be repeated after three months, when an increase in dosage may be more rapid; even a third cure after a year, with another fairly rapid increase in concentrations. Of course, all depends on the patient's condition. He laid important stress on individualization during treatments and considered that the greatest advantages of the bee venom treatment are:

1) No harmful consequences.
2) Improvement of general condition and feeling.
3) Disappearance of psychic depression.
4) Improvement in appetite and sleep.
5) Increase of weight.

M. Roch

Professor Roch, of the Medical Faculty of Geneva, wrote an article in 1928 in which he treated the subject of bee venom more from a theoretical than a practical viewpoint, giving the results of his physiological and toxicological experiments. He mentioned the good clinical results obtained with the substance by others in the treatment of rheumatism and arthritis, but seemed to be rather skeptical about it. He referred, for instance, to Terc and Keiter, almost doubting their published results, but said he had to take Professor Langer's word that "these men are no charlatans."

In 1933, Roch showed an entirely different attitude, and published fourteen cases treated with bee venom:

10 cases of Sciatica - 7 very good, and 3 fair results 2 very good results
2 cases of Lumbago - 2 very good results
2 cases of Chronic Rheumatism - 2 improvements

Among others he reported a case of a young man of 20, who had been discharged from military service on account of severe, very painful chronic neuralgia of the left side. Salicylates, massage, light, diathermy, spa, and injections of Naïodine were of no avail. After three months' suffering, he was admitted to the hospital. Roch started treatments with Apicosan. A week later, there was great improvement, and 20 days later patient left the hospital, cured and delighted, able to resume his work.

Roch had best success in neuralgia, though in rheumatism and arthritis, his results were also very favorable. He noticed that outside of antineuralgic and antirheumatic effects, Apicosan had tonic, distinctly cardiotonic, effects.

Roch referred to his personal experience, which he also reported to the Congress of Rheumatism in Paris. He thought it is rather exceptional that a physician himself should use the method which he liberally ministers to his patients. Osteoarthritis of the knee had been the diagnosis and he tried everything without help or even improvement. Osteosarcoma was then suspected. Before he consented to amputation, he requested Dr. M. A. DuBois to give him a series of Apicosan injections. Not only did he find the treatment tolerable but the result was so excellent that he abandoned the thought of an osteosarcoma.

Perrin and Cuènot

Professor Maurice Perrin, of the Medical Faculty of Nancy, France, and his assistant Alain Cuènot, published the results of 19 cases of arthritis deformans, articular rheumatism, arthritis, rheumatoid pains, lumbago and sciatica, treated with bee venom. They introduced these case records and the remarkable results they obtained to the Third International Congress for Rheumatism (October 1932). Their results were so excellent that they made the statement that bee venom has a remote action in the system, especially on the parts attacked by rheumatism. They admitted that they had started their research work of treating rheumatism with bee venom with a certain skepticism, but now they were convinced of the possibility of attaining success in cases which so far had resisted all the other usual medications. Today they are the chief exponents of apitherapy in France.

Perrin and Cuènot gave, in their introduction, a detailed general history of bee-venom treatment. They thought bee venom and the bark of the willow tree (which contains salicylic acid) the two oldest remedies known. Even Hippocrates, Celsus, Galen, used the venom of the bees for therapeutic purposes. Both Perrin and Cuènot undertook a thorough study of the subject, particularly with regard to the hypersensitivity of some patients toward the venom. They explained this as a proteotoxic shock but as the effective element of bee venom is not a protein, they admit that they are entirely in the dark as to its curative power, mentioning that the injectable bee venom which is made in Germany contains no albumin or protein, has no hemolytic action, does not produce proteotoxic shock, and still has its therapeutic efficiency preserved. They had, however, no occasion to treat any patient with this product.

They used live bees in their treatments and described the procedure. They applied them usually on the affected parts; for instance, in arthritis, over the affected joints; in sciatica, on the extensor surface of the femur, etc., cleansing the skin with ether, as alcohol is destructive to bee venom.

TREATMENTS WITH INJECTABLE BEE VENOM

Perrin and Cuènot prepared a special bee venom solution for winter use, which is described in Chapter IV.

Perrin and Cuènot attributed four effects to the venom:

1) A general tonic effect. Patients all felt stronger; were more agile; more alert, less out of breath; their sleep and appetite greatly improved; and the authors were not surprised that beekeepers all live to a robust old age. They thought the venom has also a cardiotonic action, like digitalis.
2) Local irritant action, like that of a mustard plaster, scarification, or a hot-point needle.
3) Anti-infective power.
4) Antirheumatic and analgesic effect of first order.

An exacerbation of the pain, usually followed by amelioration, was often noticed. I quote some of their cases, which may be of interest:

Arthritis Deformans.-There was improvement after 59 stings.

Julia H., 31 years. The pain and deformity started in 1924, and gradually became worse. Patient was treated with salicylates, mesothorium, antistreptococcus serum, intramuscular milk injections, iodides, physiotherapy-all without improvement.

In the winter of 1930-31, large doses of syrup of iodide and cod liver oil were given as a tonic. A diffuse eczema developed on the chest and legs, which lasted for three weeks. After this dermatosis, though she had been bedridden for 22 years, she was able to go about, but soon again became worse.

In July, 1931, patient was bedridden, in very poor health, with severe pain, insomnia, and raised temperature.

July 11, 1931, three bees were applied, with normal reaction.

July 15th, 17 stings. After the 15th sting, malaise, and after the 17th, she fainted. Three hours later, vomiting, vertigo, buzzing of the ears, itch, urticaria. Patient was very agitated and slept poorly. Next day symptoms ameliorated. Three days later, all malaise disappeared, with hardly any local reaction. Violent paroxysm in the joints.

July 20th, 6 stings. Four or five hours later, profuse perspiration, malaise, pain in the joints, and slight urticaria. Next day, much improved.

July 23rd, 10 stings over left knee. Rheumatic joints active, considerable focal reaction.

July 24th, 10 stings on shoulder. After an hour, strong general reaction syncope, intense urticaria.

July 30th, 5 stings.

August 4th, 8 stings.

Altogether, she received 59 stings. By the middle of September, she had less pain, was making very good progress, sleep had improved. In October, she was out of bed and around the house. Was able to undress and go to bed by herself. In November, was able to go shopping, even made a trip to the city, which she had not been able to do since 1923.

Very Advanced Arthritis Deformans. Sixty-one stings were given. Quick improvement resulted.

Jeanne M., 61 years old. Suffered from the ailment since her thirtieth year. Previous ten years, had been laid up, hardly able to move. She received 61 stings in one month. Intense focal reactions, recrudescence of pains. Next month, slept much better, had less pain, but two months later same condition as before treatment.

The writer thinks that the publication of such cases is very regrettable, especially the fact that no reason is given for the interruption of the treatment.

Rheumatic Pain in Both Knees. Adele G., 75 years. First session, applied 1 sting; second, two days later, 6 stings; third, 6 stings; after which pain entirely disappeared.

Jean W. Arthritis in the right knee. 50 stings. No recurrences for years.

Ernst L., 31 years. Intolerable pain in left knee for a week. 4 bees applied, loco dolenti. Next day pain completely disappeared.

Rheumatism in the Knee. Ailment of several years' standing. 12 stings applied, next day pain was gone. Three months later, recurrence. After 12 stings, pain entirely disappeared within 24 hours.

Traumatic Arthritis Subsequent to a Chronic Dislocation of the Shoulder. Robert K., 61 years. His shoulder had been dislocated 10 years previously. Immediate reduction, but pain persisted. He could not use right arm. In three sessions, 30 bees were applied, in situ. Pain disappeared. After three years, pain returned. Applied 10 stings. Pain stopped entirely. Two years later, pain appeared again but 10 stings removed it.

Pierre L., 25 years. Intense pain in both knees, slight bilateral hydrarthrosis. Was treated with salicylates and rest, without improvement. 5 stings were applied over each knee. Next day, all pain gone.

Pierre D., 67 years. Muscular rheumatism in his right arm, especially in biceps. Had it for 35 years. 5 stings applied. All pain disappeared. Free from pain for last three years.

Jean B. Left shoulder dislocated in 1931. Since that time joint painful, though dislocation was reduced. In May, 1932, 5 stings applied on site. Next day, all movement of arm free. Fully recovered.

Post-traumatic Pain in the Shoulder. Joseph P., 60 years. No fracture or dislocation, but severe bruise. Persistent pain. Treated with acupuncture. No relief. 6 stings, loco dolenti. Three days later, 15 more. All the pain gone.

Lumbago. Stephano X., 32 years. Two stings applied on the lumbar region, which produced freer muscular movements. Slept well. Next day, 5 more stings. Pain disappeared. Perfectly relieved.

Sciatic Neuritis.-Paul B., 52 years. Suffered from sciatica for five years. Treated in 1923. Ailment so painful, he was unable to walk. Six stings were applied daily over the nerve for one month. Pain gradually left him for the first time in five years.

F. Thompson

Thompson, of London, formerly demonstrator of Physiology in the London Hospital Medical College, in an article which appeared in *The Lancet* of August 1933, stated it was his opinion that muscular rheumatism, lumbago, sciatica, fibrosities, and complications after acute or subacute rheumatism were curable in about 80 percent of the cases, by a course of bee stings. He himself, after suffering for 20 years, was cured in this way in six weeks, and from that time kept a hive in the yard by his consulting room for the benefit of others willing to submit to the treatments.

Thompson thought that in the more chronic forms of arthritis and periarthritis the results are not so encouraging, though the method is not unworthy of trial when all other remedies have failed, as one does occasionally see surprising results. The following treatment was suggested:

229

at first, one bee sting, administered on a convenient place and the toxic effects noted; if not abnormal, the treatment is repeated twice weekly for the first week, two stings twice weekly for the second week, three the third, and so on. By the end of the sixth week, immunity is obtained and relief from the symptoms as well. If reaction is unfavorable to the first sting, treatment should be discontinued; otherwise patient may continue it himself at the nearest apiary. If living in the country, he should be encouraged to keep bees.

Thompson said, "I have used Kretschy's 'Immenin' for therapeutic purposes without any good results."

References to articles by workers named in this chapter are given after Chapters II and IV.

Chapter XII Medico-Legal Aspects of Bees and Their Injuries

Bees have considerable medico-legal interest. In the oldest law books, bees and honey are frequently mentioned. The ancient Egyptian, Greek, and Roman archives contain legal references to both. Solon, the great Athenian law-giver and reformer (594 B.C.), often refers in his laws to bees. (Plutarch, Solon. 23.) Plato (first half of the 4th Century B.C.), repeatedly mentioned the existing laws, especially with respect to swarming and poisoning of bees.

Pseudo-Quintilian (1st Century A.D.) was alluding to bees in the 13th of his Declamationes majores: A poor man brought suit for damages against his rich neighbor, who had given him orders to remove the bees because they hurt his flowers. After he refused, the rich man sprinkled poison over the flowers which killed the bees. Neither the rich man's reply nor a description of the poison is recorded. (Fraser.)

Justinian (533 A.D.), in his Institutiones (II-1-14)-which is one of the most important documents in all jurisprudence-defined the law about swarming bees. It is rather interesting to note that our present laws which refer to swarming are almost identical, even though those of Justinian were written nearly fifteen centuries ago. According to the Justinian code, bees are wild by nature. A swarm on your tree is not considered to be your property until you have hived it, no more than the birds which build their nests in your trees. If any one else hives it, he becomes the rightful owner. Anybody is permitted to remove honeycombs made by wild bees, but if some one enters upon your property, of course you have the right to prevent his entrance, or to charge the intruder with trespass.

"If the swarm will not be stayed, but, hasting on still, goes beyond your bounds; the ancient Law of Christendome permitteth you to pursue them withersoever, for the recovery of your owne. If your swarm goes so fast and so far that you lose sight and hearing of them, you also lose your right and property in them." According to the oldest Germanic laws anybody was privileged to pursue and capture a swarm, except on territories owned by the king.

The German archives mentioned the adjudication of a complaint which was lodged before the tribunal of Worms, when a child was killed by bees. The judgment ordered that the hive should be taken to the public square and the bees and hive burned.

MEDICO-LEGAL ASPECTS OF BEES AND THEIR INJURIES

In laws of the Middle Ages, frequent allusions are made to bees, especially with reference to swarming. For instance, Alfred the Great, King of the Saxons (under whose leadership the English gained their first decided naval advantage over the Vikings and who made many judicial and educational reforms), did not forget the bees in his laws. He ruled that when a swarm of bees was on its way, the church bells must ring so that the nearest neighbor might take them. We also read that in the Middle Ages, as a punishment law-breakers were tied, hand and foot, their bodies smeared with honey, exposed to the sun, and left to the mercy of the bees until they were stung to death.

In old Saxony, to damage a bee hive or steal one was considered a great crime. If the hive were stolen from an enclosure, the penalty was death. In old Bavarian law books, we find that very severe punishment was meted for adulterating honey. Honey was held in high esteem, and if anybody committed the crime of adulterating it, his punishment was the loss of one hand or the payment of a fine of 65 pfennigs (Hovorka).

Bee stings may play quite an important part in compensation cases. Sugar refineries, conserve and candy factories, are often exposed to annoyances by bees. A bee sting, such a painful surprise, may also cause serious accidents. Automobile, motorcycle, and bicycle accidents are, indirectly, more frequently caused by bee stings than we imagine, often even with fatal outcome. It can be easily understood why a driver of an automobile or motorcycle, stung suddenly by a bee on the face or hands, may lose control of the vehicle. Roch, of Geneva, reported that he himself witnessed a serious accident. A young man was riding a motorcycle when he suddenly turned a somersault and collapsed. Closer examination revealed that he had been stung by a bee on the neck, possibly on the jugular vein. In the report of the Swiss Casualty Company of Lucerne, we find that in 1920 and 1921 alone, in a country of only four million inhabitants, they had 1,785 claims and paid out 184,000 francs in indemnities for injuries due to bee stings. We even find that bees were linked with unlawful acts. Casper, *Traité de Médic. Legale* II, p. 125, mentioned two cases. In one case, the parents of a twenty-one months' old illegitimate child exposed it to bee stings with the purpose of getting rid of it. Another one was that of a nurse who put a bee into the mouth of an infant, also with criminal intent.

The most interesting legal document referring to bees is a 33-page report of Dr. M. A. Delpech to the Police Prefect of Paris. So many complaints had been lodged with the authorities in Paris about injuries, damages, and losses caused by bees that the Police Prefect commissioned

232

Delpech, a member of the Academy of Medicine and Public Health Counsellor, to report to him about the situation, and to suggest some legislation, because so far there had been no laws which regulated the maintenance of beehives and fixing of responsibility for injuries. The complaints were innumerable. Some people were unable to go into their gardens, open their windows, or go to the well for water, without being attacked or stung by bees.

Most complaints were from sugar refineries. Some reported enormous losses, such as one hundred quarts of syrup a day. Besides, the bees molested and harassed the laborers, and disturbed them at their work. One of the sugar refiners, M. C. Say, complained that his yearly losses amounted to at least 25,000 francs. Not only did the bees take with them a quantity of sugar, but some fell into the melted syrup. The worst part of it was that the bees had always chosen the best quality of syrup, preferring certain colors. The conserve manufacturers complained that during the hot summer days legions of them invaded their factories. The laborers, who worked almost stripped, were often compelled to take off several days to nurse their painful injuries. Some refineries complained that their neighbors kept as many as 120 to 150 hives. A well-populated hive contains about 40,000 workers, so that in a hundred hives there were approximately 4,000,000 worker bees. As there were not enough flowers to provide them with food, they were compelled to look for substitutes.

Girls' schools remonstrated that the bees distracted the attention of the pupils. The visiting bees often intruded under their skirts. One school reported that, without exaggeration, almost every pupil had been stung. Another school submitted a list of 104 pupils who had been more or less severely injured on the neck, face, and hands. Some of them had had to stay home for two or three days, others even a week, nursing their injuries. One of the pupils who had been stung on the hand suffered quite a severe inflammation, which left her with a bad scar. Orphan asylums reported that, daily, about a dozen inmates were stung. In addition, there were numerous complaints about serious and fatal accidents to men and beasts. Horses, dogs, cattle, and poultry were killed.

Delpech collected proofs of fifteen injuries caused by bees which ended fatally, and of seven grave accidents. In his final report, he suggested that amateur beekeepers deserve consideration, but the instalment, by professionals, of larger apiaries should be prohibited.

MEDICO-LEGAL ASPECTS OF BEES AND THEIR INJURIES

In general, the laws pertaining to bees greatly vary according to countries. In the United States, there are very few laws, and the decisions in litigations for injuries or damages caused by bees are adjudicated, as a rule, from the legal opinions handed down in previous cases. The essential principles are that bees are considered wild by nature (ferae naturae) but when hived they are subject to ownership (domitae naturae). One may acquire property in wild animals, including bees, by reclaiming and making them tame by art, industry, and education (per industriam), or by so confining them within his own immediate power that they cannot escape and use their natural liberty.

Most of the lawsuits have been for damages for personal injury or harm to property, like horses, sheep, dogs, poultry, etc. Many other suits have been for annoyances caused by bees, where they were considered a nuisance. The acquisition of a stray swarm and the question of a beekeeper's right to follow his own swarming bees have led to many litigations. Bees are not considered by law as fierce or dangerous. In case of injury, it is essential to prove negligence; otherwise the owner of the bees is not liable for any accident or injury caused by them.

The case of Earl vs. Van Alstine is often referred to. The defendant, Van Alstine, owned fifteen hives, which he kept in his yard, adjoining the public highway. Earl, the plaintiff, passed on the highway with a team, when the bees attacked the horses, and, as a result, one of them died. The deciding judge gave his opinion as follows: "There are two questions which have to be decided: (1) Is the owner of the bees liable for any injury they do? (2) Did the defendant keep the bees in such an improper place as to render him liable?" The court decided in favor of the defendant, that he was perfectly justified in keeping bees on his property. From the various testimonies given, it appeared that bees had been kept in the same place for eight or nine years, and no proof was offered that the slightest injury had been done by them previously. One witness testified that he had passed and repassed the property frequently, with teams of horses and otherwise, without ever having been molested.

Many other similar verdicts have been rendered. The main point is that the owners must keep the hives where they will be least troublesome. A city, of course, has the right, called "police power," to pass ordinances restricting certain persons from exercising their constitutional rights, if such restriction is for the public health and welfare.

MEDICO-LEGAL ASPECTS OF BEES AND THEIR INJURIES

The case of Arkadelphia vs. Clark, in 1889, is a well-known litigation, which lasted a long time. Clark kept bees, but the City of Arkadelphia adopted an ordinance that it should be unlawful for any person to own, keep, or raise bees within the city limits, and declared it a nuisance. Clark was given notice to remove his bees, but he refused to comply. He was fined day after day for ten successive days. He did not pay his fine, and was committed to jail. The court decided, in a long argument, that the city had no right to make such an ordinance; all ordinances arbitrary in their terms and unreasonable, unnecessarily encroaching on private rights, are void. Clark won on final decision.

In another case, Olmsted vs. Rich, the evidence showed that the beekeeper had a large number of hives on property adjoining the plaintiff's, and during the spring and summer the bees interfered with enjoyment of the plaintiff's premises. The bees drove the owner, his servants, and his guests from the garden and grounds, stinging them and making the premises unfit and unsafe for residential purposes. The verdict was against the beekeeper, granting a permanent injunction, which was affirmed on appeal.

In the Johannesburg Star (December, 1933), we read the following account:

"Bloemfontein, South Africa.

"Judgment was delivered today in the Orange Free State Provincial Division of the Supreme Court by Mr. Justice P. U. Fischer in the case of Mrs. Wasserman v. the Union Government. The plaintiff, Mrs. Wasserman, sued the Government on behalf of her minor children for £2,000, as damages stated to have been sustained as the result of her husband, a member of the Police Force stationed at Frankford, being stung to death by bees on November 1.

"From the evidence it appeared that a swarm of bees had nested between the wooden lining and corrugated iron wall of an office in the building, and he was instructed by the sergeant in charge to assist him in locating the nest. He mounted a tub and put his head through a window above which was the bees' exit, and was immediately stung by two bees, on the upper lip and above the right temple, as a result of which he died within 20 minutes, notwithstanding immediate medical assistance.

"The pleadings alleged negligence in not removing the bees, or otherwise rendering the premises safe for those employed therein.

"The Court found that the defendant was in no way responsible for the presence of the bees in the building, and as there was no act of commission, the Government could not be held liable. The Court further found that, assuming the order to locate the bees was a lawful order, the deceased nevertheless was aware of and voluntarily incurred the risk of damages. In those circumstances the plaintiff was held not to have made out her case, and absolution from the instance was granted."

CHAPTER REFERENCES

BLAAS, C. M. Die Biene in Deutscher Volkssitte, und Meinung, Bericht. und Mitteil. des Alterthumvereins, Wien., XXIV.

DELPECH, A. Les dépots de ruches d'abeilles existant sur differents points de la ville de Paris, Ann. d'Hyg. Par., III, Janvier, 1880.

FRASER, H. M. Beekeeping in Antiquity, 1931.

HOVORKA, D., UND KRONFELD, U. Vergleichende Volksmedizin, 1908.

KNORTZ, K. Insecten in Sage, Sitte und Literatur, 1910.

MORLEY, M. W. The Honey Makers, 1899.

ROOT, A. J., AND ROOT, E. R. The ABC and XYZ of Bee Culture, 1917.

Chapter XIII Questionnaire

Several bee journals were good enough to extend to me the courtesy, for which I am duly appreciative, of printing in their publications a questionnaire, inserted with the idea and expectation of gaining additional useful information about the subject.

George S. Demuth and E. R. Root, Editors of *Gleanings in Bee Culture*, as an introductory article in their November, 1933, issue, commented on the questionnaire as follows:

BEE STINGS FOR RHEUMATISM

"For years bee stings have been used as a remedy for arthritis and rheumatism, but largely without sufficient scientific proof of their efficiency. Now comes Dr. Bodog F. Beck, of New York City, with a request that beekeepers help him in his investigation of this interesting and important subject. On page 673 in this issue, he gives a list of questions he would like to have beekeepers answer. If a large number of answers are sent in, Dr. Beck will have some important data that may lead to establishing the bee-sting remedy as a standard for certain types of rheumatism and arthritis. We hope that our readers will respond generously to Dr. Beck's request."

QUESTIONNAIRE TO BEEKEEPERS

1. If, before your occupation of beekeeping, you were stung by bees, were you, or were you not, sensitive to the injury? Kindly state to what degree.

2. If you were sensitive, did the sensitivity continue, lessen, disappear, or increase during your close contact with bees?

3. In case you became immune to the effect of bee sting injuries, what length of time did it require?

4. Please give your local and general symptoms of (a) a normal sting; (b) an unusually severe sting.

5. What is your favorite remedy for treating both the local and general effects of bee stings?

6. Did you ever suffer from rheumatism or arthritis before you kept bees? If so, taking for granted that you were stung by bees, have you been

relieved, cured, or have you had a recurrence? Please give details as to time and other important aspects.

7. Did you acquire either of the above ailments during the time you were exposed to bee stings?

8. Do you know of a case of paralysis or cancer improved or cured by bee stings? If so, kindly give details.

9. Do you know of any fatal cases resulting from bee sting injuries? If so, give approximate number of bee stings and other details. Give initials of victim, also place where it occurred, to avoid error of recording the identical case more than once.

10. Have you any additional interesting or instructive general facts to report?

I received hundreds of replies from almost every state of the nation and from England, Canada, from many European countries, and also from Hawaii, Australia, New Zealand, South Africa, etc. The interest evidenced by those who replied was gratifying and encouraging, and the information secured, very instructive and valuable. The letters alone would make an interesting volume. The consideration, courtesy, and enthusiasm of the beekeeping fraternity and apiphiles, volunteering all possible assistance, were a real revelation. Many of the letters-we might just as well call them dissertations—would be worth publishing in their entirety. Beekeeping was portrayed by some as a hobby, a diversion, a pastime, or a healthy outdoor avocation; by others as a profession, a profitable vocation, producing honey and wax, or a means of utilizing the blissful services of the bees for pollinating the fruit trees of their orchards. One made the statement that the expression "beekeeper" is all wrong. "We don't keep the bees-the bees keep us"; another, "They are my real pets."

All the letters were written in an extremely friendly and accommodating spirit. The questionnaire had hardly been published before I was flooded with replies, all eager to assist me in furthering and championing the idea, expressing in a sincere tone their delight that a physician should take up a problem which they all considered worthy of attention and thorough research, wishing me good luck and success in my investigation. I cannot omit voicing here my thanks for the great willingness and cordiality with which such a large number literally showered upon me all the information they could supply.

QUESTIONNAIRE

The letters, for the most part, represented the plain, unpretentious rural population. The majority of the writers were farmers, beekeepers, and laborers, and still their writings afforded a delightful and refreshing study. The notes were not intended for publication, were written offhand, unpremeditated, but we cannot fail to observe and admire in their choice of words, in their well-drawn narratives, the ready pen, even a certain literary merit, and all-around common sense, often sprinkled with waggish, wit snapping humor, though some of the replies were scribbled in pencil on rather unconventional farm stationery.

The various points in which I was most interested were:

1. The initial sensitivity of the individuals; the time and manner in which they acquired immunity, and its degree.

2. The circumstances which influenced normal and severe bee sting injuries, and their symptoms.

3. Information and evidence as to the curative and preventive value of bee venom in arthritis and rheumatism.

4. Fatalities from bee sting injuries.

INITIAL SENSITIVITY OF THE INDIVIDUALS; THE TIME AND MANNER IN WHICH THEY ACQUIRED IMMUNITY, AND ITS DEGREE

(a) With respect to individual sensitivity, we were able to compute the following statistics from the answers received:

Slightly sensitive	10%
Sensitive	36%
Very sensitive	54%

(b) Regarding their acquired immunity:

Continued sensitivity	16%
Diminished sensitive	76%
Absolute immunity	8%

(If we compare these percentages with those of Langer and Flury, the differences are almost negligible.)

(c) With regard to the period required by beekeepers to gain a fairly permanent state of immunity, our figures show:

1-5 years	69%
6-10 years	14%
10-20 years	8%
Longer period	9%

The descriptions of the manner in which the initial sensitivity was revealed varied only slightly. Some reported moderate sensitivity, others a rather expressed, or even great sensitivity to bee stings at the beginning of their exposures, but the majority grew accustomed to the effects, becoming less and less sensitive, and gradually acquired a certain degree of immunity. They all made the same statement-with very few exceptions-that during the summer they became more or less immune to the stings, and by fall, reached their maximum nonsensitive state. The next spring, not having been exposed to stings during the winter, they were again relatively sensitive, but this renewed sensitivity gradually receded once more during the summer, each consecutive year losing less and less of their acquired immunity, until, a certain number of years, it assumed a fairly permanent state. How little rheumatics react to bee stings is illustrated in the following letter:

E. C. B., of Brookville, Illinois, wrote: "I am 38 years old and I have just taken up beekeeping this year. I was surprised that I am practically immune to swelling after being stung by the bees. I received one sting on the lower left eyelid this summer and all effects had left my eye. I had an attack of inflammatory rheumatism when I was 13 and another the following year, and one when I was 18 years old. I am inclined to believe that the fact that I am subject to rheumatism is the reason I am immune to bee stings."

How various constitutional states influence sensitivity to bee stings is proved by the following interesting communication:

C. E. D., of Crawford, Colorado, wrote: "My mother, wife, and sister, all three have been able to stand bee stings without any trouble before they became mothers. After they had children, these women became very sensitive and remained so. Regardless of where they are stung, their throats swell so much that they have great difficulty in breathing for half an hour or so. Their hearts are also affected. They all see to it that they don't get stung very often. Is this a coincidence or does motherhood have that effect generally?"

CIRCUMSTANCES WHICH INFLUENCE NORMAL AND SEVERE BEE STING INJURIES, AND THEIR SYMPTOMS

Considering this question, we note that in 76 percent of the cases of bee sting injuries the sensitivity diminished and in 69 percent immunity was acquired the first five years, the stings having afterwards hardly any effect. The majority made the identical statement, that they felt the stings as much or even less than average mosquito bites-in a word, the effects were negligible. This applied both to the local and general reactions.

Of course, topographical conditions and low constitutional states changed the modalities and influenced them to a marked degree, often causing inconsistent or even diametrically opposite symptoms.

The topographical conditions were very important, for instance, around the eyes, nose, ears, lips, or neck, or near the finger nails. They all seem to agree that the bridge of the nose is the most sensitive area.

G. A. F., of Seattle, Washington, wrote that he started beekeeping when he was 18 years old, and kept bees continually for 45 years. Though he was very sensitive at the beginning, the sensitivity gradually wore off. The stings caused practically no swelling, but once when he was stung on the nose, between the nostrils, the pain was terrific, producing steady sneezing for five minutes together with the discharge of a large quantity of mucus from the nose (apparently an allergic effect-Author) and he shed more tears than "an Irishwoman at a wake." The full effects disappeared in a half hour. He is now past 64, never had arthritis or rheumatism, and stated that when sitting on the floor he is able to get up without touching it with his hands or elbows. He further reported that he has great faith in bee venom, never wears a veil or gloves, is stung frequently, but "welcomes quite a number of stings every year," his complexion is florid, he has been underweight all his life, and had never required the services of a physician. G. E. C., of Beaver Falls, New York, answered the question as follows:

"I think that if one gets stung on the partition of the nose-or whatever you call it-it is almost sure death. Well, I got stung right there, and I can tell you it was some. experience. I thought I was a goner, but still live to tell the tale. I was hoeing in the garden when one lit on my lip, crawled up my nostril, backed out, went off apparently satisfied, came right back, and binged me right there. I sneezed and coughed, my body was all red, and prickled all over." (See the fatal case of Alexander S. Baker.)

The reports often mention the fact that in run-down conditions, in poor health, a considerably increased sensitivity was noticeable, which is only natural, as sensitivity to bee venom depends to a great extent on the constitutional state.

A. E. C., of South Africa, wrote as follows:

"I was stung at odd times by bees and the application of the bluing bag took the pain and swelling away, or rather I should say there was no swelling.

"Then I developed an inflammation of the kidneys, and after two years' constant medical treatment I was stung by a bee on the neck. Very serious symptoms developed, and the doctor was in attendance all night. There was a rash like scarlet fever over my body, especially my limbs. My face was congested, and my heart failing.

"Since then, I have been stung three times, once on the lip and the swelling was so excessive, both internally in the throat, palate, mouth, etc., that apart from the heart collapse I was in danger of suffocation. The swelling spread even to the glands under my arm.

"The second time I was stung on the forehead, where the hair joins the face, and the third time, on the leg. My collapses were more serious, but the swellings were not so severe. On all three occasions, the rash appeared about five to ten minutes after I was stung and great numbness in my limbs, excessive 'pins and needles' sensation, until my hands became ice cold and numb. I was shivering on a hot tropical midday, in spite of hot water bottles, blankets, and eiderdown. My heart was missing every third beat. Ephedrine made my symptoms more severe. I was given heart massage, large quantities of brandy, bicarbonate of soda, heart stimulants, and hot fomentations were applied constantly, one after another, as hot as they could be borne."

INFORMATION AND EVIDENCE AS TO CURATIVE AND PREVENTIVE VALUE OF BEE STINGS IN ARTHRITIS AND RHEUMATISM

With regard to the effect of bee venom as a cure for arthritis and rheumatism, the reports were unanimous: some had rheumatism before keeping bees and lost it; others never had it and never acquired it. All were in arthritis or rheumatism. An enumeration of all information on the subject agreement on the point that it is known that beekeepers do not suffer from would fill a book, itself. I quote some reports (alphabetically):

QUESTIONNAIRE

C. S. B., of Shelton, Washington, sent the following letter:

"I had rheumatism when I was a small boy. The doctor who treated me told my mother I would be badly afflicted in later years. I am a farmer and have worked hard during the last 50 years, making my home in Western Washington. As one who is predisposed to rheumatism from boyhood, I can offer some testimony along this line of information. I handled bees for the last 50 years. I feel a pleasant glow after a sting and after the poison takes effect. Some will smile at this statement. I feel the stings are a benefit to me. Last June, I felt a twang of rheumatics in my left shoulder. I picked a bee up, pressed it against my arm, picked up another, pressed it into the hollow of my elbow until it had done its duty, picked up another and pressed it just above my elbow. In three days, I felt no rheumatic symptoms. I am 78 years old, full of pep and vim, and fully believe bee stings are a great benefit to me."

C. E. Call, a veterinary surgeon of Rosedale, Indiana (I had better mention here that any time I cite a full name, it is with permission tendered), wrote:

"I wish to say that some 20 years ago, after exposure while attending to a case of obstetrics (in March), I contracted a very bad case of inflammatory and articular rheumatism. The third morning after my exposure, I failed to get up, and was bed fast for four weeks and had to be turned on a sheet. For five years, I went to bed every spring with rheumatism. I went to the springs, took salicylates, antirheumatic remedies, boiling, sweating, and all the trimmings. I became interested in bees and began working them as a sideline to my veterinary practice. I have had no rheumatism for 15 years-or ever since I began with the bees, and I give the bees credit for curing me, and they didn't charge me even a cent for it, either. I run about 75 colonies. The bees work for me all summer, and board themselves.

"I find that a sting of the hybrids is more potent than that of the Italian or gentler races."

G. H. C., of Enosburg Falls, Vermont:

"I never knew a person who worked with bees more or less for years, to have rheumatism. I have worked with bees and handled them without protection most of the time for the last fifty years, and had thousands of stings. A case of rheumatism will never swell from bee stings,

243

as one poison works against the other." (This belief seems to be very popular, as it is often mentioned.)

Alice D., of Manitoba, Canada, wrote an interesting communication about honey used in inflammation of the eyes, and also stated that she had painful arthritis for two or three years, but after receiving several stings at the time, the swelling gradually disappeared and had given her very little trouble since. Arthritis is sometimes troublesome in late winter in hands, wrists, and elbows, but disappears when working with the bees. She also reported that she had heard of a fatality in the neighborhood from one sting, but did not get any particulars. However, she understood that it was a person with a very weak heart.

L. M. D., of Edmeston, New York:

"I am 67 years old and handled bees for a long time. Yes, I had rheumatism before caring for the bees and I am now free from it and consider bee stings the cure."

A. R. F., of Levy, Arkansas:

"I had rheumatism and took medicine for it six months with no result. One Sunday morning, I was stung on the chest by six or eight bees and in less than 10 days I was fully cured."

B. H., of Ste. Martine, Chateauguay County, Quebec, Canada:

"I have been keeping bees for nearly 25 years and as for my experience about bee stings, I must tell you that last summer I had such a sore back that I could hardly walk. No liniments helped me. Finally, I thought I would try my own bees. It takes a good many stings to make me swell. I took about 12 or 15 bees and applied them myself on my back. I at once felt better. An hour later, I decided to take another dose, and the next morning about 15 more. The day after I could walk and dance.

"I made another experiment two weeks later on a friend of mine who had been suffering from rheumatism in the arm for several weeks, especially the last two days he could hardly sleep. I asked him if he would object to bee stings for a sure cure. He said "I'll stand anything to get rid of my soreness." I at once got about a dozen bees, went to his home, just like a family doctor-but I must tell you everyone in the house ran out for fear of being stung. I proceeded to give him 10 stings in the arm. That was Sunday afternoon, and Monday morning he went to work on the job he had left two weeks before."

QUESTIONNAIRE

G. B. H., of Creston, Iowa:

"Before taking up beekeeping in 1917, I had suffered from some form of rheumatism. After working with the bees and receiving several stings, all traces of the trouble left me. In 1928, I sold all my bees and for several years, up to 1930 and 1931, I continued to visit other beekeepers and to do some work with the bees just for the fun of it, which, of course, resulted in a few stings. From 1931 until the winter of 1932, I had no contact with bees and during this winter of 1932 developed a very painful attack of arthritis in my right elbow. The pain was so bad that I could only lift my arm with difficulty or grip any object. The latter part of February, I was talking with a boy whom I had interested in bees a few years ago and told him to get a few bees for me the first warm day they were out. The boy came to my home with 10 bees in a queen cage. Before retiring that night, I caused four of the bees to sting me about the elbow, leaving the stings in for several minutes. The next night two of the remaining bees were dead, but I repeated with the other four just as I had done the previous night, making eight stings in all.I noticed relief within twenty-four hours and in just a few days all traces of pain had gone, with no return up to date."

G. H. H., of Taunton, Massachusetts:

"The first year I kept bees, I was practically immune to stings in three months. I had suffered more or less with sciatic rheumatism for 20 years before keeping bees. I can truthfully say that the bees have kept rheumatism away from me for the last seven years. Whenever I feel anything like it, I always go to the bees and let them do their stuff."

A. C. K., of Grand Rapids, Michigan:

"I suffered from rheumatism in my right hand ever since an auto accident five years ago, and I have not been bothered since I was stung by the bees the first time."

E. B. K., of Lititz, Pennsylvania:

"About 38 years ago, I had rheumatism and had a doctor trying all he knew. I was on it for a whole year and I still got worse. Then after a year of pain, I told my wife I would try the bees. I went to my carpenter shop, made a cage to go into the entrance of the beehive, and soon had enough in it. I made them sting me from the right hip down to the foot. I had only 30 stings, the pain left me right away, and ever since had no rheumatism. I certainly do stand up high and shout very loud for bee stings."

QUESTIONNAIRE

L. K., of Greentown, Indiana:

"Yes, I have had two attacks of rheumatism before keeping bees. Both have been severe enough to swell up my ankles and knees, and practically disable me for four to six weeks. Since keeping bees I never had a return of the trouble. Occasionally, have symptoms of a rheumatic attack coming, think I am in for another siege, but in a few days it blows over and does not return."

H. M. M., of Boyertown, Pennsylvania:

"I am in the bee business and working at my bees some 59 years. I am 80 years old, lean and tall, about the same shape as my grandfather, but he had always to fight rheumatism and several of my cousins died from it, but I don't know what rheumatism is, and I am sure the bee stings will keep it from me. Dr. L. E. claims the same thing. Yes, bee stings will prevent and cure rheumatism."

G. S. McR., of Thief River Falls, Minnesota :

"When I was a boy between the ages of 10 and 17, I had a number of attacks of rheumatism, one of which was so severe in the muscles of my chest that it affected my heart action, and made me swoon away as if dead. From 17 to 21, I worked with bees and had no recurrences. In the winter of 1911, I worked in a creamery in Fargo, North Dakota, where it was wet, and then had to do some delivering on the outside, without changing my clothes. In the spring, after quitting the creamery, I had rheumatism in my feet so bad I could not walk. I got over this during the summer. I am now 43 and have worked with bees every summer for 13 years, started with a few hives and increased them to I have been stung several times each season. I have been entirely free from rheumatic pains during these years, except one fall I felt slight pains in my shoulder and I went into the bee cellar and made two or three bees sting me on the back of the hand. In a day or two, I had no more pains."

C. M. P., of Excelsior, Minnesota:

"I am nearly 75 years old. Until I was 23, I lived in Ohio where father kept bees, and was often stung. From Ohio I moved to South Dakota, where at the time there were no bees. Before coming to Minnesota, maybe 25 years ago, I contracted rheumatism, which at times was very acute. I took up beekeeping. My first experience was an accident with the bees, and it seemed I had a thousand stings. I was almost black, covered with them, and each one gave me a full dose of rheumatic cure. I certainly responded to the

246

dose, which was so effective that from the time I have no rheumatism worth mentioning, though for the last ten years I had only a few stings, my son looking after the bees."

J. W. P., of Puyallup, Washington, wrote the following, relative to the curative effect of bee venom:

"It happened 40 years or more ago. The facts and details are as clearly in my mind as at the time it happened. I am past 60 now. I bought my first swarm of bees of Mr. Wm. Stolley, an educated German beekeeper, living near Grand Island, Nebraska. He invited me to visit him often and proved to be a most efficient teacher of beekeeping. It was then that he told me what had happened that summer to one of the county commissioners in Hall County, of which Grand Island was the county seat. This county commissioner had suffered from rheumatism for a long time. He had tried several doctors, but none of them did him any good. He kept growing worse, until he get around only with the use of crutches. He was a friend of Mr. Stolley, who pleaded with him time and again to let him try the bee sting cure. Finally, when the doctors could give him no more hope, he agreed to do as Mr. Stolley said. He was brought to Mr. Stolley's apiary each week and Mr. Stolley administered several stings each visit, increasing the number each time. Before the summer was gone, this man walked without crutches and went about his business as before. Mr. Stolley told me he had cured other cases the same way.

"I remember reading in my earlier beekeeping experience-I think it was A. J. Root who said, 'You'll very seldom find a beekeeper who is troubled with rheumatism.' During all my experience, I have found this to be true. I cannot recall a single case where a beekeeper had rheumatism."

C. W. S., of Oklahoma City, Oklahoma:

"At the age of 35, before being exposed to bee stings, I was bothered with rheumatism of the left shoulder, and, also, with kidney trouble. I am now 71 years old, and entirely free from these ailments."

E. E. S., of Weslaco, Texas:

"I was affected with rheumatism in both shoulders. Since I have taken up commercial beekeeping, I was not bothered with it any more."

QUESTIONNAIRE

H. A. S., of Bordentown, New Jersey:

"I suffered from rheumatism and lumbago before I kept bees, but I consider myself cured and so far had no recurrence. Started beekeeping in 1920."

L. M. S., of Harrison, Ohio:

"I am glad to tell you what I know from personal experience, which covers a period of 40 years. One time I bought some hives at a public sale, and gave some to a boy friend, a neighbor, who had inflammatory rheumatism. Being green, even with extra clothes on, he received some good stinging, which made him sick. He had some whiskey, and went to sleep. Some time later he told me: 'I'll be d, if I don't believe bee stings were good for rheumatism.' I told him I knew they are good. He did not have any since, and the same boy is now a husky policeman in Chicago.

"A man worked for me six years ago in Montana. One day, working with the bees, he took off his veil, because it was too hot for him. He was properly stung on the face and hands. He told me sometime later that this was the first winter he didn't have any rheumatism and he wondered why."

A. T. W., of Arcadia, Nebraska, answered Question 6 about rheumatism:

"Yes, that is why I began to handle bees. Had rheumatism so I could hardly get around to do my work (have always been a farmer). About 20 years ago, I read that bee stings were good for my affliction. I secured four colonies of mongrel bees-and just 15 seconds later, the stinging began. I believe those four colonies could have won the World War. I veiled my face, and allowed them to attack my hands, arms, and legs. At the end of the second season, I felt the rheumatism only occasionally in periods of bad weather. At the same time, I became immune to any painful effects of the stings, I felt cured, and had no recurrences for the past 16 years.

"I am nearly 67, take care of all of my outdoor work without ill effects. I introduced, since, pure bred queens which reduced the temper of the bees. I get stung occasionally. I am busy every day with my farm and stock raising, I never had a day's sickness (except rheumatism), I never took aspirin, bromo quinine, or pills, never had a doctor except for life insurance, never use tobacco or liquor, not even 3.2, and I feel like a four-year old. I am eating honey for the last 57 years and use sugar only sparingly.

QUESTIONNAIRE

"I might add that a half-brother of mine, Dr. G. R. M., of Kemmerer, Wyoming, told me several years ago that he uses 'Apis' successfully in the treatment of rheumatism."

C. A. Z., of Livonia, Missouri:

"As I have worked with bees for more than half a century, since 1879, I have had a wide and varied experience with bees and their stings. I can give you some information that will be of value to you in compiling your book on stings for rheumatism. Now at my age (?), my hands and fingers are as limber as a child's and I do not suffer the agony I have seen others. My wife was so bad with rheumatism in the knees that she had to walk with a cane. I had her helping me with the bees and she got an unusual lot of stings on the affected parts. It was not long until she was walking without a cane and she has not suffered from rheumatism since.

"About five years ago, a traveling salesman came to my house and asked if I cared if he let the bees sting him. He said he was suffering from rheumatism. He, also, stated that five years previous he had rheumatism so bad that they carried him to a bee yard on a stretcher and applied the stings. This was the first time it recurred. So he went to the yard, helped himself and got the stings, and when he departed, seemed to be relieved. I have not seen him since."

It seems superfluous and really of little or no advantage to cite more of the answers, as it would just lead to repetition.

The belief that bee stings cure rheumatism is much more widespread in this country than I had ever thought. Many beekeepers relate how often strangers visit them, asking for bees or for permission to go near the hives, so as to be stung for curative purposes. Some apiarists seem to take especial pride in it and boast of their "roadside clinics." One was quite concerned because the doctors intend to compete with his bees.

With reference to Number 5 of the Questionnaire, "What is your favorite remedy for treating local and general effects of bee stings?" a great majority answered that their most popular remedy was "nothing," that is, "Forget it and go on with your work." The next most popular local remedy seems to be household ammonia, in the form of compresses. They all agree on one point-to remove the sting. Some put on hot water, hot fomentations; others, ice or running cold water. The different remedies used were: alcohol, spirits of camphor, soda, salt, aspirin, honey, onions, mud, crushed weeds, blue bag, machine oil, etc. Some suggested a few puffs of hot smoke, which will also help to prevent the sting from becoming a target for the rest of the bees. Others just blew on the sting.

For treating the general effects, the most popular remedies were: hot coffee, whiskey, or brandy, and aromatic spirits of ammonia. In severe intoxication, all reported that the doctors used adrenalin chloride or 1:1000 epinephrine, administered hypodermically.

About the question of paralysis, J. B., of Trenton, New Jersey, wrote:

"The man's name was C. He had a stroke of apoplexy, his left side was totally lame. Since having bees, he has been completely cured. He is still alive, and in fine health."

On the subject of cancer, there was only one reference to a beekeeper who died from cancer. H. E. C., of Honolulu, Hawaii, wrote:

"A thin, light skinned Englishman, who owned the bees I am now operating in Oahu, worked among them for a number of years, receiving the usual number of stings. On account of the thinness and lightness of his skin, the doctors said the tropical sun gave him cancer. At any rate, he died from it. His name was L. St. J. G."

Many others mention the fact, that according to their knowledge, cancer is almost unknown among beekeepers.

The reports on fatal bee sting injuries are fully treated in Chapter VI, Section 3.

Chapter XIV Concluding Remarks

I started this volume with apologies, so I do not intend-though I am almost tempted to repeat the same practice.

I realize the fact that the treatise does not seem to be complete without an enumeration of my own case records, but I received so many personal and written requests and enquiries about the technic employed in the administration of the treatments with injectable bee venom that I do not wish to delay publication any longer. I have inserted in the text most of my technical experiences and clinical observations, and I reserve the privilege— to avoid any further delay-of publishing my records at a later date. In the meantime, both the number of my treated cases will increase and I shall also gain a further opportunity for study. As it is, I have quoted so many cases of foreign coworkers that they will be sufficiently illustrative to enable the reader to form an opinion about the curative value of bee venom. In fact, I am convinced that the inclusion of additional case records with the already abundant material would be more disturbing than helpful.

Originally, I had planned to include in this volume other subjects, *viz.*, anatomy, physiology and biology of the bee, prevention of bee sting injuries, medicinal use of wax and honey, etc., which undoubtedly have medical interest but no close connection with bee venom therapy. As an afterthought, I decided to include these with others of a more popular aspect in a second volume, which will soon leave the press.

There is still much research work to be done in connection with this remedial agent. To be sincere, even if the publication of this book might be considered premature, I do not feel any regret, because the fact alone that the material is placed at the disposal of the medical profession is rather comforting to me. It will give me only a great satisfaction if I succeed in arousing interest and gain coöperation in interpreting many more ambiguities. Whoever has read this volume will fully comprehend the wide field offered to any student of medicine, whether a clinician, biochemist, serologist, or pathologist. It is an immensely absorbing and fascinating worthwhile study.

The domestic production of an efficient and reliable injectable bee venom is an urgent desideratum. So far, the preparations on the market are not entirely dependable; for unknown reasons their potency occasionally varies, with the result that it is then inadequate. In spite of all our successes, we still seem to be far off from the time when we can claim that our injectable substance is "just as good" as the "original" venom of our little friend, the bee.

In conclusion, I am not only hopeful, but confident that the salutary effects of the modern application of this age-old remedy-properly administered will prove a great boon and blessing in our endeavors to check the progress, and eventually to quell the ravages of these "world diseases."

If the reader's interest in this volume is tantamount only to a fraction of the pleasure it has given me to present it, I have been amply rewarded for all my efforts.

Composite Bee Venom Therapy Bibliography

ABDERHALDEN, E. Allgemeine Technik und Isolierung der Monoamidosäuren, Berlin, 1922.

ADRIAN, E. Über Arthropathia psoriatica, Mitt. a. d. Grenzgeb. d. Med. u. Chir. Jena, 1924.

ADRIAN, E. D. The nervous mechanism of pain, Univ. Coll. Hosp. M., 1929.

AINLEY-WALKER, E. W. Bee Stings and Rheumatism, Brit. M. J. Lond., Oct. 1908.

ALLEN, F. M. Studies concerning Glycosuria and Diabetes, Boston, 1913.

ALTSCHUL. Real-Lexicon für homöopath, Arzneimittellehre, Therapie und Arzneibereitungskunde, Sonderhausen, 1864.

AMERICAN BEE JOURN. Bees and Medicine, Febr. 1925.

ANONYME. Le venin de l'abeille, Bull. mens. de la Federat. Nat. d'apiculture de France, Dec. 1932.

ASBERGER, A. Über den Zusammenhang des Psoriasis mit Gelenkerkrankungen, 1927.

ASCHNER, B. Klinik und Behandlung Menstruationstörungen, Stuttg. u. Leipz., 1931.

ARISTOTLE, Historia Animalium, IV (Bekker, J. 1837).

ARTHUS, M. Réchérches experimentales sur le venin des abeilles, Compt. rend. de Soc. de Biol. Par., 182, 1919.
De L'Anaphylaxie à l'immunité, 1921.

AUBRY (quoted by G. Legal), Thèse de Paris, 1922.

BANNATYNE, G. A. Rheumatic arthritis, its pathology, morbid anatomy and treatment, London, 1904.

BARCROFT, J. The respiratory function of the blood, Cambridge, 1914.

BARKER, L. F. Differentiation of the diseases included under chronic Arthritis, Am. J. M. Sc. Phila., Jan. 1914.

BARTHOLOMEW, G. M. D. Bee Stings, Journ.-Lancet, July, 1929.

BAUDISCH, H. Bienenstitch, Prag. Med. Wchnschr., 31, 1906.

BAYLEY DE CASTRO, A. The Effects of Bee Venom, Indian M. Gaz. Calcutta, 62, 1927.

BECKER, S. Behandlung rheumatischer Erkrankungen mit injizierbaren Bienengiftpräparat Immenin, Therap. d. Gegenw. Berl. u. Wien, 6, 1931.

BEHAN, R. J. Pain, 1922.

COMPOSITE BIBLIOGRAPHY

BEHRENS, D. Erkrankungen und Todesfälle durch Insectenstiche, Inaug. Diss. Würzb., 1920.

BENSON, R., and SEMENOV, H. Allergy in its relation to Bee Stings, J. of Allerg., I, 1930.

BERG, R. Ein Fall von Idiosyncrasie gegen Wespengift, Berl. klin. Wchnschr., 1204, 1920.

BERGMANN, N. Über Psoriasis und Gelenkerkrankungen, Diss. Berl., 1913.

BERLIOZ, L. Mémoire sur les maladies chroniques, les evacuations sanguines et l'acu-puncture, Rev. des Alcaloides, Oct. 1928.

BERT, P. Gaz. Méd. de Par., 771, 1865.

BERT ET CLOEZ. Venin des Hymenoptères, Compt. rend. de Soc. de Biol. Par., Juillet,1865.

BERTARELLI, E., U. TEDESCHI, A. Experimentelle Untersuchungen über das Gift der Hornisse, Centralbl. f. Bakteriol. (etc.) Jena, Bd. 68, 1913.

BESREDKA, A. Are antivirus specific? J. Immunol. Balt. & Cambridge, Eng., 23, 1932.

BEVEN, J. O. Acidosis following Bee Stings, Lancet, Lond., II, 850, 1920.

BIBLIOTEQUE MÉDIC. Des accidents produits par la piqûre L'Hymenoptères, 66, 1819.

BILLARD, G. La Phylaxie, Par., 1931.

BLAAS, C. M. Die Biene in Deutscher Volkssitte und Meinung, Bericht. und Mitteil des Alterthumvereins, Wien., XXIV.

BOINET, E. Deux cas de guérison du lupus par les piqûres d'abeille, Marseille Med., 60, 1923.

BOINET, M. De l'utilisation des piqûres d'abeilles pour le diagnostic differentiel entre la mort apparente et la mort réelle. Congres de l'A. F.A.S. à Nimes en 1912.

BOLLINGER. Infektion durch Tiergifte, Ziemssen's Handbuch der spec. Pathol., 652, 1876.

BOUCHACOURT, L. Sur la valeur thérapeutique du venin des abeilles, et sur l'apithérapie, La Med. Internat. Illustr., Mai, 1934.

BOURDILLON, H. Psoriasis et Arthropathie, Thèse 328, Par., 1888.

BRANDT UND RATZEBURG. Die Honigbiene, Mediz. Zoologie, I, 1829.

BRAUN, L. J. B. Notes of desensitization of a patient hypersensitive to bee stings, South African M. Rec. Capetown, 23, 1925.

BROWN, G. Med. J. Australia, Sydney, Dec. 1931 (quoted by Cleland).

BROWN, TH. R. On the Chemistry, Toxicology and Therapy of snake poisoning, Johns Hopkins Hosp. Bull. Balt., 105, 1899.

COMPOSITE BIBLIOGRAPHY

BÜCHNER'S REPETITORIUM FÜR PHARMACIE, 6, 420, 1857.

BUCKY, G., UND MÜLLER, E. F. Strahlende Energie, Haut und autonomes Nerven system, München. Med. Wchnschr. 22, 1925.

BURTON, E. T. Answer to Ainley-Walker, Brit. M. J. Lond., II, 1369. 1908.

CAFFE. Schmidt's Jahrbücher, 12, 1852.

CAJORI, CROUTER, AND PEMBERTON. The alleged rôle of lactic acid in arthritis and rheumatoid conditions, Arch. Int. Med. Chicago, 34, 1924. The physiology of synovial fluid, Arch. Int. Med. Chicago, 37, 1926.

CALMETTE, A. Le venin des serpents, Paris, 1896.
Les venins, les animaux venimeux et la serotherapie antivenimeuse, Paris, 1907.

CARLET, M. Memoirs sur le venin et l'aiguillon de l'abeille, Ann. Sc. Nat. Zool., 9, 1890.

CARLET, M. G. Sur le venin d'Hymenoptères et organ. excreteurs, Compt. rend. Ac. d. Sc. Par., 98, 1884.

CARRIER, E. B. Studies on the physiology of capillaries, Am. J. Physiol. Baltim., 61, 1922.

CARTON, P. Menace de mort par une piqûre d'abeille, Vie et Santé, 3, Août, 1927.

CASPER. Traité de Médic. Legale, II, 125.

CATOLA. Crises vasomotrices céphalique et menièreformes par venin d'abeille, Rev. neurolog. Par., 35, 1928.

CAWSTON, F. G. Acute Poisoning from Bee Stings, J. Trop. M. (etc.) Lond., Dec. 1930.

CECIL, R. L., AND ARCHER, B. H. Classification and treatment of chronic Arthritis, J. Am. M. Ass., 87, 1926.

CHOPRA, R. N., AND CHOWAN, J. S. Snake venoms in Medicine, Indian M. Gaz. Calcutta, 67, 1932.

CLELAND, J. B. Insects in their relationship to injury and disease in man in Australia, Med. J. Australia, Sydney, Dec. 1931.

COATES, V., AND DELICATI, L. Rheumatoid Arthritis and its treatment, London, 1931.

COHN, S. Beiträge zur Kenntniss des Bienengiftes, Inaug. Dissert. Würzburg, 1922.

COHNHEIM, J. Gesammelte Abhandlungen, Berlin, 1885.

CONRADI, A. F. Osservationi di puncture di api susseqita da fenomen. extraordinari, Animal. Univers. di Medicina, 257, 1822.

COOKE, R. A. Cutaneous Reactions in Human Hypersensitiveness, Proc. N. York Path. Soc., XXI, 1921.

COMPOSITE BIBLIOGRAPHY

CORNIL, L. A propos d'un cas d'accidents toxiques graves consecutifs a une piqûre d'abeille et rapellant les phenomènes d'anaphylaxie, Bull. Soc. Pathol. comp. Mars, 1917.

COUCH, L. B. Formic Acid in Rheumatic Conditions, Med. Rec. N. Y., June, 1905.

CRAIG, H. K. Rheumatism, N. York M. J. (etc.), Sept. 1917.

CRUICKSHANK, J. The bacterial flora of the intestines in Health and chronic Disease. Brit. M. J. Lond., Sept. 29, 1928.

CZYHLARZ AND DONATH. Ein Beitrag zur Lehre von Entgiftung. Centralb. f. innere Med., 13, 1900.

D'ABREU, A. R. Effects of Bee Venom, Ind. M. Gaz. Calcutta, Nov. 1926.

DALE, SAMUEL. Pharmacologia seu manuductio ad materiam medicam, London, 1737.

DAVIS, F. P. Medical Summary, 1908.

DEEKS, W. E. Suggestions on the nature and treatment of rheumatism, N. York M. J. (etc.), March, 1906.

DELPECH, A. Les depots de ruches d'abeilles existant sur differents points de la ville de Paris, Ann. d'Hyg. Par., III, Janvier, 1880.

DEMARTIS, T. P. Abeille Méd. Par., 30, July 25, 1859.

DENYS, J., ET VAN DE VELDE, H. Sur la production d'une antileucocidine chez les lapins vaccines contre le Staphylocoque Pyogène, Cellule, Lierre et Louvain, 1895.

DENYS, J. A propos d'une Critique dirigée contre le pouvoir bactericide des humeurs, Cellule, Lierre et Louvain, 1924.

DERRICK, E. A striking general reaction to a Bee Sting, Med. J. Australia, June, 1932.

DEUTSCH, D. Histamin zur Therapie rheumatischer Erkrankungen, Med. Klin. Berl. u. Wien, 41, Oct. 1931.

DEVAUCHELLE, Utilisation des piqûres d'abeilles dans le rheumatisme. Chasseur franc., October 1923.

DITTON, D. Bienenstichvergiftungen, Aerztl, Sachverst. Ztg. Berl. 22, 1930.

DOLD, H. Immunisierungsversuche gegen das Bienengift, Ztschr. f. Immunitätforsch. u. exper. Therap. Jena, 26, 1917.

DONNELLY, J. F. D. Wasps and Bee Stings, Nature, 435, 1898.

DOUGLAS, N. Birds and Beasts of the Greek Mythology.

DUPUYTREN, G. Leçons orales de clinique chirurgicale, 85, 1839.

EDWARDES, T. The Lore of the Honey Bee, Lond. 1925.

COMPOSITE BIBLIOGRAPHY

ELLIS, R. V., AND AHRENS, H. G. Hypersensitiveness to airborne bee allergen, J. Allergy 3, 1930.

ESSEX, H. E., MARKOWITZ, J., AND MANN, F. C. The physiological Action of the venom of the Honey Bee, Am. J. Physiol., Baltimore, 94, 1930.

FABRE, P. L'intoxication par les piqûre d'hymenoptères, J. des Pract., 802, 1903.
Le Venin des Hymenoptères, Bull. Acad. de Méd. Par., 1905.
Sur les phenomènes d'intoxication dus aux piqûres d'hymenopt. Paris, 1906.

FALK, N. Psoriasis arthropathica, Arch. f. Dermat. u. Syph. Wien u. Leipz., 129, 1921.

FARNSTEINER, K. Der Ameisensäuregehalt des Honigs, Ztschr. f. Untersuch. d. Nahrungs u. Genussmittel, Berl., 1908.

FAUST, E. S. Die tierischen Gifte, 1906.
Vergiftungen durch tierische Gifte, Handbuch der Inner. Mediz. (Mohr. u. Staehlin), Bd. 4, Th. II, Aufl. II.
Über Ophiotoxin aus dem Gifte d. Cobra di Capello, 1907.
Darstellung und Nachweis tierischer Gifte, Handbuch biolog. Arbeits-methoden, IV, 7, 1923.
Handbuch d. experiment. Pharmakolog., Bd. II, 2, 1924.

FEHLOW, W. Die Bienengiftbehandlung rheumatischer Erkrankungen, Deutsche Med. Wchnschr. Berl. u. Leipz., 2, 1934.

FENGER, H. Anatomie und Physiologie des Giftapparates bei der Hymenopteren, Arch. f. Naturgeschicht, 7.

FISCHER, A. Blute funde bei rheumatischen Erkrankungen, Rheumaprobleme, 1929.

FITZSIMONS, F. W. Snake Venoms, their therapeutic uses and possibilities, Capetown, 1929.

FLANDIN, Ferreyrolles et de Lepinay: Traitment des algies par l'acupuncture chinoise, Bull. et mem. Soc. Méd. d. Hôp. de Par., May, 1933.

FLEXNER, S., AND NOGUCHI, H. Snakevenom in relation to Hemolysis, Bacteriolysis and Toxicity, J. Exper. M. N. Y., 6, 1902.

FLURY, F. Über die Bedeutung der Ameisensäure als naturl. vorkommen. Gift, Bericht. deutsch. pharmazeut., Ges. 1919.
Über die chemische Natur des Bienengiftes, Arch. f. exper. Path. u. Pharmakol. Leipz., 85, 1920.
Über den Bienenstich, Naturwissenschaft, II, 1923.
Lehrbuch der Toxicologie, 1928.

FONTANA, F. Abhandlung über das Viperngift, Berl., 1787.

FORCHHEIMER. Therapeusis of Int. Diseases, Billings a. Irons, II, 150, 1917.

COMPOSITE BIBLIOGRAPHY

FORSBROOK, W. H. C. A dissertation on Osteo-arthritis, Lond., 1893.

FOSTER, B. The synthesis of acute rheumatismus, Clin. Med. Long., 1874.

FRANCK, E. Bienenstich Vergiftung oder Herzleiden als Ursache plötzlich. Todes., Aerztlich. Sachverst. Ztg., 18, 1930.

FRASER, H. M. Beekeeping in Antiquity, 1931.

FREEDLANDER, S. O., AND LENHART, C. H. Clinical observations on the capillary circulation, Arch. Int. Med., Chicago, 29, 1922.

FREEDMAN, T. Non-specific vaccine Therapy with Omnadin, South African M. Rec. Capetown, 6, 1932.

FREUND, E. Lehrbuch für Gelenkserkrankungen, Wien, 1929.

GAGE, W. V. The relation of capillary caliber to normal and patholog. sensation and function, Med. Rec. N. Y., Sept. 1917.

GALEN. Kühn, Leipz., 1820.

GAUTIER, A. Les Toxines microbiennes et animales, 1896.

GAY, F. P. Tissue Resistance and Immunity, J. Am. M. Ass., Oct. 1931.

GEIGER, C. W., AND ROTH, J. H. Bee Stings of the Uvula, J. Am. M. Ass., Aug. 1923.

GELPKE, L., UND SCHLATTER, C. Unfallkunde, 82, 1917.

GIBB, D. F. Anaphylaxis from Pollen, introduced by a Bee Sting, J. Canada M. Ass., Oct. 1928.

GLOVER, J. A. A report on Chronic Arthritis, Ministry of Health Rep. 52, Lond.,1928.

GOETZ, A. Generalisierte Urticaria, Deutsch. Med. Wchnchr. Berl. u Leipz. 55, 1929.

GOLDSCHMIDT, S., AND LIGHT, A. B. A method obtaining from veins blood similar to arterial blood in gaseous content, J. Biol. Chem. N. Y., 64, 1925.

GOODMAN, N. M. Anaphylaxis from Bee Stings, Lancet, Lond., Sept. 24, 1932. Goss, E. L. A Bee Sting, Journ.-Lancet, 46, 1926.

GOSS, E.L. A Bee Sting, Journ.-Lancet, 46, 1926.

GOULLON, H. Das Beinengift im Dienste der Homeopathic, Leipzig, 1880.

GREGG, A. L. Anaphylaxis from Bee Stings, Lancet, Lond., March 1932.

GRÜNSFELD, M. Das injizierbare Bienengiftpräparat Immenin von Standpunkte des praktischen Arztes, Wien. Med. Wchnschr., 8, 1932. Bee poison at the bedside, Bee-World, 12: 2-3, 1931.

GUNN, J. A. Snake Venoms, Cambridge Univ. Med. Soc. Mag., 1, 1929.

HANSEN, A. A. A fatal Bee Sting on leg, Ugesk. f. Laeger Kjøbenk, 83, 1921.

COMPOSITE BIBLIOGRAPHY

HARMER, J. M., AND HARRIS, K. E. Observations on the vascular reaction in man in response to histamine, Heart, Lond., XIII, 1926.

HELD, F. Beiträge zur medizinischer Bedeutung des Bienengiftes, Inaug. Diss. Wurzb., 1922.

HERING, C. American Provings, 1853.
Condensed Materia Medica, Apis mellifica, 1877.
The guiding symptoms of our Materia Medica, Philadelphia, 1879.
Kurzgefasste Arzneimittellehre, 3d Ed., Berl., 1889.

HINSDALE, A. E. The writings of A. E. Hinsdale, J. Am. Inst. Homeop. N. Y., 22, 1929.

HOHENHEIM, VON, TH. (Paracelsus). Schriften, Leipz., 1921.

HOLTZ, H. Anatomische Studien des Bienenstachels, Nordl. Bienenzeit, 1883.

HOPKINS, F. G. The problems of specificity in biochemical catalysis, Oxford, 1931.

HOVORKA, D., UND KRONFELD, U. Vergleichende Volksmedizin, 1908.

HOWALD, S. Tod eines Bienenzüchters nicht infolge eines Bienenstiches, Schweiz. Bienen Ztg., 31, 1895.

HUNTER, W. A. Med. J. Australia, Sidney, Dec. 1931 (quoted by Cleland).

HUSEMANN, F. Handbuch der Toxicologie, I, 273, 1862.

HUWALD, G. Klinisch-biologisch. Befunde bei Verletzung der Cornea durch Bienen stiche, Graefe's Arch. f. Ophthalmol., 50, 1904.

HYATT, J. D. The Sting of the Honey Bee, Amer. Quart. Microsc. J., I, 1878.

JOBLING, PETERSON, EGGSTEIN. Mechanism of anaphylactic shock, J. Exper. M. N. Y., Oct. 1915.

JONES, W. R. Bee Sting Treatment, Northwest Med. Seattle, 25, 1926.

JUBLEAU, Le traitment du rheumatisme par piqûres d'abeille, Chronique Méd., Mai, 1925.

JÜHLING, J. Die Tiere in deutscher Volksmedizin, Alter und Neuer Zeit.

JUSTINIAN. Institutiones II.

KAFKA, J. Therapeutische Erfahrungen über das Bienengift, Berl. 1858.

KARSCH, F. Über eine Doppelrolle des Stachels der Honigbiene, Entomolog. Nachricht, 1884.

KEITER, A. Rheumatismus und Bienenstichbehandlung, 1914.
Bienenstichkur, Umschau & Therap. Mon. Bericht., 1913.

KLEINE, F. K. Über Entgiftung in Tierkörper, Ztschr. f. Hyg. Infektionskrankh. Leipz., 36, 1901.

KNORTZ, K. Insecten in Sage, Sitte und Literatur, 1910.

COMPOSITE BIBLIOGRAPHY

KOBERT, R. Practical Toxicology, 1910.
Beiträge zur Kenntniss der Saponinsubstanzen, 1904.

KOEHLER, A. Zur Funktion des Bienenstachels, Arch. f. Bienenkund., III, 1921.

KRAEPELIN, C. Untersuchungen über den Bau, Mechanism. und Entwickelungs geschicht. des Stachels der bienenartig. Tiere, Zeitschr. f. wiss. Zool., XXIII.

KREBS, W. Bericht über die Erfolge mit Apicosan, Ztschr. f. ärztl. Fortbild., April 1929.

KRETSCHY, F. Die moderne Bienengifttherapie, Ztschr. f. Wissensch. Bäderkunde, 2, 1928.
Das Bienengift in seiner historischen Entwicklung als Therapeutikum, Bienen Vater, 6: 185, 928.

KRITSCHEWSKY, J. L. A contribution to the theory of anaphylactic shock, J. Infect. Dis., Chicago, 1918.

KROGH, A. The supply of oxygen to the tissues and the regulation of the capillary circulation, J. Physiol., 52, 1918.

KROGH AND VIMTRUP. The Capillaries, Special Cytology, I, 1932.

KRONER, J. Die Behandlung der chron. Polyarthritis im Spätstadium, München. Med. Wchnschr., 39-40, 1930.
Spätstadien rheumatischer Erkrankungen und ihre Behandlung, RheumaJahrbuch, 1929.

KYES, P. Über die Wirkungsweise des Cobragiftes, Berl. klin. Wchnschr., 38-39, 1902.

KYES, P., UND SACHS, H. Zur Kenntniss der Cobragiftactivierenden Substanzen, Berl. klin. Wchnschr., 2-4, 1903.

LACAILLADE, C. W., JR. The Determination of the Potency of Bee Venom, Am. J. Physiol. Baltimore, 105, Aug. 1933.

LAIGNEL-LAVASTINE ET KORESSIOS. Traitment des Algies cancereuses par le venin de Cobra, J. Med. de Par., 30, July 27, 1933.

LAMARCHE. Le traitment du rheumatisme par les piqûres d'abeilles, Ann. Méd. de Caen., Febr. 1908.

LANGER, J. Über das Gift unserer Honigbiene, Arch. f. Exper. Path. u.
Pharmakol. Leipz., 38, 1897.
Der Aculeatenstich, Arch. f. Dermat. u. Syph., 43, 1898.
Abschwächung und Zerstörung des Bienengiftes, Arch. internat. de
Pharma codyn. Grand et Par., 6, 1899.
Versuche zur Anwendung von Bienenstich und Bienengift als
Heilmittel bei chron.-rheum. Erkrankungen des Kindesalters, Jahrb. d.
Kinderh. Leipz., 81, 1915.
Über Bienenstich, Vortrag d. deutsch. bienenwirtschaftl., Centr.
Vereins, Prag., 1895.
Bienengift u. Bienenstich, Bienenvater, Jahrg., 33, 10, 1901.
Die Entgiftung des Bienengiftes, Vortr. deutsch. bienenwirtschaftl.
Centr. Ver., 1898.
Neure Ergebnisse über Bienenstich, Vortr. Stuttgart, 1930.
Zur Frage der tötlichen Bienenstiche, Vortr. Wandersammlm deutsch.
Bienen write, 1927.
Das histolog. Bild des Aculeatenstiches, Arch. f. Derm. u. Syph. Leipz.
u Wien, 1932.
Die Fixation des Bienengiftes an der Stichstelle, Biochem. Ztschr.
Berl., 1932.
Beurteilung des Bienenhoniges und seiner Verfälschung mittels biolog.
Eiwess differenzier, Arch. f. Hyg. München u. Berl., 71, 1910.

LEDERLE, P. Über das Gift der Honigbiene, Bienen Zeit., 204, 1919.

LEGAL, G. Contribution a l'étude des Conditions des Gravité des Piqûres
d'Hymenopt. Thèse Méd., 1922.

LEGIEHN, D. Eigenthümliche Wirkung eines Bienenstiches, Berl. klin.
Wchnschr., 787, 1889.

LEWIS, TH. Studies of Capillary Pulsation, Univ. Coll. Hosp. Mag., IX, 2,
1924. The blood vessels of the human skin and their response, Lond.,
1927.

LIVINGSTONE, A. T. The capillary and venous circulation in relation to
disease, N. York M. J. (etc.), Nov. 29, 1919.

LLEWELLYN, L. J. Aspects of Rheumatism and Gout, Lond., 1927.

LOEBEL, R., U. SIMO, A. Über ambulatorische Behandlung chron.
Gelenkskrankheiten, Neuralgien, Myalgien mit unspecif. Reiztherapie,
Med. Klin. Berl. u. Wien, 10, 1930.

LOEVENHART, A. S. Certain aspects of biological oxidation, Arch. Int. Med.,
Chicago,152, 1915.

LOMBARD, W. P. The blood pressure in arterioles, capillaries and small veins,
Am. J. Physiol., 29, 1912.

LUKOMSKI, M. Gaz. d. Hôp. Par., 107, Sept. 1864.

COMPOSITE BIBLIOGRAPHY

LYSSY, R. Réchérches expermientales sur le venin des Abeilles, Arch. internat. de Physiolog. Liege & Par., 16, 1921.

MARBARET DU BASTY, P. G. Des accidents produits par la piqûre des Hymenopt. port aiguillon, Thèse de Par., 2875, 1875.

MABERLY, F. H. Brief Notes on the Treatment of Rheumatism with Bee Stings, Lancet, Lond., July 23, 1910.

MACKAY, H. Severe toxemia following Bee Stings, Canada M. Ass. J., Nov., 1924.

MAINGGOLAN, F. J. Use of Omnadin in bites of wasps, bees and other insects, Geneesk. Tijdschr v. Nederl. Indie, 824, 1932.

MATHESON, R. Medical Entomology, 1933.

MEASE, D. Grave accidents produced by the sting of bees and other insects, Am. J. M. Sc., Phila., 1836.

MEIGS, G. S. The relation between allergic intracutaneous reaction and symptoms of Anaphylaxy, J. Inf. Dis., Chicago, 15, 3, 1904.

MELTZER, S. J., AND LANGMANN, G. Is living animal tissue capable of neutralizing the effects of Strychnine and Venom? Med. News, Nov. 1900.

MERL, TH. Bienenkörper als Ameisensäureträger, Ztschr. f. Untersuch. d. Nahrungs u. Genussmittel, Berl. 42, 1921.

MEYERHOF, O. Chemical dynamics of life phenomena, 1924.

MITCHELL, S. WEIR. Research upon the venom of the rattlesnake, etc., Wash., 1861.
Cat-Fear, Ladies Home Jour., March, 1906.

MOLINÉRY. Le traitment du rheumatisme par les piqûres d'abeilles, Chron. Méd., Mars, 1925.

MONAELESSER, A. Effets du venin de Cobra modifié sur les tumeurs cancereuses, Par., 1933.

MORGENROTH, J., UND CARPI, W. Über ein Toxolecithid des Bienengiftes, Berl. klin. Wchnschr., 43, 1906.

MORGENTHALER, O. Die Bienengiftbehandlung bei rheumatischen Erkrankungen Schweiz, Bienen Zeit., 55: 482, 1932.

MORLEY, M. W. The Honey Makers, 1899.

MUCK, O. Eine ubersehene Bienengiftstudie, Wien. Tierärztlich. Monatschr., 1, 1922.

MUFFET, B. T. The Theatre of Insects, London, 1658.

MULLER, E. F. Strahlende Energie, Haut und autonomes Nervensystem, München. Med. Wchnschr., 22, 1925.

COMPOSITE BIBLIOGRAPHY

MURAKAMI, K. Influence of Bee's poison on blood picture, blood corpuscles and cholesterol content of blood in rabbit, Okayama Igakkai Kwai Zasshi, 40, 1928.
Influence of Bee's poison on protein and carbohydrate metabolism, Okayama Igakkai Zasshi, 40, 760, 1928.

NATT, A. G., AND BOYD, L. J. The Pathology and Pharmacology of Apis Mellifica, J. Am. Inst. Homeop., 16, 1923.

NEISSER, M., U. WECHSBERG, F. Über Staphylotoxin, Ztschr. f. Hyg. Infectionskrankh., 36, 1901.

NETOLITKY, F. Insekten als Heilmittel, Pharmazeut. Post, Wien, 1, 1916.

NEUWIRTH, E., UND WEISS, E. Zur Behandlung chronischer Arthritiden der Frauen mit Schlamm, Arch. Med. Hydrolog., 3, Nov. 1933.

NICHOLS, E. H., AND RICHARDSON, F. L. Arthritis deformans, J. Med. Research, Bost., 16, 1909.

NIETLISPACH, W. Insektenstich und Unfall., Zürich.

NOBL, G. Zur Kenntniss der Psoriasis Arthropathie, Arch. f. Dermat. u. Syph. Wien u. Leipz., 123, 1916.

NOGUCHI, H. Snake Venoms, 1909.

NOTHNAGEL. Speciel. Pathol. u. Therap., Bienengift, Bd. I, 1910.

NOWOTNY, H. Immeninbehandlung chron. entzündlich. Processe, München. Med. Wchnschr., 29, 1932.

O'MAHONEY, W. W. Virtues of bee venom, Irish Bee J., 33: 37, 1933.

PAP, L. Endocrine arthralgia, Orvosi hetil, Budapest, Oct. 1931.

PARISIUS, W., UND HEIMBERGER, H. Acute Myelosen nach Bienenstichen, Deutsch. Arch. f. klin. Med., 143, 1924.

PASSOW, PR. Über Apicosanbehandlung bei Iritis rheumatica, Klin. Monatsbl. f. Augenh, 79, 1927.

PATTON, W. S., AND EVANS, A. M. Insects, Ticks, Mites and Venomous Animals, I, II.

PAUL, G. Das Wesen der Hautimpfung und ihre Bedeutung für die Bekämfung des chron. Rheumatismus, Wien. Med. Wchnschr., 14, 1927.

PAVY, F. W. On Carbohydrate metabolism, etc., London, 1906.

PAWLOWSKY, E. N. Gifttiere und Ihre Giftigkeit, 1927.

PEMBERTON, R. The significance and use of diet in treatment of chron. arthritis, N. York State M. J., 26, 1926.
Arthritis and Rheumatoid Conditions, their Nature and Treatment, 1930.

PERITZ, G. Der Muskelrheumatismus, Ergebn. der Ges. Med., 3, 1922.

COMPOSITE BIBLIOGRAPHY

PERRIN, M., ET CUÈNOT, A. La metathèse, modalité nouvelle de la protection contre le toxique, ses application pratique, Bull. gen. de Thérap. (etc.), Soc. de therap., Par., 4, Avril 1931.
Contribution a l'étude du pouvoir anatoxique et de la phylaxie, J. de Physiol. et Path. gen. Par., I, Sept. 1931; II, Dec. 1931; III, Mar. 1932.
A propos de 13 observations, nouvelles d'hypersensibilité au venin d'abeilles, Rev. Méd. de l'Est, 60, 1932.
Le traitment de l'Hypersensibilité au Venin d'Abeilles, Bull. gen. Therap. (etc.), Par., 183, 1932.
Rheumatisme et Venin d'Abeilles, Rev. Méd. de l'Est, Apr. 1933.

PESCHEL, E. Psoriasis und Gelenksrheumatismus, Diss. Berl., 1897.

PHILOUZE. Du venin des abeilles, Ann. Ste. Lineenne de Meine et Loire, IV, 1860.

PHISALIX, C. Récherches sur le venin d'abeilles, Compt. rend. Soc. de Biol. Par., 1904.

PHISALIX, M. Symptômes graves determines chèz une femme jeune par la piqûre d'une seule abeille, Bull. du Mus. d'Hist. Nat., 7, 547, 1918.
Animaux Venimeux et Venins, 1922.

PLATEAU, F. Venins D'abeille, Art. Dict. Physiol. de Ch. Richet, 1895.

PLINY. C. Plinius secundi naturalis historia, Teubner, 1870.

PODOLSKY, E. The Use of Bees in Medicine, N. York M. J. (etc.), Nov. 1930.
Medicine Marches On, 1934.

POGANY, J. Die Wirkung des Histamins auf die Blutgefässe des Menschen, Zeitschr. f. ges. Exper. Med. Berl., 75, 1931.

POLLACK, H. Über Apicosanbehandlung bei Iritis rheumatica, Klin. Monatsbl. f. Augenh., 81, Nov. 1928.

POZZI-ESCOT, E. The Toxins and Venoms and Their Antibodies, 1906.

QUINCY, JOHN. Pharmacopoeia officinalis, extemporanea or Complete English Dispensatory, London, 1733.

RICHARDSON, B. W. The cause of coagulation of the blood, Astley Cooper Prize Ess., 1856.

RICHET, C. Anaphylaxie, Par., 1913.
Diction. de Physiolog. Abeille, 1895.

RILEY, W., AND JOHANNSEN, O. A. Handbook of Medical Entomology, Ithaca, 1915.

ROCH, M. Les Piqûres d'hymenoptères au point de vue chimique et thérapeut., Rev. méd. de la Suisse Rom. Genève, Nov. 1928.
Le venin d'abeille dans le traitment des sciatiques, Rev. Méd. de la Suisse Rom. Genève, Febr., 1933.

ROLLESTON, H. Idiosyncrasies, London, 1927.

COMPOSITE BIBLIOGRAPHY

ROOT, A. J. AND E. R. The ABC and XYZ of Bee Culture, 1917.

ROSENBACH, O. Energetick und Medizin, 1904.

ROWNTREE, L. J., AND ADSON, A. W. Bilateral lumbar sympathetic ganglionectomy and ramisectomy for polyarthritis of the lower extremities, J. Am. M. Ass., 88, 1927.
Polyarthritis, further studies of the effects of sympathetic ganglionectomy and ramisectomy, J. Am. M. Ass., July, 1929.

ROWNTREE, ADSON, AND HENCH, P. S. Preliminary results of resection of sympa thetic ganglia and trunks in 17 cases of chronic "infectious" arthritis, Ann. Int. Med., Nov. 1930.

RUHMANN, W. Die örtliche histamin Einwirkung bei Muskelrheuma, München. Med. Wchnschr., Dec. 1931.

RYLE, J. A. Anaphylaxis from Bee Stings, Lancet, Lond., March, 1932.

SACHS, H. Hemolysine, Ergebn. d. Allg. Path. u. path. Anatom. (etc.) Wiesb., 735, 1901.

SAJO, K. Ortliche Empfänglichkeit für Bienengift, II, Kosmos, Stuttg., 1914.

SALMON, WM. Pharmacopoeia Londoniensis or New London Dispensatory, Lond., 1716.

SCHMIDT. Jahrbücher der Medizin, 76, 1852.

SCHMIDT, A. Der Muskelrheumatismus (Myalgie), 1918.

SCHOLZ, W. Bienenstich in den weichen Gaumen, Deutsch. Med. Wchnschr. Berl. u. Leipz., 51, 1926.

SCHWAB, R. Eine neue Applikationsmethode des Bienengiftes rheumatischen Erkrankungen (Forapin), München. Med. Wchnschr., 81, 1934.

SOLIS-COHEN, S., AND GITHENS, TH. S. Pharmacotherapeutics, Mat. Med. and Drug Action, 1928.

SOLLMAN, A. Die Bienenstachel, Ztschr. f. Zoolog., XIII, 4.

SOLLMAN, T., AND PILCHER, J. D. Endermic Reactions, J. Pharmacol. a. Exper. Therap., Baltimore, 9, 1917.

SOZINSKEY, TH. S. Medical Symbolism, 1891.

SPALIKOURSKY. Piqûres des Abeilles, Rev. Scientif., 1899.

SPANGLER, R. H. The Treatment of Epilepsy with hypoderm. inject. of rattlesnake Venom, Crotalin, N. York M. J. (etc.), Sept. 1910, 1911, 1912.

STANLEY, H. M. In Darkest Africa, 1890.

STERN, H. Sixteen years experience with formic acid as a therapeutic agent, J. Am. M. Ass., Apr. 1906.

STOVER, G. H. Antitoxic Relation betw. Bee Poison and Honey, Johns Hopkins Hosp. Bull., Nov., 1898.

COMPOSITE BIBLIOGRAPHY

STRASSER, PR. Report of the 43d Balneolog. Congress, 1928.

STREBEL, J. Bienen und Wespenstichverletzungen des Auges, Klin. Monatsbl. f. Augenh., 86, 657, 1931.

STUMPER, C. R. Venins des fournis, Comt. rend. Acad. d. Sc. Par., 174, 1922.

SYLVESTER, H. M. Formic acid in its therap. relation to joint diseases, J. Am. Inst. Homeop., 222, 1929.

TAGUET, CH. La Cure des Algies et des tumeurs malignes, Jour. de Méd. de Par., 3, Aout, 1933.

TASCHENBERG, O. Die Giftige Tiere, 1909.

TERC, PH. Über eine merkwürdige Beziehung des Bienenstiches zum Rheumatismus, Wien. med. Presse, 35, 1888.
Der Bienenstich als Heilmittel gegen den Rheumatismus, Steirischer Bienenvater, I, 1904.
Das Bienengift in der Heilkunde, Steirischer Bienenvater, V, 1907.
Die Beziehung des Bienenstiches zum Rheumatismus und zur entstellenden Gelenksgicht, 1910.

TERTSCH, R. Das Bienengift im Dienste der Medizin, 1912.

THOMPSON, F. About Bee Venom, Lancet, Lond., 2, Aug. 19, 1933.

THRAENHART. Bienenstichbehandlung gegen Rheumatismus, Schweiz. Bien. Zeit., 1921.

UMBER, F. Zur Nosologie der Gelenkserkrankungen, 1929.

VAN HASSELT, L. Handbuch der Giftlehre, II.

VAUGHAN, V. C. Protein Split Products in Relation to Immunity and Disease, 1913.

VAUGHAN, W. T. Allergy and Applied Immunology, 1931.

VIGNE, P., ET BOUGALA. Amelioration dans un cas de lèpre et dans un cas d'ulcère de jambe par les piqûres d'abeilles, Marseille Méd., 60, 1923.

VORMANN. Perforation des Augenliedknorpels mit Verletzungen des Augenapfelbindehaut durch einen Bienenstich, München. Med. Wchnschr., 71, 1924.

VRIES, W. DE. Das Bienengift und seine Anwendung bei rheumatischen Erkrankungen, Bienen Zeit., 47, 281, 1932.

WALDHEIM, VON, F. S. Ignaz Philipp Semmelweis, Wien & Leipz., 1905.

WALTER, H. E. The Human Skeleton, 1918.

WASSERBRENNER, K. Über Behandlung von rheumatischen Erkrankungen mit Bienengift, Wien. Klin. Wchnschr., 35, 1928.

WATERHOUSE, A. T. Bee Stings and Anaphylaxis, Lancet, Lond., II, 946, 1914.

WEGELIN, C. Tod durch Bienenstich, Schweiz. Med. Wchnschr., 32, Aug. 12, 1933.

WEIL, R. The Nature of anaphylaxis and relationship betw. anaphylaxis and immu nity, J. Med. Research, Boston, XXVII, 4, 1913.

WEINERT, H. Über Bau und Bedeutung des Wehrstachels der Bienen u. Wespen, Wissenschaftlich. Wchnschr., 15, 1920.

WELLS, G. H. Chemical Pathology, 1925.
The Chemical Aspects of Immunity, 1929.

WEST, S. The Form and frequency of cardiac complications in rheumatic fever, Practitioner, Lond., 1888.

WILDE, P. The Physiology of Gout, Rheumatism and Arthritis, London, 1921.
The Pyretic Treatment of Rheumatism and Allied Disorders, Lond. 1928.

WOLF, C. W. Apis Mellifica, or The Poison of the Honey Bee considered as a Therapeutic Agent, Berlin, 1858.

WOODYATT, R. F. Diabetes (Wells' Chem. Path.).

WOODYATT AND SAMSUM, J. Biolog. Chem. N. Y., 30, 1917.

WYATT, B. L. Chronic arthritis, fibrosities, Diagnosis and treatment, 1933.

YOANNOVITCH, G., AND CHAHOVITCH, X. Le traitment des tumeurs par le venin des abeilles, Bull. Acad. de Méd. Par., Juin, 1932.

YOUNG, C. A. Bee Sting of the Cornea, Am. J. Ophth., 208, 1931.

ZANDER, E. Beiträge zur Morpologie des Stachelapparates der Hymenopteren, Ztschr. f. wiss. Zoolog., 56, 1899.

ZANGOLINI. Symptômes d'empoisonnement par piqûres d'abeilles, Gaz. Méd. de Par.,1857.

ZIMMER, A. Die Behandlung der rheumat., Krankheiten, Leipz., 1930.

ZIMMERMANN, W. Bienen und Wespenstich-Vergiftungen, Samml. von Vergiftungs-fälle., Bd. 5. June 1934.

ZINSSER, H. The more recent developments in the study of anaphylactic phenomena, Arch. Int. Med. Chicago, 16, 1915.

ANNOTATED GLOSSARY

Includes contemporary references.

---

1 Dhakal A, Sbar E. Jarisch-Herxheimer Reaction. [Updated 2023 Apr 24]. In: StatPearls [Internet]. Treasure Island (FL): StatPearls Publishing; Jan 2024. https://www.ncbi.nlm.nih.gov/books/NBK557820/

2 Agatston, Arther, Why America Is Fatter and Sicker Than Ever July 3, 2012. Circulation; Vol. 126, No.1. https://www.ahajournals.org/doi/10.1161/CIRCULATIONAHA.112.098566

3 Joel Achenbach, Dan Keating, Laurie Mcginley, And Akilah Johnson, Dying Early America's Life Expectancy Crisis, An Epidemic of Chronic Illness is Killing Us Too Soon. October 3, 2024. The Washington Post. Retrieved at https://www.washingtonpost.com/health/interactive/2023/american-life-expectancy-dropping/

4 Bogdanov Stefan, Bee Venom: Production, Composition, Quality, Bee Products Science, ResearchGate, April 2016. (PDF) Bee Venom: Production, Composition, Quality (researchgate.net).

5 Kubala, Jillian, MS, RD, Bee Venom: Uses, Benefits, and Side Effects, Healthline, June 24, 2019.

6 Park S., Baek H., Jung K.H., Lee G., Lee H., Kang G.H., Lee G., Bae H. Bee venom phospholipase A2 suppresses allergic airway inflammation in an ovalbumin-induced asthma model through the induction of regulatory T cells. Immun. Inflamm. Dis. 2015;3:386–397. doi: 10.1002/iid3.76

7 Ye M., Chung H.S., Lee C., Yoon M.S., Yu A.R., Kim J.S., Hwang D.S., Shim I., Bae H. Neuroprotective effects of bee venom phospholipase A2 in the 3xTg AD mouse model of Alzheimer's disease. J. Neuroinflamm. 2016;13:10.

8 Question Video: Recalling the Effect of Histamine on Blood Vessels | Nagwa. https://www.nagwa.com/en/videos/957174525150/

9 Shi P, Xie S, Yang J, Zhang Y, Han S, Su S, Yao H. Pharmacological effects and mechanisms of bee venom and its main components: Recent progress and perspective. Front Pharmacol. 2022 Sep 27;13:1001553. doi: 10.3389/fphar.2022.1001553. PMID: 36238572; PMCID: PMC9553197.

10 Charles Mraz – Health and the Honey Bee, American Apitherapy Society, Inc. https://apitherapy.org/uk/charles-mraz-3/

11 Britannica, The Editors of Encyclopedia. "Lyme disease". Encyclopedia Britannica, 16 Mar. 2024, https://www.britannica.com/science/Lyme-disease. Accessed 29 March 2024

12 Meriläinen L, Herranen A, Schwarzbach A, Gilbert L. Morphological and biochemical features of Borrelia burgdorferi pleomorphic forms. Microbiology (Reading). 2015 Mar;161(Pt 3):516-27. doi: 10.1099/mic.0.000027. Epub 2015 Jan 6. PMID: 25564498; PMCID: PMC4339653.

13 Anderson C, Brissette CA. The Brilliance of Borrelia: Mechanisms of Host Immune Evasion by Lyme Disease-Causing Spirochetes. Pathogens. 2021 Mar 2;10(3):281. doi: 10.3390/pathogens10030281. PMID: 33801255; PMCID: PMC8001052.

14 Holtorf Medical Group How Does Lyme Disease Evade the Immune System? February 5, 2021. https://holtorfmed.com/articles/lyme-disease/how-does-lyme-disease-evade-the-immune-system/

15 Joan, Slonczewski (students), Borrelia burgdorferi and Lyme Disease Pathogenesis, MicrobeWiki, BIOL 238 Microbiology, Kenyon College, 2016.

16 Jensen Gs, Cruickshank D, Hamilton De. Disruption of Established Bacterial and Fungal Biofilms by a Blend of Enzymes and Botanical Extracts. J Microbiol Biotechnol. 2023 Jun 28;33(6):715-723. doi: 10.4014/jmb.2212.12010. Epub 2023 Mar 10. PMID: 37072676; PMCID: PMC10331947.

17 Ross, Md, Treat Lyme, retrieved at https://www.treatlyme.net/guide/bee-venom-therapy-lyme

18 Lobel, Ellie, Bee Venom Therapy for Lyme Disease, March 19, 2020.

19 Allen, H. B., Shaver, C. M., Etzler, C. A., & Joshi, S. G.. Autoimmune diseases of the innate and adaptive immune system including atopic dermatitis, psoriasis, chronic arthritis, lyme disease, and Alzheimer's disease. Immunochem Immunopathol, 1(112), 2. 2015.)https://www.researchgate.net/profile/Herbert-Allen-2/publication/292962946_Autoimmune_Diseases_of_the_Innate_and_Adaptive_Immune_System_including_Atopic_Dermatitis_Psoriasis_C hronic_Arthritis_Lyme_Disease_and_Alzheimer's_Disease/links/56b0b 79708ae8e372151d7a7/Autoimmune-Diseases-of-the-Innate-and-Adaptive-Immune-System-including-Atopic-Dermatitis-Psoriasis-Chronic-Arthritis-Lyme-Disease-and-Alzheimers-Disease.pdf

20 David S. Cassarino, Martha M. Quezado, Nitya R. Ghatak, Paul H. Duray; Lyme-Associated Parkinsonism: A Neuropathologic Case Study and Review of the Literature. Arch Pathol Lab Med 1 September 2003; 127 (9): 1204–1206. doi: https://doi.org/10.5858/2003-127-1204-LPANCS

21 Hyde Jenny A., 2017, Borrelia burgdorferi Keeps Moving and Carries on: A Review of Borrelial Dissemination and Invasion, Frontiers in Immunology, 8, DOI=10.3389/fimmu.2017.00114, https://www.frontiersin.org/journals/immunology/articles/10.3389/fim mu.2017.00114

22 Kingston, Ann, The Truth About Lyme Disease, Macleans Online, Posted March 24, 2014. Retrieved at https://www.hoffmancentre.com/wp-content/uploads/pdfs/lyme/The%20Truth%20About%20Lyme%20Dise ase.pdf

23 Macdonald Alan B.,Plaques of Alzheimer's disease originate from cysts of Borrelia burgdorferi, the Lyme disease spirochete, Medical Hypotheses, Volume 67, Issue 3, 2006, Pages 592-600, ISSN 0306-9877, https://doi.org/10.1016/j.mehy.2006.02.035.

24 Rooney, P., & Perrin, D. America's Health Care Crisis Solved (1st ed.). Wiley. 2008.

25 Bellik, Yuva. Bee Venom: Its Potential Use in Alternative Medicine. Anti-Infective Agents in Medicinal Chemistry (Formerly? Current Medicinal Chemistry - Anti-Infective Agents). 2015.13. 3-16. 10.2174/2211352513666150318234624.

26 Broadman, Joseph M.D, Bee Venom Therapy, Health Resources Press, 1997.

27 Eteraf-Oskouei, Tahereh, AU - Najafi, Moslem, TI - Uses of Natural Honey in Cancer: An Updated Review, PT - JOURNAL ARTICLE, DP - 2022/3/9, TA - Adv Pharm Bull, PG - 248-261, VI - 12, IP - 2, SO - Adv Pharm Bull 2022/3/9;12(2):248-261, AID - 10.34172/apb.2022.026 [doi], 4099 - https://apb.tbzmed.ac.ir/Article/apb-30355

28 Chan-Zapata I, Segura-Campos MR. Honey and its protein components: Effects in the cancer immunology. J Food Biochem. 2021 May;45(5):e13613. doi: 10.1111/jfbc.13613. Epub 2021 Mar 26. PMID: 33768550.

29 Masad RJ, Haneefa SM, Mohamed YA, Al-Sbiei A, Bashir G, Fernandez-Cabezudo MJ, Al-Ramadi BK. The Immunomodulatory Effects of Honey and Associated Flavonoids in Cancer. Nutrients. 2021 Apr 13;13(4):1269. doi: 10.3390/nu13041269. PMID: 33924384; PMCID: PMC8069364.

30 Kim Y.-M., Lee J.-D., Park D.-S. The Anti-Cancer Effect of Apamin in Bee-Venom on Melanoma cell line SK-MEL-2 and Inhibitory Effect on the MAP-Kinase Signal Pathway. J. Acupunct. Res. 2001;18:101–115.

31 Liu J, Xiao S, Li J, Yuan B, Yang K, Ma Y. Molecular details on the intermediate states of melittin action on a cell membrane. Biochim Biophys Acta Biomembr. 2018 Nov;1860(11):2234-2241. doi: 10.1016/j.bbamem.2018.09.007. Epub 2018 Sep 10. PMID: 30409519.

32 Perkins, Harry, Honeybee Venom as An Anti-Cancer Treatment Continues, Harry Perkins Institute of Medical Research. May 30, 2020. Retrieved at https://perkins.org.au/honeybee-venom-as-an-anti-cancer-treatment-continues/

33 Dong Ju Son a, Jae Woong Lee a, Young Hee Lee a, Ho Sueb Song b, Chong Kil Lee a, Jin Tae Hong; Therapeutic application of anti-arthritis, pain-releasing, and anti-cancer effects of bee venom and its constituent compounds. Elsevier Pharmacology & Therapeutics, Volume 15, Issue 2, August 2007 Pages 246-2701. https://doi.org/10.1016/j.pharmthera.2007.04.004

34 Kwon Ny, Sung Sh, Sung Hk, Park Jk. Anticancer Activity of Bee Venom Components against Breast Cancer. Toxins (Basel). 2022 Jul 5;14(7):460. doi: 10.3390/toxins14070460. PMID: 35878198; PMCID: PMC9318616.
https://www.ncbi.nlm.nih.gov/pmc/articles/PMC9318616/

35 Małek A, Strzemski M, Kurzepa J, Kurzepa J. Can Bee Venom Be Used as Anticancer Agent in Modern Medicine? Cancers (Basel). 2023 Jul 21;15(14):3714. doi: 10.3390/cancers15143714. PMID: 37509375; PMCID: PMC10378503.

36 Socarras Km, Theophilus Pas, Torres Jp, Gupta K, Sapi E. Antimicrobial Activity of Bee Venom and Melittin against Borrelia burgdorferi. Antibiotics (Basel). 2017 Nov 29;6(4):31. doi: 10.3390/antibiotics6040031. PMID: 29186026; PMCID: PMC5745474. Retrieved from https://www.ncbi.nlm.nih.gov/pmc/articles/PMC5745474/

37 Wehbe R, Frangieh J, Rima M, El Obeid D, Sabatier J-M, Fajloun Z. Bee Venom: Overview of Main Compounds and Bioactivities for Therapeutic Interests. Molecules. 2019; 24(16):2997. https://doi.org/10.3390/molecules24162997

38 Amna Ahmed, Zujaja Tul-Noor, Danielle Lee, Shamaila Bajwah, Zara Ahmed, Shanza Zafar, Maliha Syeda, Fakeha Jamil, Faizaan Qureshi, Fatima Zia, Rumsha Baig, Saniya Ahmed, Mobushra Tayyiba, Suleman Ahmad, Dan Ramdath, Rong Tsao, Steve Cui, Cyril W C Kendall, Russell J de Souza, Tauseef A Khan, John L Sievenpiper, Effect of honey on cardiometabolic risk factors: a systematic review and meta-analysis, Nutrition Reviews, Volume 81, Issue 7, July 2023, Pages 758–774, https://doi.org/10.1093/nutrit/nuac086

39 Olas B. Bee Products as Interesting Natural Agents for the Prevention and Treatment of Common Cardiovascular Diseases. Nutrients. 2022 May 28;14(11):2267. doi: 10.3390/nu14112267. PMID: 35684067; PMCID: PMC9182958.

40 Zahran F, Mohamad A, Zein N. Bee venom ameliorates cardiac dysfunction in diabetic hyperlipidemic rats. Exp Biol Med (Maywood). 2021 Dec;246(24):2630-2644. doi: 10.1177/15353702211045924. Epub 2021 Sep 22. PMID: 34550826; PMCID: PMC8669171.

41 Hassan, A.K., El-kotby, D.A., Tawfik, M.M. et al. Antidiabetic effect of the Egyptian honey bee (Apis mellifera) venom in alloxan-induced diabetic rats. JoBAZ 80, 58 (2019). https://doi.org/10.1186/s41936-019-0127-

42 Khulan TS, Ambaga M and Chimedragcha CH, Effect of Honey Bee Venom (Apis mellifera) on Hyperglycemia and Hyperlipidemia in Alloxan Induced Diabetic Rabbits, Journal of Diabetes and Metabolism, 2015:6;3, DOI: 10.4172/2155-6156.1000507.

43 Lima WG, Brito JCM, da Cruz Nizer WS. Bee products as a source of promising therapeutic and chemoprophylaxis strategies against COVID-19 (SARS-CoV-2). Phytother Res. 2021 Feb;35(2):743-750. doi: 10.1002/ptr.6872. Epub 2020 Sep 18. PMID: 32945590; PMCID: PMC7536959.

44 Kasozi KI, Niedbała G, Alqarni M, Zirintunda G, Ssempijja F, Musinguzi SP, Usman IM, Matama K, Hetta HF, Mbiydzenyuy NE, Batiha GE, Beshbishy AM, Welburn SC. Bee Venom-A Potential Complementary Medicine Candidate for SARS-CoV-2 Infections. Front Public Health. 2020 Dec 10;8:594458. doi: 10.3389/fpubh.2020.594458. PMID: 33363088; PMCID: PMC7758230.

45 Yang W, Hu FL, Xu XF. Bee venom and SARS-CoV-2. Toxicon. 2020 Jul 15;181:69-70. doi: 10.1016/j.toxicon.2020.04.105. Epub 2020 Apr 30. PMID: 32360140; PMCID: PMC7190514.

46 Du W, Han S, Li Q, Zhang Z. Epidemic update of COVID-19 in Hubei Province compared with other regions in China. Int J Infect Dis. 2020 Jun;95:321-325. doi: 10.1016/j.ijid.2020.04.031. Epub 2020 Apr 20. PMID: 32325276; PMCID: PMC7169896.

47 Manuela B. Pucca, Felipe A. Cerni, Isadora S. Oliveira, Timothy P. Jenkins, Lídia Argemí, Christoffer V. Sørensen, Shirin Ahmadi, José E. Barbosa and Andreas H. Laustsen, Bee Venom—A Potential Complementary Medicine Candidate for SARS-CoV-2 Infections, frontiers, volume 8, 2020. https://doi.org/10.3389/fpubh.2020.594458.

48 Hristina Vlajinac, Eleonora Dzoljic, Jadranka Maksimovic, Jelena Marinkovic, Sandra Sipetic & Vladimir Kostic. Infections as a risk factor for Parkinson's disease: a case–control study, International Journal of Neuroscience, 123:5, 329-332, 2013 DOI: 10.3109/00207454.2012.760560 .

49 Kim K.H., Lee S.Y., Shin J., Hwang J.T., Jeon H.N., Bae H. Dose-Dependent Neuroprotective Effect of Standardized Bee Venom Phospholipase A2 Against MPTP-Induced Parkinson's Disease in Mice. Front. Aging Neurosci. 2019;11 doi: 10.3389/fnagi.2019.00080

50 Hartmann A, Muellner J, Meier N, Hesekamp H, van Meerbeeck P, et al. Correction: Bee Venom for the Treatment of Parkinson Disease – A Randomized Controlled Clinical Trial. PLOS ONE 11(9): e0162937, 2016. https://doi.org/10.1371/journal.pone.0162937

51 Andreas Hartmann, Bee Venom as a Neuroprotective Agent in Parkinson's Disease, The Michael J. Fox Foundation for Parkinsons Research, https://www.michaeljfox.org/grant/bee-venom-neuroprotective-agent-parkinsons-disease

52 Karishma Abhishek, Bee Venom - Osteoarthritis and Parkinson's Disease, Parkinson's Resource Organization, June 20, 2022. https://www.parkinsonsresource.org/news/articles/bee-venom-osteoarthritis-and-parkinsons-disease/

53 Miklossy, Judith Et Al. 'Borrelia Burgdorferi Persists in the Brain in Chronic Lyme Neuroborreliosis and May Be Associated with Alzheimer's Disease.' 1 Jan. 2004: 639 – 649. Retrieved from https://content.iospress.com/articles/journal-of-alzheimers-disease/jad00387

54 Nicolson, Garth. (2008). Systemic Intracellular Bacterial Infections (Mycoplasma, Chlamydia, Borrelia species) in Neurodegenerative (MS, ALS, Alzheimer's) and Behavioral (Autistic Spectrum Disorders) Diseases. Townsend Letter. 295. 74-84.

55 Jang S, Kim KH. Clinical Effectiveness and Adverse Events of Bee Venom Therapy: A Systematic Review of Randomized Controlled Trials. Toxins (Basel). 2020 Aug 29;12(9):558. doi: 10.3390/toxins12090558. PMID: 32872552; PMCID: PMC7551670.

56 Choi GM, Lee B, Hong R, Park SY, Cho DE, Yeom M, Park HJ, Bae H, Hahm DH. Bee venom phospholipase A2 alleviates collagen-induced polyarthritis by inducing Foxp3+ regulatory T cell polarization in mice. Sci Rep. 2021 Feb 10;11(1):3511. doi: 10.1038/s41598-021-82298-x. PMID: 33568685; PMCID: PMC7876016.

57 Khalil A, Elesawy BH, Ali TM, Ahmed OM. Bee Venom: From Venom to Drug. Molecules. 2021 Aug 15;26(16):4941. doi: 10.3390/molecules26164941. PMID: 34443529; PMCID: PMC8400317.

58 Merriam-Webster.com Dictionary "Wheal.", Merriam-Webster, https://www.merriam-webster.com/dictionary/wheal. Accessed Mar 28, 2024.

59 Van der Valk JP, Gerth van Wijk R, Hoorn E, Groenendijk L, Groenendijk IM, de Jong NW. Measurement and interpretation of skin prick test results. Clin Transl Allergy. 2016 Feb 23;6:8. doi: 10.1186/s13601-016-0092-0. PMID: 26909142; PMCID: PMC4763448.

www.ingramcontent.com/pod-product-compliance
Lightning Source LLC
Chambersburg PA
CBHW050224270326
41914CB00003BA/559